Pregnancy, Childbirth and The Newborn

Pregnancy, Childbirth and The Newborn

Editor: Cora Bailey

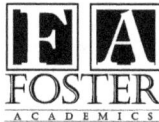

FOSTER
ACADEMICS

www.fosteracademics.com

www.fosteracademics.com

FA
FOSTER
ACADEMICS

Cataloging-in-Publication Data

Pregnancy, childbirth and the newborn / edited by Cora Bailey.
p. cm.
Includes bibliographical references and index.
ISBN 978-1-63242-662-8
1. Pregnancy. 2. Childbirth. 3. Newborn infants. 4. Obstetrics. 5. Pediatrics. I. Bailey, Cora.
RG551 .P74 2019
618.2--dc23

Foster Academics,
118-35 Queens Blvd., Suite 400,
Forest Hills, NY 11375, USA

ISBN 978-1-63242-662-8 (Hardback)

Contents

Preface

This book was inspired by the evolution of our times; to answer the curiosity of inquisitive minds. Many developments have occurred across the globe in the recent past which has transformed the progress in the field.

Pregnancy is an important period in a woman's life. To have a healthy pregnancy, a healthy newborn and to prevent complications during childbirth, regular checkups, exercise, a healthy diet and dietary supplements are of the utmost importance. Childbirth can occur by a Caesarean section or through vaginal passage. Caesarean sections are recommended for babies in the breech position, for twins or in cases of extreme distress. Pain control, active management of labor, fetal monitoring, etc. are integral to delivery management. The care of the newborn infant is vital to its health and well-being. Adequate breastfeeding and food consumption, good hygiene and care are essential to an infant's health. Low weight or premature infants, or infants with congenital malformations, intrauterine growth restriction, birth asphyxia, pulmonary hypoplasia or sepsis can have a better chance of survival and normal neurological and physiological development if provided with due care and monitoring. The fields of perinatology and neonatology are actively involved in the medical care of the mother and the infant respectively. This book contains some path-breaking studies in pregnancy and childbirth. It discusses the fundamentals as well as modern approaches of childbirth. It will help the readers in keeping pace with the rapid changes in this field.

This book was developed from a mere concept to drafts to chapters and finally compiled together as a complete text to benefit the readers across all nations. To ensure the quality of the content we instilled two significant steps in our procedure. The first was to appoint an editorial team that would verify the data and statistics provided in the book and also select the most appropriate and valuable contributions from the plentiful contributions we received from authors worldwide. The next step was to appoint an expert of the topic as the Editor-in-Chief, who would head the project and finally make the necessary amendments and modifications to make the text reader-friendly. I was then commissioned to examine all the material to present the topics in the most comprehensible and productive format.

Editor

"We know it's labour pain, so we don't do anything": healthcare provider's knowledge and attitudes regarding the provision of pain relief during labour and after childbirth

Mary McCauley[1*], Valentina Actis Danna[1], Dorah Mrema[2] and Nynke van den Broek[1]

Abstract

Background: Most women experience pain during labour and after childbirth. There are various options, both pharmacological and non-pharmacological, available to help women cope with and relieve pain during labour and after childbirth. In low resource settings, women often do not have access to effective pain relief. Healthcare providers have a duty of care to support women and improve quality of care. We investigated the knowledge and attitudes of healthcare providers regarding the provision of pain relief options in a hospital in Moshi, Tanzania.

Methods: Semi-structured key informant interviews ($n = 24$) and two focus group discussions ($n = 10$) were conducted with healthcare providers ($n = 34$) in Tanzania. Transcribed interviews were coded and codes grouped into categories. Thematic framework analysis was undertaken to identify emerging themes.

Results: Most healthcare providers are aware of various approaches to pain management including both pharmacological and non-pharmacological options. Enabling factors included a desire to help, the common use of non-pharmacological methods during labour and the availability of pharmacological pain relief for women who have had a Caesarean section. Challenges included shortage of staff, lack of equipment, no access to nitrous oxide or epidural medication, and fears regarding the effect of opiates on the woman and/or baby. Half of all healthcare providers consider labour pain as 'natural' and necessary for birth and therefore do not routinely provide pharmacological pain relief. Suggested solutions to increase evidence-based pain management included: creating an enabling environment, providing education, improving the use of available methods (both pharmacological and non-pharmacological), emphasising the use of context-specific protocols and future research to understand how best to provide care that meets women's needs.

Conclusions: Many healthcare providers do not routinely offer pharmacological pain relief during labour and after childbirth, despite availability of some resources. Most healthcare providers are open to helping women and improving quality of pain management using an approach that respects women's culture and beliefs. Women are increasingly accessing care during labour and there is now a window of opportunity to adapt and amend available maternity care packages to include comprehensive provision for pain relief (both pharmacological and non-pharmacological) as an integral component of quality of care.

Keywords: Pain relief, Analgesia, Maternity care, Quality of care, Labour, Childbirth, Healthcare providers

* Correspondence: Mary.McCauley@lstmed.ac.uk
[1]Centre for Maternal and Newborn Health, Liverpool School of Tropical Medicine, Pembroke Place, Liverpool L3 5QA, UK
Full list of author information is available at the end of the article

Background

Most women experience pain during labour and after childbirth. The World Health Organization (WHO) includes pain management as a standard of quality of care, highlighting that all aspects of health care should be given timely, appropriately, and should respect a woman's choice, culture and needs [1].

The Sustainable Development Goal three highlights health and well-being, and the Global Strategy for Women's, Children's and Adolescent's Health emphasises that all women have the right to, and should obtain, the highest attainable standard of health, including physical and psychological care [2, 3].

The severity of pain and its detrimental impact on the health and well-being of mothers during labour and after childbirth has resulted in health policy development in many high-income countries such as the United Kingdom (UK), where pain relief options (both pharmacological and non-pharmacological) are routinely discussed during antenatal contacts and then offered during intrapartum care by a trained healthcare provider, as per the individual woman's choice [4–6].The provision of effective routine pain relief results in a more positive experience of labour and childbirth for the woman [4, 7].

Women report feeling empowered and in control when they have been enabled to make informed decisions [8], including the choice of how to cope with and alleviate their pain during labour and after childbirth [9]. In low resource settings, pain management options (especially pharmacological options) are not well-established and the provision of pain relief options often depends on the health system capacity, the knowledge and attitudes of healthcare providers and availability and cost of medications [10–14]. Healthcare providers can play a positive role by educating women about the options available and supporting their choice in coping with labour pain; or a negative role by demonstrating disrespectful care, withholding care and lack of communication [11, 12, 14] .

Globally, 78% of women give birth with the assistance of a skilled birth attendant [13]. With increasing numbers of women accessing maternity care in low resource settings, there are many potential opportunities for healthcare providers to improve the quality of care for women. There are international policies and guidelines to increase quality of care (including pain management) but, at present, there is little practical implementation. It is imperative that healthcare providers are enabled to provide respectful maternity care that goes beyond the provision of basic emergency care and includes pain management (especially pharmacological) as a component of health and well-being during labour and after childbirth [3, 13].

There have been several studies regarding pain management during labour and after childbirth in low resource settings to assess women's knowledge and views on the acceptability and use of different pain management options during labour [15–24]. However, there is lack of research exploring how the perspectives of healthcare providers can affect the provision of pain relief options and the quality of care experience for women during labour and after childbirth.

This study sought to assess the knowledge and attitudes regarding the provision of pain relief during labour and after childbirth among healthcare providers who provide routine maternity care in Tanzania. In addition, we explored enabling factors and barriers as well as healthcare providers' recommendations regarding how pain relief options (both pharmacological and non-pharmacological) could be integrated as important components of respectful maternity care in low resource settings.

Materials and methods

Study design and setting

A qualitative descriptive design was used. Data collection was conducted between May and June 2017, using semi-structured key informant interviews (KII) and focus group discussions (FGD). Participants were recruited from the Departments of Obstetrics and Gynaecology and Anaesthesia of a hospital in Moshi, Tanzania. KII and FGDs were held in a location convenient for the participants that would ensure privacy.

Participants

All participants were healthcare providers and were chosen purposively, based on their involvement with maternity care and level of experience. Anaesthetic nurses and doctors working in the obstetric theatres were included to broaden the scope of the topic. FGDs were conducted with nurse-midwives to explore views of the same cadre and to enable triangulation of the data. Snowballing and opportunistic techniques were employed to identify healthcare providers and ensure participants were recruited sequentially until saturation was met.

Topic guide

A topic guide was developed and piloted in the Kilimanjaro Christian Medical Centre, with five participants to refine and improve its quality. For example, the introduction was amended to ensure that the participants were aware that we sought to assess their general views and not their own personal experiences (if any) regarding the use of pain relief options (both pharmacological and non-pharmacological) during labour and after childbirth. The topic guide served as a flexible tool to facilitate the interviewer in obtaining the participants' answers whilst ensuring that the interview remained on topic. The topic guide also acted as a cue to ask more probing questions to further understand participants' knowledge and awareness. In addition to sociodemographic topics, the guide included four main subject areas: 1) knowledge and awareness of pain management options; 2) pain management practice in place; 3) perceptions and beliefs regarding different types of pain relief options (both pharmacological and non-pharmacological) and 4) recommendations to develop a comprehensive pain management service as part of better quality maternity care.

Data collection

Prior to interview, all eligible participants were approached and given verbal and written information regarding the study including a brief overview of the research aims and interview questions. An interview appointment was then scheduled at a convenient time for the participant. All participants were interviewed in English, with the average interview lasting 30 min. All interviews were conducted face-to-face, recorded on a digital recording device and transcribed upon completion. Triangulation of results by method of data collection (KII and FGDs) and data sources (nurses-midwives, obstetric doctors, anaesthetic doctors and nurses) was used to increase validity [25]. All efforts were made to emphasise confidentiality to ensure the participants felt comfortable to provide honest answers. Interviewing participants with varied levels of experience from different departments in the hospital (antenatal clinic, labour ward, obstetric theatre, postnatal ward), provided a wide range of opinions and increased transferability.

Analysis

Transcribed interviews were initially open coded and then reviewed by a second researcher for sense checking and to avoid bias. Codes were identified and grouped into categories by the first researcher and then reviewed by a second researcher, enabling the first abstraction of data [26]. Thematic framework analysis of the categories was then undertaken by the first researcher and independently by a second researcher. The separate results were then brought together and refined to agree on the key themes. This strengthened the results and helped to remove potential bias [27].

Ethics

Full ethical approval was granted by the Liverpool School of Tropical Medicine, UK (LSTM14.025) and the Kilimanjaro Christian Medical College Research Ethics and Review Committee, in Moshi, Tanzania (N. 2047). Written informed consent was obtained from all participants of the study.

Results

Participants' characteristics

Thirty-four healthcare providers participated, 24 in KII and 10 in two FGDs. Seventeen were doctors with different levels of experience (general junior doctor, specialist registrar, consultant) and 17 were midwives or nurse-midwives. Five healthcare providers were recruited from the Department of Anaesthesia and all worked in the obstetric theatres. Most participants were female (n = 24), aged between 26 and 35 years and had up to five years' experience of providing maternity care.

Emerging themes

The main emerging themes included: 1) enabling factors and opportunities; 2) barriers and challenges; and 3) context specific recommendations from healthcare providers on how to improve pain management.

Enabling factors and opportunities

Factors facilitating the provision of pain relief for women in labour and after childbirth included: healthcare providers' positive attitude to help women; awareness of both pharmacological and non-pharmacological various methods of pain relief; the common use of non-pharmacological pain relief methods during labour; and the routine use of opioids after Caesarean section.

Positive attitudes and awareness of pain relief

Most healthcare providers expressed positive attitudes regarding pain management during labour as part of routine maternity care (Table 1: Q.1, Q.2, Q.3). Many healthcare providers reported a good knowledge of non-pharmacological methods of pain relief including: comforting and counselling the women, provision of psychological support, back massage, breathing techniques, encouraging the presence of a companion in the early stages of labour and encouraging the mother to walk or have a bath (Table 1: Q.4, Q.5). Other methods such as transcutaneous electric nerve stimulation, yoga, acupuncture and water birth were mentioned (Table 1: Q.6, Q7). Most healthcare providers were also aware of both pharmacological options including oral medications (paracetamol, diclofenac and ibuprofen); opioids (codeine, tramadol, pethidine and morphine), nerve and pudendal block, and epidural and spinal anaesthesia. Only a few healthcare providers were aware of nitrous oxide inhalation as a pain relief option.

Current use of pain relief

Most healthcare providers reported that they did routinely offer non-pharmacological options, such as counselling women about the nature and severity of labour pain and trying to provide psychological support and reassurance (Table 1: Q.8). Many healthcare providers

Table 1 Healthcare providers' quotes of enabling factors

THEME 1: Enabling factors for providing pain relief		
Sub-theme	Quote	
Positive attitudes	Q 1	"If there are pain relief drugs to give the mothers, let it come and be provided to the mothers so that they deliver peacefully. I could see that it's better and good, and it will be helpful to the mother." (Nurse-midwife, KII)
	Q 2	"I think [pain relief] should be part of management for those women who would wish to get that service." (Specialist registrar in O&G, KII)
	Q 3	"I think it is good to provide [pain relief] because the labour pain is too much, and you go through the pain for hours and hours." (Consultant Obstetrician and Gynaecologist, KII)
Knowledge of pain relief options	Q 4	"We are taught to allow the woman to walk; that could help to minimize the pain, also if there is a chance, the woman must be massaged on the back." (Nurse-midwife, KII)
	Q 5	"You can do back rubbing, or [...] ambulation, like sitting and walking or positioning; there is also partner involvement and [...] bathing." (Consultant Obstetrician and Gynaecologist, KII)
	Q 6	"I was reading in the internet that in some settings they have water birth delivery, that this is something to reduce pain." (Midwife, KII)
	Q 7	"There is acupuncture, that can be used to relief the pain, but we don't have anyone who is familiar with it." (Midwife, FGD)
Current practice	Q 8	"To the mother in labour pain, I reassure her, I massage her [...] I tell her to breath in and out to get relief and sometimes when she is tired, I encourage her; if she's feeling like to bath, then I encourage her to bath." (Nurse-midwife, KII)
	Q 9	"If she comes with a husband, or mother or mother-in-law, sometimes it is helpful, as you can call the relative [...] to talk with the woman sometimes it helps to release the suffering." (Specialist registrar in O&G, KII).
	Q 10	"Once the woman is contracting more and the cervix is not growing well with the contractions, we give buscopan or hyoscine, so at least the pain is a little bit reduced and the cervix is moving on." (Midwife, KII)
	Q 11	"During labour, I think mostly we use buscopan and paracetamol." (Specialist registrar in O&G, KII)
	Q 12	"For Caesarean sections, the protocol is pethidine for 24 h, thereafter we do give the paracetamol." (Midwife, KII)
	Q 13	"When you have an episiotomy, it must be lignocaine, local analgesia and sutured." (Consultant Obstetrician and Gynaecologist, KII)

commonly encouraged the support of a companion during the early stages of labour (Table 1: Q.9).

Many healthcare providers reported that they offered women paracetamol for pain; and buscopan and hyoscine were prescribed (erroneously) to distend the cervix (Table 1: Q.10, Q.11). Many healthcare providers reported that there was a protocol for management of pain after Caesarean section including pethidine for 24 h, followed by oral paracetamol and/or oral diclofenac according to the severity of pain (Table 1: Q.12). In cases of perineal or vaginal tears, or if an episiotomy was performed, some healthcare providers reported that an infiltration of lignocaine was recommended prior to suturing (Table 1: Q.13).

Within these themes, there was an underlying willingness of healthcare providers to provide better care, especially during labour, including to do more to alleviate pain and more frequently. However, there were barriers to the facilitation.

Barriers and challenges

Barriers affecting the provision of pain relief options (both pharmacological and non-pharmacological) included: 1) health system barriers (lack of staff, equipment and protocols); 2) limited education and opportunity to practice pain relief methods (especially pharmacological); and 3) negative beliefs, fears and malpractice.

Health system barriers

Many healthcare providers highlighted the difficulty in providing 'one-to-one' individualised care for women because of the shortage of nurse-midwives compared to the high number of labouring women (Table 2: Q.14, Q.15). Although family members could stay with the woman in the early stages of labour in the antenatal ward, their presence was restricted in the labour room due to limited space and out of respect for the privacy of other women in labour room (Table 2: Q.16). Some healthcare providers were aware that labouring in water was a non-pharmacological option for pain relief but many explained that there were no facilities to implement this option in such settings.

Many healthcare providers were aware of epidural medication but the limited number of trained anaesthetists and the lack of essential equipment (needles, catheters, drugs) meant this service was unavailable (Table 2: Q.17, Q.18). Most healthcare providers reported a lack of posters, leaflets and information materials regarding pain management options available for them or for the women.

Limited education and opportunity to practice pain relief methods

Various healthcare providers expressed a lack of specific education regarding different pain management (especially

Table 2 Healthcare provider quotes regarding barriers

THEME 2: Barrier to providing pain relief

Sub-theme	Quote	
Shortage of staff	Q 14	"Let's say we have four patients to monitor labour and all of them are in pain so you, you are the only one who is there in room 3 [pre-labour room], this is your location, you are the only healthcare provider, so how could you manage to help everyone; go and massage everyone who is in such pain, who is experiencing more pain?" (Midwife, KII)
	Q 15	"[…] I mean the shortage of nurses, or staff become a major challenge because you may find, maybe you're allocated to a certain room, five or ten mothers are in labour, you are, you're there by yourself …it becomes difficult." (Nurse-midwife, FGD)
Privacy	Q 16	"We need to keep the privacy, and if you have a lot of relatives around and only a small curtain, there is no privacy to patients, no secret for them…we need more space." (Nurse-midwife, KII)
Limited education and opportunity	Q 17	"I think maybe there a lack of trained personnel for [epidural], because it is not used here and no-one is experienced to teach us." (Specialist registrar in Anaesthetics, KII)
	Q 18	"I think shortage of resources, especially we don't have the catheters and monitors, you know for every patient you need a continuous tocographic machine for every patient, we don't have these resources." (Specialist registrar in O&G, KII)
	Q 19	"Teaching about pain management is not part of formal classes in medical school, because even when we learnt about labour, the slides on pain management was just one so, no, not much emphasis on pain management." (Specialist registrar in O&G, KII)
	Q 20	"I've read about epidural, but I've no experience with epidural." (Specialist registrar in O&G, KII)
	Q 21	"I know there are different methods of labour analgesia and epidural is one of them; but you can also give nitrous oxide but I've not much experience because I've just observed in some few centres abroad but I've not been trained on that." (Consultant Obstetrician and Gynaecologist, KII)
Negative beliefs, fears, malpractices	Q 22	"There is a belief that this pain, we need to know how much pain this patient is experiencing at least at the beginning of the labour to be able to assess and evaluate the progress of labour." (Junior doctor, KII)
	Q 23	"Once you give someone pethidine (she) may be dizzy, may feel like sleeping, so once someone is dizzy, and feel like sleeping all the time, how does she push?" (Midwife, KII)
	Q 24	"…the other thing is pain relief can cause harm to babies, they can sedate them, you'll have an inactive baby, you can't use it…"

Table 2 Healthcare provider quotes regarding barriers (Continued)

THEME 2: Barrier to providing pain relief

		(Consultant Obstetrician and Gynaecologist, KII)
	Q 25	"…Whatever is available, like the opioids analgesics, they are not really recommended before a woman gives birth because that will also give respiratory depression to the babies, so before they deliver there is very little you can do…" (Specialist registrar in O&G, KII)
	Q 26	"They will go through labour and pain must be there so to deliver a baby, if there is no pain that means, there can't be a baby without pain." (Nurse midwife, KII)
	Q 27	"I've not practiced pain relief during labour because we assume that it should be there, and we take it as a normal, [but] of course it's not normal but we take it as if every woman should experience this." (Specialist registrar in O&G, KII)
	Q 28	"It happens sometimes the woman may get a tear; we normally give infiltration before starting repairing but some healthcare providers, they just stitch it without giving it, even if the mother is screaming, they just say "shut up her", and just proceed, so it happens." (Specialist registrar in Anaesthesia, KII)
	Q 29	"During episiotomy, sometimes they do not actually provide the lignocaine, local anaesthesia during the cutting but it is written in the book, it is written there." (Nurse-midwife, FGD)
Limited availability of protocols	Q 30	"We don't have a proper, pain management protocol for women who are delivering normally; we don't give them analgesia." (Specialist registrar in O&G, KII)
	Q 31	"For those of who had vaginal deliveries once they complain of severe pain we just give them diclofenac injection, maybe a start dose and observe; if the pain continues we give paracetamol." (Junior doctor, KII)
	Q 32	"I have not seen a protocol anywhere, but we've just learned it from our senior that this is how we do things, this is how we manage this." (Junior doctor, KII)

pharmacological options) during medical or midwifery undergraduate education (Table 2: Q.19). Healthcare providers expressed doubts regarding the efficacy of non-pharmacological methods.

With regards to pharmacological options, some healthcare providers explained that their experience was limited to the use of oral medication only; whereas training on nerve block, epidural and the use of nitrous oxide was not available (Table 2: Q.20, Q.21).

Negative beliefs, fears and malpractices
Some healthcare providers said they were concerned about missing important signs during labour if pharmacological

pain relief was provided. The severity of pain during labour was considered an indicator of the progress of labour and, if removed, would hinder the correct evaluation of labour (Table 2: Q.22). Many healthcare providers explained that pharmacological pain relief interferes with the progression of labour and that all drugs (especially opioids) have detrimental side effects for the mother and/or the baby (Table 2: Q.23, Q.24, Q.25). In addition, almost half of all healthcare providers considered labour pain a 'natural' process, that does not require both pharmacological treatment or management (Table 2: Q.26). Moreover, most healthcare providers explained that it was the belief of the local community that labour pain must be present and that nothing can be done to relieve it (Table 2: Q.27).

Many healthcare providers mentioned the use of opioids was limited to women who had a Caesarean section. Some healthcare providers also reported that pharmacological pain relief was not part of the routine protocol for women who have had a vaginal delivery because it was assumed that these women did not have significant pain. Thus, oral paracetamol or diclofenac was given only if the woman requested it (Table 2: Q.30, Q.31).

Some healthcare providers reported witnessing colleagues suture perineal or vaginal tears without using lignocaine, despite its availability and the woman screaming in pain (Table 2: Q.28, Q.29). Misconception regarding the correct use of the options available (for example the use of buscopan to distend the cervix, fear of opioids, and limited use of non-pharmacological methods) was found to be a cross-cutting theme among the barriers.

Recommendations on how to improve pain relief management

Many healthcare providers provided suggestions on how pain management (both pharmacological and non-pharmacological options) could be improved, by creating an enabling environment, providing antenatal education, and emphasising research and protocols. Most healthcare providers highlighted the need to expand the teaching of the correct use of pharmacological options including opioids and epidural analgesia as part of undergraduate and postgraduate education (Table 3: Q.33). Increasing the number of staff in the labour ward would allow the staff to improve non-pharmacological support for each woman and more nurses and clinicians should receive specialist training in anaesthesia (Table 3: Q.34, Q.35). Monthly staff educational meetings were suggested as opportunities to discuss new pharmacological methods and approaches, increasing awareness and discussion in the wider team of healthcare providers. Healthcare providers emphasised the need to develop context-specific pain management protocols (Table 3: Q.36). Some healthcare providers suggested

Table 3 Healthcare provider quotes regarding solutions

THEME 3: Recommendations for providing pain relief

Sub-theme		Quote
Education for healthcare providers	Q 33	"I think we need to get education and to be educated on how and what specific pain relief should be given during labour pain, because sometimes you just start, you don't know what to give. If we get that education I think it will be very helpful to us." (Specialist registrar in Anaesthetics, KII)
	Q 34	"I suggest our health facility should liaise with the Government to promote more healthcare providers to go to anaesthetic school, because what we're having here now it is a problem of shortage of this kind of profession." (Nurse-midwife, FGD)
Increased staff numbers	Q 35	"We really need the number of staff to be the same as the number of women who are labouring." (Specialist registrar in O&G, KII)
Cultural appropriate protocols	Q 36	"It's better if everyone in the Department comes with something, then we discuss, we share, we know why we are doing this, in our setting, rather than copy from somewhere else." (Specialist registrar in O&G, KII)
Research	Q 37	"I think we should do a study on women […] you can ask them what they really want during labour, if they really want analgesia or don't. That will give us the way to set the service." (Specialist registrar in Anaesthetics, KII)
Education for women	Q 38	"To improve our health education at the clinic, to tell the mothers, they should know that during labour they will feel pain; […] because having that in your mind you can tolerate the pain." (Nurse, KII)

further research to understand how best to provide pain relief care that meets a woman's individual health needs (Table 3: Q.37). Some healthcare providers stressed the importance of educating women regarding the nature, progression and severity of labour pain during antenatal contacts (Table 3: Q.38).

Discussion
Statement of principal findings
Most healthcare providers want to provide women with pain relief options (both pharmacological and non-pharmacological) but report feeling helpless in their attempts to support women due to a lack of staff and resources, limited education regarding the use of various methods of pain relief and the complex cultural context in which labour pain is considered. There are conflicting ideas between healthcare provider's willingness to provide pain management during labour and the belief that this pain is natural and thus little can be done. Structural barriers limited implementation of pharmacological

pain relief; whereas available options (opioids) were not routinely offered or used during labour due to fear of side effects for the mother and/or the newborn baby. Education (pre-service and in-service) would be helpful to develop healthcare providers' confidence to offer more evidence-based pain relief options (both pharmacological and non-pharmacological) to all women during labour and after childbirth.

Strengths of the study

To the best of our knowledge, this is the first study to use qualitative approaches to assess healthcare providers' knowledge and attitudes regarding the provision of pain relief during labour and after childbirth in a low resource setting.

This study has highlighted key areas that need to be addressed to support the provision of routine pain relief options (both pharmacological and non-pharmacological) for women during labour and after childbirth. A range of healthcare providers who worked in different departments were interviewed resulting in a wide spectrum of responses. Interviews were also triangulated with information from FGDs improving the reliability of findings. All healthcare providers approached welcomed the discussion on routine pain relief during labour and after childbirth and were keen to contribute to ideas for solutions.

Limitations of the study

This study population included mainly female healthcare providers who provide routine maternity care in a large teaching hospital in an urban setting and excluded cadres of healthcare providers who do not provide maternity care or work in a rural setting and may have alternative perspectives or different insights. Similarly, community-based healthcare providers may have different perceptions and experience. Their opinions would be important to ensure women have access to good quality of care including pain relief, in the community setting.

How does this study relate to other literature?

In our study, healthcare providers routinely adopted non-pharmacological methods (breathing techniques, exercises, back massage, counselling and psychological support, companionship) as common pain management options; although most healthcare providers were doubtful regarding the efficacy of such methods. These approaches are used in many settings as a first line option, to improve the childbirth experience and increase women's sense of control and participation in the decision-making process [4, 23, 28]. However, in our study a high workload and staff shortages (especially nurse-midwives) meant that it was not always possible to offer this support to all women at all time. In our study, simple oral medication (for example paracetamol)

was the most common pharmacological pain relief option used during labour as a second line option, and opioids were reserved for women who have delivered by Caesarean section. However, in other settings, opioids are routinely offered to women in the early stages of labour [29–31]. Parenteral opioids are reported to be commonly prescribed by Indian obstetricians [10]. In Nigeria, two separate surveys confirmed the demand and acceptability of use of opioids for labouring women by various cadres of healthcare providers [32, 33] .

In our study, opioids were not offered to women during labour (due to concerns regarding the side effects and/or potential subsequent fetal compromise) and hyoscine and buscopan was given despite lack of evidence of benefit [34]. The reasons for this practice requires further study.

Some healthcare providers reported that they had witnessed colleagues suture perineal and vaginal tears without the use of local anaethetic, despite the availability of this pharmacological pain relief option. This practice is abuse against women, and goes against the principles of respecful maternity care, which requires healthcare providers to be gentle, respectful and establish effective communication with women to ensure they are informed regarding any interventions during labour and childbirth [14]. This sub-standard care or 'malpractice' must be addressed urgently [14]. Epidural analgesia during labour is widely available in well-resourced settings in high-income countries, but is often absent in the public sectors in low resource settings (as in our study) due to lack of an enabling environment. In India, the cost of the epidural service, the length of time required for monitoring and lack of staffing were the main barriers to the provision of epidural to women [35, 36]. In other studies, Indian obstetricians report a lack of education and training on epidural as a pharmacological pain management option in their training programmes [35, 36]. These challenges were similar to those reported in our study, where healthcare providers were not in a position to implement this service due to financial constraints [37] and a limited number of appropriately trained healthcare providers and/or anaesthetists (0.05 anaesthetists for every 100,000 people) [38].

Our study found that cultural beliefs have an influence on the attitudes of healthcare providers with many considering labour pains to be 'natural'. In a similar study in Ethiopia, McCauley et al. [12] found that 24% of healthcare providers felt that pain should not be relieved and that labour pain was 'natural'. In Bangladesh, 60% of healthcare providers believed strongly that 'women should endure the natural pain of labour' without pain relief being offered [39]. There is a need to better educate healthcare providers regarding the optimum use of available pharmacological options, including the physical and psychological consequences of protracted and unrelieved pain in women during labour and after childbirth [9, 14, 40]. We note that there are limited recommendations for the education, discussion, and provision for routine pain relief during labour and after childbirth in the recent updated WHO guidelines [41]. Amended antenatal care packages that include health education and health promotion regarding pharmacological and non-pharmacological pain relief options would be beneficial.

Conclusion

Many healthcare providers in low resource settings do not routinely offer effective pharmacological pain relief during labour and after childbirth, despite some available resources. Most healthcare providers are open to helping women and improving quality of care during labour and after childbirth using an approach that respects a women's culture wishes and beliefs. This study provides an understanding of the complexity of factors regarding the attitudes of healthcare providers to offer pain relief and provides recommendations to ensure pain management (both pharmacological and non-pharmacological) options are an integral part of maternity care. Women are increasingly accessing care during labour and there is a window of opportunity now to adapt and amend available maternity care packages to include comprehensive provision for pain relief as a component of quality of care.

Abbreviations
FGD: Focus group discussion; KII: Key informant interviews; LSTM: Liverpool School of Tropical Medicine; O&G: Obstetrics and gynaecology; UK: United Kingdom; WHO: World Health Organization

Acknowledgements
A huge thank you to all the staff working at the Kilimanjaro Institute of Public Health and at the Kilimanjaro Christian Medical Centre in Tanzania. Thank you to Dr. Sia E Msuya and Dr. Patricia Swai who provided invaluable support in organising data collection and obtaining ethical approval. Thank you to Dr. Pendo Mlay (Head of Department of Obstetrics and Gynaecology) and Dr. Kaino Mwemezi (Head of the Department of Anaesthesia) for their support during data collection. A special appreciation for Dr. Florence Mgawadere, for her contributions and support during data collection. Thank you to all healthcare providers who participated in this study and who continue to work in sometimes very difficult situations, striving to provide good quality of care. We sincerely applaud them and their work.

Funding
This study was funded by a grant from the Global Fund, Contract number 20168770.

Authors' contributions
MMC and VAD conceived the study idea, study design and developed the topic guide. VAD conducted the interviews, transcription, data analysis, and interpreted and presented the results. DM contributed to data collection and data analysis. MMc co-ordinated and supervised the research activities, contributed to the interpretation of results and wrote the manuscript. NvdB has reviewed the results and contributed to the manuscript. All authors have read, edited and approved the final manuscript for submission.

Competing interests
The authors declare that they have no competing interests.

Author details
[1]Centre for Maternal and Newborn Health, Liverpool School of Tropical Medicine, Pembroke Place, Liverpool L3 5QA, UK. [2]Kilimanjaro Christian Medical Centre, Moshi, Kilimanjaro, Tanzania.

References
1. Yanti Y, et al. Students' understanding of "women-Centred care philosophy" in midwifery care through continuity of care (CoC) learning model: a quasi-experimental study. BMC Nurs. 2015;14(1):22.
2. United Nations. Sustainable Development Goals 2016 ; Available from: http://www.un.org/sustainabledevelopment/health/. [cited 08 May 2017]
3. World Health Organization (2015) *The Global strategy for women's, children's and adolescents' Health (2016–2030),* pp. 5–6
4. National Institute for Health and Care Excellence (NICE), Intrapartum care for healthy women and babies. 2014.
5. The American College of Obstetricians and Gynecologists. Obstetric Analgesia and Anesthesia. Obstet Gynecol. 2017;129(4):e73.
6. The Royal Australian and New Zealand College of Obstetricians and Gynaecologists (2016) *Standards of Maternity Care in Australia and New Zealand:* The Royal Australian and New Zealand College of Obstetricians and Gynaecologists, Available at: https://www.ranzcog.edu.au/RANZCOG_SITE/media/DOCMAN-ARCHIVE/Standards%20in%20Maternity%20Care%20%28C-Obs%2041%29%20Review%20March%202016.pdf. (Accessed 11 Aug 2017).
7. Lally JE, et al. Pain relief in labour: a qualitative study to determine how to support women to make decisions about pain relief in labour. BMC Pregnancy Childbirth. 2014;14:6.
8. Lally JE, et al. More in hope than expectation: a systematic review of women's expectations and experience of pain relief in labour. BMC Med. 2008;6:7.
9. Hodnett ED. Pain and women's satisfaction with the experience of childbirth: a systematic review. Am J Obstet Gynecol. 2002;186(5 Suppl Nature):S160–72.
10. Bhuvaneshwari K, Chellammal K. And Rengasamy, Attitude of obstetricians regarding labour analgesia and limitations in practising it. Int J Reprod, Contracept, Obstet Gynecol. 2017;6(2):388–91.
11. Mahiti GR, et al. Women's perceptions of antenatal, delivery, and postpartum services in rural Tanzania. Glob Health Action. 2015;8:28567.
12. McCauley M, Stewart C, Kebede B. A survey of healthcare providers' knowledge and attitudes regarding pain relief in labor for women in Ethiopia. BMC Pregnancy Childbirth. 2017;17(1):56.
13. World Health Organization. Skilled Attendants at Birth. 2017 [cited 12 Sep 2017]; Available from: http://www.who.int/gho/maternal_health/skilled_care/skilled_birth_attendance_text/en/.
14. White Ribbon Alliance, Respecful Maternity Care: the universal right of childbearing women. 2011.
15. James JN, Prakash KS, Ponniah M. Awareness and attitudes towards labour pain and labour pain relief of urban women attending a private antenatal clinic in Chennai. Indian J Anaesth. 2012;56(2):195–8.
16. Raven J, et al. The quality of childbirth care in China: women's voices: a qualitative study. BMC Pregnancy Childbirth. 2015;15:113.
17. Abasiattai A, Olatunbosun O, Edubio M. Awareness and desirability of antenatal attendees about analgesia during childbirth in a university teaching hospital in southern Nigeria. Int J Rep, Contra, Obstet Gynecol. 2016;5(5):1540–4.

18. Anarado A, et al. Knowledge and willingness of prenatal women in Enugu southeastern Nigeria to use in labour non-pharmacological pain reliefs. Afr Health Sci. 2015;15(2):568–75.

19. Nabukenya MT, et al. Knowledge, attitudes and use of labour analgesia among women at a low-income country antenatal clinic. BMC Anesthesiol. 2015;15(1):98.

20. Waweru-Siika W. Perception of labour pain among rural women presenting to a tertiary hospital in Kenya. East Afr Med J. 2015;92(3):120–5.

21. Ogboli-Nwasor EO, Adaji SE. Between pain and pleasure: pregnant women's knowledge and preferences for pain relief in labor, a pilot study from Zaria. North Niger Saudi J Anaesth. 2014;8(Suppl 1):S20–4.

22. Ndikom CM, Olejiya TE. Perceived need and use of pain relief during labour among childbearing women in Ibadan, Nigeria. Afr J Midwifery Womens Health. 2015;9(3):125.

23. Oyetunde MO, Ojerinde OE. Labour pain perception and use of non-pharmacologic labour support in newly delivered mothers in Ibadan, Nigeria. Afr J of Midwifery & Women's Health. 2013;7(4):164.

24. Sawyer A, et al. Women's experiences of pregnancy, childbirth, and the postnatal period in the Gambia: a qualitative study. Br J Health Psychol. 2011;16(3):528–41.

25. Carter N, et al. The use of triangulation in qualitative research. Oncol Nurs Forum. 2014;41(5):545–7.

26. Gale NK, et al. Using the framework method for the analysis of qualitative data in multi-disciplinary health research. BMC Med Res Methodol. 2013; 13(1):117.

27. Pope C, Ziebland S, Mays N. Qualitative research in health care: Analysing qualitative data. BMJ. 2000;320(7227):114–6.

28. World Health Organization, Companion of choice during labour and childbirth for improved quality of care, in 2016. 2016.

29. Mohammad-Hasan A, et al. Intravenous paracetamol versus intramuscular pethidine in relief of labour pain in primigravid women. Niger Med. 2014; 55(1):54–7.

30. Wee MYK, et al. A comparison of intramuscular diamorphine and intramuscular pethidine for labour analgesia: a two-Centre randomised blinded controlled trial. BJOG: An International Journal of Obstetrics and Gynaecology. 2014;121(4):447–56.

31. Ullman R, et al. Parenteral opioids for maternal pain relief in labour. Cochrane Database Syst Rev. 2011;9:CD007396.

32. Ogboli-Nwasor E, et al. Pain relief in labor: a survey of awareness, attitude, and practice of health care providers in Zaria. Niger J Pain Res. 2011;4:227–32.

33. Lawani LO, et al. Obstetric analgesia for vaginal birth in contemporary obstetrics: a survey of the practice of obstetricians in Nigeria. BMC Pregnancy and Childbirth. 2014;14(1):140.

34. Sirohiwal D, Dahiya K, De M. Efficacy of hyoscine-N-butyl bromide (Buscopan) suppositories as a cervical spasmolytic agent in labour. Aust N Z J Obstet Gynaecol. 2005;45(2):128–9.

35. Taneja B, Nath K, Dua CK. Clinical audit on the existing attitudes and knowledge of obstetricians regarding labour analgesia. Indian J Anaesth. 2004;48(3):179.

36. Hussain S, Maheswari P. Barriers for labour analgesia in South India; knowledge and attitude of relevant stakeholders: a hospital-based cross-sectional study. Indian J Anaesth. 2017;61(2):170–3.

37. Dyer RA, Reed AR, James MF. Obstetric anaesthesia in low-resource settings. Best Pract Res Clin Obstet Gynaecol. 2010;24(3):401–12.

38. Epiu I, et al. Challenges of anesthesia in low and middle-income countries: a cross-sectional survey of access to safe obstetric anesthesia in East Africa. Anesth Analg. 2017;124(1):290–9.

39. Tasnim S. Perception about pain relief during Normal labour among health care providers conducting delivery. Med Today Tomorrow. 2009;22(1):20–3.

40. MacKinnon AL, et al. Birth setting, labour experience, and postpartum psychological distress. Midwifery. 2017;50:110.

41. World Health Organization. WHO recommendations on antenatal care for a positive pregnancy experience. Geneva: World Health Organization; 2016.

2

Perceived causes of adverse pregnancy outcomes and remedies adopted by Kalenjin women in rural Kenya

Roselyter Monchari Riang'a[1,2*] , Anne Kisaka Nangulu[1,3] and Jacqueline E. W. Broerse[2]

Abstract

Background: There have been few studies about the basis on which women in developing regions evaluate and choose traditional rather than western maternal care. This qualitative study explores the socio-cultural perceptions of complications associated with pregnancy and childbirth and how these perceptions influence maternal health and care-seeking behaviours in Kenya.

Methods: Kalenjin women ($n = 42$) aged 18–45 years, who were pregnant or had given birth within the last 12 months, were interviewed. A semi-structured interview guide was used for data collection. A further nine key informant interviews with Traditional Birth Attendants (TBAs) who were also herbalists ($n = 6$), community health workers (CHWs) ($n = 3$) and a Maternal and Child Health (MCH) nursing officer ($n = 1$) were conducted. The data were analysed using MAXQDA12 software and categorised, thematised and analysed based on the symbolic dimensions of Helman's (2000) ill-health causation aetiologies model.

Results: Pregnancy complications are perceived as the consequence of pregnant women not observing culturally restricted and recommended behaviour during pregnancy, including diet; physical activities; evil social relations and spirits of the dead. These complications are considered to be preventable by following a restricted and recommended diet, and avoiding heavy duties, funerals, killing of animals and eating meat of animal carcasses, as well as restricting geographical mobility, and use of herbal remedies to counter evil and prevent complications.

Conclusion: Delay in deciding to seek maternal care is a result of women's failure to recognise symptoms and maternal health problems as potential hospital cases, and this failure stems from culturally informed perceptions of symptoms of maternal morbidity and pregnancy complications that differ significantly from biomedical interpretations. Some of the cultural maternal care and remedies adopted to prevent pregnancy complications, such as restriction of diet and social mobility, may pose risks to the pregnant woman's health and access to health facilities whereas other remedies such as restricting consumption of meat from animal carcasses and heavy duties, as well as maintaining good social relations, are cultural adaptive mechanisms that indirectly control the transmission of disease and improve maternal health, and thus should not be considered to be exclusively folk or primitive.

Keywords: Pregnancy, Perceptions, Care-seeking behaviour, Maternal health, Kalenjin, Uasin-Gishu, Kenya

* Correspondence: monchari2002@yahoo.com; r.m.rianga@vu.nl
[1]School of Arts and Social Sciences, Moi University, P.O. Box 3900-30100, Eldoret, Kenya
[2]Athena Institute, Faculty of Science, Vrije Universiteit Amsterdam, De Boelelaan 1085, 1081 HV Amsterdam, The Netherlands
Full list of author information is available at the end of the article

Background

Utilization of professional maternal health services is crucial in improving maternal, foetal and newborn health outcomes. It is estimated that 90% of pregnancy-related maternal deaths can be prevented with timely medical interventions during Antenatal Care (ANC) appointments, emergency obstetric care, safe abortion, delivery and Postnatal Care (PNC) period [1]. As a result, the World Health Organization (WHO) recommends at least four ANC visits, postnatal check-ups within 2 days of birth, and that all deliveries be attended delivered by skilled health providers and that ANC begin as soon as a woman becomes pregnant for essential interventions to be effectively administered [2].

However, maternal deaths remain high in low- and middle-income countries (LMICs) with a maternal mortality rate (MMR) of 239 per 100,000 live births [3]. Untimely, underuse or lack of professional medical interventions have been established as the main contributing factors [4, 5]. Globally, during the period 2007–2014, 64% of pregnant women attended the WHO-recommended minimum of four ANC contacts, with 78% of births being attended by a skilled health professional [6]. Low access to professional maternal care services is worse in LMICs. The Kenya Demographic Health Survey (KDHS) statistics, for instance, indicated that although nearly 90% of women seek ANC in health facilities, 58% of pregnant women made four or more ANC visits, while 20% made their first visit within the first trimester [7]. Many women wait until the last trimester to do this while others make only one visit, thus limiting the benefits that would have been extended to them under the free government maternal care programme [8–10]. Overall, 44% of births in Kenya are attended by skilled birth attendants [11]. The underuse of professional maternal health services is reportedly higher in rural areas [7] and the situation is worse in some parts of the country. For instance, in Uasin Gishu County of Kenya (where this study was conducted), only 22% of pregnant women attended at least four ANC sessions, while only 30% of all births are attended by skilled health staff [12].

In contrast to the limited uptake of professional maternal health services in Kenya and other LMICs, most women make extensive use and reliance on traditional maternal care and remedies, even when they are suffering serious emergency obstetric complications. A study by Kaingu et al. [10] in Machakos County Kenya, for instance, identified a total of 10 pregnancy-related complications and symptoms, including being threatened spontaneous abortion, labour complications and post-partum haemorrhage that are being managed at the mother's home by Traditional Birth Attendants (TBAs). They further identified 55 plant species that were being used as medicinal herbs for the management and treatment of pregnancy complications. TBAs, mothers-in-law and older female relatives are important community resource persons whom pregnant women routinely consult throughout the course of pregnancy and childbirth, especially in rural areas in LMICs [7, 8, 11]. The situation is made particularly challenging by the fact that most informal maternal care providers, especially in the rural areas, have no formal training in maternal care and child delivery, instead they rely on their traditional knowledge, which is not well known in the literature. There is little evidence that this situation will soon improve because even when mothers seek care at the health facilities, studies indicate that they tend to integrate both western and indigenous knowledge in their understanding of health and medicine [13].

Indigenous knowledge is an integral part of life in rural communities. This knowledge has a great influence on how communities perceive health, illness, causes of disease and consequently their care-seeking behaviours [14, 15]. These traditional healthcare practices could be useful or detrimental. Rather than ignoring and condemning it, this knowledge should be explored, strengthened through research and scientific evidence, documented and disseminated, especially to healthcare providers, so that they can be informed about the actual practices in which women engage during pregnancy and childbirth. To this end, the present study aims to gain insight into traditional antenatal care practices adopted by pregnant women and their implications for maternal health and access to biomedical care interventions. Examining the socio-cultural context of pregnancy and childbirth is important to understanding maternal mortality and health-seeking behaviours.

Theoretical framework

This study was guided by symbolic interaction and functionalist perspectives. The research findings are analysed through the lens of symbolic interactionism in order to understand how the Kalenjin perceive and respond to adverse pregnancy outcomes. It was established that the Kalenjin women's responses and behaviours regarding pregnancy complications are directed by the meanings they attribute to these complications. These meanings are constructed and learned through social interactions with other members of society. What is important to realise, however, is that these meanings are based on what is culturally believed to be true and not what is 'objectively true' from the perspective of western biomedical models. Hence, these meanings may override and conflict with biomedical realities of health and thus require contextualised interpretations and interventions. Women act in ways that accord with the meaning that they attribute to adverse pregnancy outcomes. Understanding these symbolic meanings, therefore, will assist in comprehending the Kalenjin women's responses and behaviour towards adverse pregnancy outcomes.

The discussion of the research results was also guided by the functionalist perspectives. These cultural explanatory models of illness, even if based on scientifically incorrect premises, frequently have an internal logic and consistency, which often helps the victim of illness to "make sense" of what has happened, why it has happened and the appropriate disease prevention and treatment therapy to adopt. On the other hand, some of these causal explanations of pregnancy-related illness are deliberate attempts to reduce pregnancy complications but are based on an understanding of disease transmission that differs from the western biomedical models. When the underlying unconscious adaptive significance is effective, these pregnant women will continue adopting the practice even though they may not be aware of the adoptive value of what they are doing, which contributes to the selective retention of these prevention and treatment remedies. For this reason, it is necessary to take into account these unintended, adaptive benefits of various pregnancy practices and belief systems in any attempt to unravel complex patterns of treatment during pregnancy.

However, ethnomedical explanatory models of illness are not always in people's best interest. Some belief systems and ritual practices appear to have maladaptive effects, which pose medical risks to those practising them. It is therefore important to understand these practices in any given intervention.

Methods
Study setting and data collection
The major focus of this qualitative study was on the cultural interpretation of pregnancy complications and the preventive and treatment remedies adopted. This study is part of broader research investigating the socio-cultural context of maternal nutrition and health in rural Uasin Gishu County in western Kenya. Data were collected between April and August 2015 from Kalenjin women, either pregnant or with a child of less than 1 year, seeking care at the government health facilities in the Maternal and Child Health (MCH) care section.

The Kalenjin is the main ethnic population in Uasin Gishu County and comprises eight sub-ethnic groups (the Kipsigis, Nandi, Tugen, Keiyo, Marakwet, Pokot, Sabaot and the Terik) that share a common dialect and similar cultural traits. Among the Kalenjin speakers, each sub-ethnic group has its own distinctive dialect. The Nandi occupies the largest settlement in Uasin Gishu County, followed by the Keiyo.

All 90 public health facilities in the county were included in the sampling frame. Quota and purposive sampling techniques were employed in the selection of a representative sample of health facilities for the study. The selection criteria included ensuring that the health facilities in all the six-quotas (sub-counties) are proportionately represented in the sample. All the health facilities must be in the rural area (outside the municipality territory) and have a catchment population mainly comprising at least 90% Kalenjin patients to enhance cultural homogeneity. This means that areas dominated by other non-Kalenjin ethnic groups and those within the municipal boundaries were eliminated. The last criterion is that the selected facilities should be spatially distributed from each other to diversify responses. In the end, a total of 23 health facilities were sampled for the study.

All the Kalenjin women who come for routine antenatal and post-partum child welfare check-ups in the sampled health facilities were included in the sampling frame. They were recruited at the MCH clinics and in maternity wards. Eligibility criteria for the study participants depended on: being pregnant or having given birth within the last year, a Kalenjin by birth, willing and able to participate in the study, able to give informed consent [16] and willing to be audio recorded. This selection criterion eliminated non-Kalenjin women and those not willing to be audio recorded. Data were collected until the information reached saturation at a sample size of 42 women [17].

Nine key informants, including six TBAs who are also herbalists, one CHW, and one nursing officer in charge of MCH, were also selected for an interview. Quota sampling and purposive sampling techniques were used in the selection of key informants [17]. One TBA from each of the six sub-counties, who was highly mentioned by women respondents who had given birth at home or took herbal remedies during pregnancy, was selected and they could be reached at home or in the market centre. The CHW and nursing officer were selected from one of the largest rural facilities in the county because they are likely to encounter a wide range of pregnancy experiences and challenges given their large catchment area. In total, six TBAs who were also herbalists, one nursing officer offering MCH care, and one CHW were recruited.

Data collection
An open-ended interview guide (Additional file 1), divided into four sections, was used to elicit the information from the Kalenjin women. The first section presented demographic characteristics of the respondents including age, educational level, parity, ethnic affiliation and gestational age at the first ANC visit, marital status, and tribal affiliation among others. The other sections contained questions about food restrictions, recommended food, activities restricted and activities encouraged during pregnancy. Every practice mentioned was probed to obtain an insight into the underlying reasons. The respondents were further questioned about their opinions regarding these cultural practices and whether they indeed practised them.

Perceived causes of adverse pregnancy outcomes and remedies adopted by Kalenjin women...

13

Face-to-face individual interviews were conducted in a private room. Each woman was interviewed once and the interview lasted between 30 and 60 min, depending on her responses. Key informant interviews (KIIs) followed later to provide clarity on the issues raised during the interviews. The KIIs lasted between an hour and 2.5 h. They were also questioned about the kind of advice they give pregnant women and health challenges they face when providing care to pregnant women. Important notes were taken and at the same time responses were audio recorded.

Ethical considerations

The study was approved by the National Commission for Science, Technology and Innovation (NACOSTI) in Kenya and a research clearance permit number: NACOSTI/P/15/2335/5353 dated 2 April 2015 was issued to facilitate the research process. As approved by NACOSTI, the permit was then presented to the Uasin-Gishu County Commissioner, County Director of Education and County Director of Health, for their approval to conduct the study in the County. Further, appointments were booked with the respective officers in charge of the various facilities visited. Participation was voluntary. The respondents were informed of the aim of the research, confidentiality and anonymity of their responses, and then gave their signed consent to participate. Permission to audio record the interview sessions was sought from each respondent. Only voices for those who consented were recorded.

Analysis

Recorded responses were transcribed and, together with field notes, were studied by way of content analysis using MAXQDA 12.0.3 software. Helman's [15] classification of lay-illness aetiologies model was adopted as the initial coding guide. Meanings attributed to various adverse pregnancy outcomes were established in the data and were classified into four major categories based on Helman's [15] symbolic classification of lay-illness causation aetiologies model: individual, natural, social and supernatural, as illustrated in Fig. 1. The categories were further classified into sub-categories and themes as interpreted below.

Individual causes These include lay theories that locate the meaning of pregnancy complications in the individual woman for "not taking care" of herself in terms of diet, dress, hygiene, lifestyle, relationships, sexual behaviour, smoking and drinking habits, physical exercise, emotions or doing something abnormal or incorrect. An adverse pregnancy outcome is, therefore, evidence of "carelessness" and the woman should feel guilty and responsible for causing it. However, in some rare circumstances, individual causes can result from external forces over which the victim had no control such as bad luck, economic power or hereditary factors.

Natural causes In this category, an adverse pregnancy outcome is thought to be caused by the natural environment, both living and inanimate. Common in this group are climatic conditions, such as excess cold, heat, wind, rain, snow, damp, cyclones, tornadoes, eclipse or severe storms. Others include accidental injuries which originate from the "natural environment", or are caused by animals, birds, insects, or infections caused by micro-organisms, such as germs, bugs or viruses.

Social causes This category involves blaming other people for causing adverse pregnancy outcomes and is a common feature of non-industrialised and smaller-scale societies, where interpersonal conflicts are frequent. The common forms of these are witchcraft, sorcery and "evil eyes". In witchcraft, certain people are believed to possess a mystical power to harm others and this power is inherited, either genetically or by membership of a particular kinship group. Sorcery, as defined by Helman

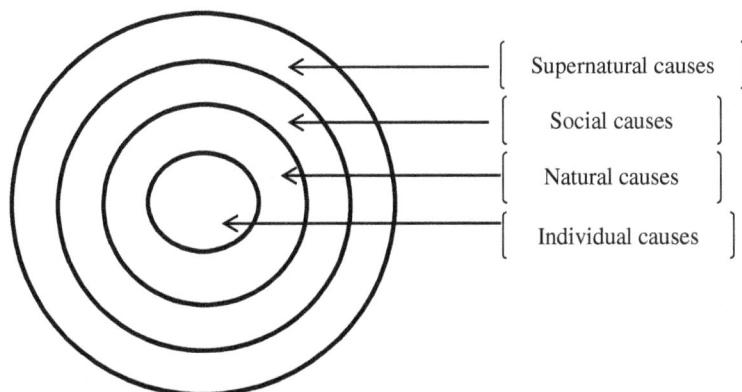

Fig. 1 Sites of illness aetiology (Helman, 2000:120)

[15], is the power to manipulate and alter natural and supernatural events with the proper magical knowledge and performance of rituals, and this is different from witchcraft. Sorcery is often practised among one's social world of friends, family or neighbours, and is often based on envy. Evil eyes, or a "wounding eye", relates to the fear of envy in the eyes of the beholder. The possessors of evil eye are usually believed to harm unintentionally and are often unaware of their powers and are unable to control them. The influence of evil eye, as explained by Helman [15], is avoided or counteracted by means of devices calculated to distract its attention, and by practices of sympathetic magic. The social aetiology of illness also includes physical injuries, such as poisoning or battle wounds, inflicted by other people. Furthermore, it can be stress or actions caused by spouse, children, friends, employer or colleagues and neighbours. It can also be contagious diseases transmitted by other people.

Supernatural causes Here a pregnancy complication is ascribed to the direct actions of supernatural entities, such as gods, spirits or ancestral shades. In the gods aetiology, illness is described as a reminder from God for a behavioural lapse or sinful behaviour. The cure in this case involves acknowledging the sins and vowing to improve one's behaviour. In the case of spiritual causes, disease-bearing spirits strike unexpectedly causing a variety of symptoms in their victims. Their invasion is unrelated to the individual's behaviour, who is therefore considered blameless and worthy of sympathetic help from others. In the case of ancestral shades causes, a pregnancy complication is ascribed to spirits of the ancestors whom they have offended and diagnosis takes place in a divinatory séance.

Results
Socio-demographic characteristics of the respondents
A total of 42 female respondents were interviewed, of whom 14 were pregnant and 28 were post-natal (Table 1). Half of the respondents had acquired primary education. All respondents were age 18 years and above and more than 26 respondents were between 20 and 29 years of age. Many respondents ($n = 30$) were married and almost all worked in the informal economy as subsistence farmers, homemakers or small entrepreneurs. Only 13 of the respondents were first-time mothers and the other 29 had 2–8 children. For the recent pregnancy, three respondents did not seek any ANC from the health facility. For those who attended ANC at the health facility, only three did so in the first trimester while the majority started after 6 months of pregnancy.

Table 1 Demographic characteristics of the respondents

Characteristic	Categories	Number of cases ($N = 42$)
Maternal status	Ante-natal	14
	Post-natal	28
Parity	First Pregnancy/child	13
	1–3	15
	4–6	11
	7–8	3
Gestational age at the first ANC visit	Never visited	3
	2 months	3
	4 months	3
	5 months	6
	6 months	16
	≥ 7 months	11
Age of respondents (years)	≤ 19	4
	20–24	16
	25–29	10
	30–34	7
	≥ 35	5
Marital status	Never married	8
	Currently married	30
	Separated	2
	Widowed	2
Educational level	Primary Education	21
	Secondary Education	16
	Tertiary Education	5
Occupation	Student/pupil	4
	Business	7
	Farming	26
	Formal employment	1
	Other	4
Sub-ethnic groups	Nandi	31
	Keiyo	4
	Marakwet	5
	Terik	1
	Kipsigis	1

Perceptions of and responses to adverse pregnancy outcomes
Several perceived causes of pregnancy complications and the remedies adopted were identified and classified into four major categories based on Helman's [15] classification of lay-illness aetiologies model as illustrated in Fig. 1. Further, sub-categories and themes that emerged were established and are presented in Table 2.

Table 2 Interpretation of pregnancy complications and remedies

Category (Cause)	Subcategory (Sub-cause)	Theme (perceived causes)	N = 42 (%)	Theme (perceived remedies)
Individual causes	Physical activities	Doing heavy duties	25(60%)	Avoid doing heavy duties
		Having sexual intercourse during pregnancy	10(24%)	Abstain from sexual intercourse during pregnancy
		Idling	9(21%)	Do light duties
		Standing or peeping at the door/window way	6(14%)	Either walk out quickly or stay
		Running or walking long distances	5(12%)	Avoid running and long walks
		Oversleeping	4(10%)	Avoid over sleeping
		Boarding a motorbike	2(5%)	Avoid using motor bikes
		Sitting and sleeping style	2(5%)	Sit with legs straight, Sleep on the side, not on back
		Dress code	2(5%)	Avoid dressing accessories around the body including necklace, belts or clothes with bands around the waist
	Diet	Eating restricted food (eggs, avocado, meat, oily food, fresh milk, cold ugali cold water, alcohol and cigarettes)	41(98%)	Avoid restricted food
		Not eating recommended food and herbal medicine (traditional vegetables, milk, liver, ugali)	41(98%)	Eat recommended food Use herbal medicine
Natural Causes	Sickness and hereditary complications	Severe cramps during menses	8(19%)	Seek herbal treatment
		Wrong foetal presentation	3(7%)	Seek TBA care to turn the foetus
		Malaria	2(5%)	Take preventive herbal remedies Only take prescribed drugs
		Amount of hair and sex of the foetus	2(5%)	Seek TBA advice/treatment
		Yellow fever	1(2%)	Seek herbal treatment
Social world	Getting in contact with dangerous people	Contact with a woman who had an abortion, or whose child died recently, or who had a wrong foetal presentation during birth, multiple births or who develops severe cramps during menses, or who have evil eyes	10(24%)	Reduce movements Avoid going to public places Use protective herbs
	Social relations	Quarrelling with/abusing someone	5(12%)	Maintain peaceful relations Confession and repentance
		Made to cry or stressed	2(5%)	Avoid emotional events
Super natural causes	Evil spirits	Eating meat of a "misfortune animal"	16(38%)	Avoid eating "evil meat"
		Killing an animal	12(29%)	Avoid killing any animal
		An animal crossing your way or meeting two snakes on your way	3(7%)	End the journey whenever one meets world animal, mostly a snake, on the way
	Gods	Laughing at a deformed person	8(19%)	Do not lough at a deformed person
	Ancestral spirits	Viewing or burying a dead person	11 (26%)	Avoid burials Do not view a dead body
		A relative committed evil actions towards the ancestor	4 (10%)	Conduct a reconciliation ritual

Individual causes

Individual cause is one of the factors that strongly emerged in this study. Under this category, pregnancy complications are seen as evidence of the pregnant woman's carelessness and as a result she should feel guilty about her incorrect practices during her pregnancy. These are particularly related to physical activities and diet.

Physical activities

One of the restricted activities that strongly emerged in the study, as reported by 60% of the respondents, is that a pregnant woman should be exempted from performing "heavy duties". Heavy duties that were commonly forbidden according to the respondents refer to activities that involve bending for long hours, carrying heavy loads, fetching water from an open well, "scooping soil" (digging), carrying soil and smearing mud houses. Other activities reported include: hand washing many clothes, splitting firewood, collecting water from the river using a heavy container (e.g. 20 kg), or carrying a heavy load of firewood. Heavy duties are believed to cause lower back pain that may cause a miscarriage, pre-term birth and excessive bleeding after birth or low birth weight. Splitting firewood is also believed to make the baby's fontanelle abnormally large, which is dangerous because it is believed to cause its death.

> *Heavy duties like digging, splitting firewood should be avoided because it drains all the energy from the lower back making it ache and become weak. This is dangerous....it can make the baby come out* [abortion].

To avoid lower back pains that cause a miscarriage, it is perceived that a pregnant woman should not only avoid heavy activities, but also seek herbal treatment. The herbs are believed to strengthen the lower back and thus minimise back pains during pregnancy and after the birth.

> *When a woman is pregnant, she should not overwork herself with housework or digging. This is why some of them come to me complaining of back pains. I give them pain relief herbs and I normally tell them to completely avoid overworking themselves.* (Herbalist 2)

Some respondents felt that fetching water from an open well is risky; a woman might lose her balance and fall into the well. Collecting water from the well is discouraged in the first 4 months of pregnancy, because at this stage, pregnancy is still considered immature hence fragile and easy to abort. Thus, such activity can be undertaken after a pregnancy is 5 months or more. A pregnant woman may also carry a light load (10 kg or less) that she can easily lift without being assisted.

> *Sometimes there are women when giving birth, legs of the baby come out first instead of the head or those who experience severe cramps during menses. Such a woman should not assist you in lifting the load to your head or back when you are pregnant. You will also give birth like her or have an abortion.*

A pregnant woman is also advised to abstain from having sexual intercourse, as reported by 24% of the respondents. However, the period of abstinence varied; to some, abstinence should begin the moment you realise you are pregnant, to others from 6 months onwards. The semen is believed to make the baby dirty, because it sticks on the baby's skin and scalp, creating a white substance. Thus, the baby must be washed with herbs for several days to clear it off. The "semen" is also believed to be dangerous for the foetus because it is thought to block the nasal passages and this could make breathing difficult and subsequently cause death. It is also thought that the "semen" can be swallowed by the foetus and remain stuck in the chest, causing a wheezing chest. The condition is believed to be more dangerous if the baby is a boy because males are considered less active in the uterus and cannot wash it off into the amniotic fluid. A woman who did not abstain from sex will be detected during birth because "she will be messy with semen" and nobody will be willing to assist her delivery, including the midwife. Instead, they will use plastic bags as gloves in assisting delivery, and the woman and her husband will be abused and ostracised.

> *.....ejaculations of the man are dangerous to the baby and messy, even those facilitating your birth might run away and leave you, they do not like looking at those things. They will be forced to use plastic bags to remove the baby and give you to wash it by yourself. They only assist you well if you give birth to a clean baby.*

Some respondents, including one of the CHWs, reported that they use condoms during pregnancy to prevent the semen from reaching the baby.

On the other hand, a pregnant woman should not be idle (21%) and should not oversleep (10%) but perform light duties. Light duties include washing a few clothes, grazing cows, weeding a small plot, or taking a nature walk. It is believed that, when a woman is idle or asleep, the foetus also becomes idle, inactive and docile because it tends to sleep a lot. A docile foetus, according to the respondents, is not strong enough to assist the mother when she is pushing during delivery, resulting in prolonged labour. Similarly, if a pregnant woman is idling or sleeping a lot makes her muscles will be weak during labour and she will not find it easy to push out the baby.

> *I was told not to sleep too much but to be active in doing light duties like grazing animals and digging but not too much of it. It makes the baby play well and be positioned in the right part of the womb; otherwise I will have trouble during birth. The pain will extend for long.*

Domestic duties like washing utensils, and when your body is okay you can go to the farm. It helps blood to flow very well, and the body to function well, but if you just stay idle it can even bring you diseases like high blood pressure and diabetes.

A pregnant woman, as reported by 14% of the respondents, should not peep through or stand in the doorway or window of a house. If she has a tendency to do this and return, during labour, the baby will also peep though the cervix, trying to come out, but instead return back into the uterus, thus prolonging labour. To avoid the chances of prolonged labour, a pregnant woman should decisively either stay inside or just walk out of the house and avoid standing in the doorway.

A pregnant woman should also avoid running or walking long distances, as reported by 12% of the respondents:

One should not run when pregnant, she can accidentally fall down causing the pregnancy to pain [contractions] *before term.*

Other restricted activities during pregnancy that were reported by less than 10% of the respondents include boarding a motorbike (the means of transport commonly used in rural areas), the dress code, sitting style and sleeping positions. High heels are considered dangerous because they might cause a woman to fall, and that could lead to pre-term contractions/miscarriage. Pregnant women should also avoid clothes with a band around the waist, such as skirts, trousers and belts. Bands around the waist are believed to make the umbilical cord twist around the baby during birth, which they believe may cause stillbirth. A pregnant woman should sit with her legs straight and apart. Sitting with her legs twisted or bent, they believe, will block the birth canal and result in obstructed labour.

Diet

Pregnancy complications were also thought to be caused by the wrong diet during pregnancy. Some foods, as reported by 98% of the respondents, were considered to jeopardise a pregnancy if consumed in excess, while others can endanger pregnancy if they are not eaten in sufficient quantity. Thus, a pregnant woman is required to eat sparingly and selectively. High-protein and energy-rich foods were believed to make the foetus grow big. A big foetus cannot be pushed out easily and will cause an obstruction, thus prolonging labour and possibly lead to caesarean section (CS). CS is believed to be a risky process in the sense that it halves the chances of mother or child survival, unlike an uncomplicated vaginal delivery. The big foetus also results in a prolonged labour and may cause tears by forcing itself out. Eggs, avocado, and oily food

were commonly reported as needing to be avoided or restricted.

I was told not to eat strong food like eggs and avocado. The baby will grow big and later will give me problems when giving birth and I can even be operated.

Other foods of this kind that should be eaten sparingly include: meat, fresh milk, cooked bananas, and cold *ugali*. TBAs/herbalists prescribe herbs to regularise the size of the baby especially if it is judged to be too big.

Consumption of alcohol and cigarettes is restricted during pregnancy because it is believed to result in low birthweight and mentally retarded babies. Furthermore, when in labour, a pregnant woman should not drink cold water. It is believed to freeze contractions and thus lead to prolonged labour.

Some foods were believed to be good for pregnancy, hence encouraged to be eaten in plenty. According to most respondents, a pregnant woman is recommended to increase her blood volume and energy. A woman with less blood volume is considered not to have strength to push out the baby, will bleed to death during labour, and might require blood transfusion, which is believed to be risky. Therefore, lots of the foods that are believed to increase the amount of blood should be eaten for the entire period of pregnancy. These include indigenous vegetables (mostly leafy greens, including pigweed, black nightshade, spider plant, spinach, white vine spinach, pumpkin leaves and cowpea leaves), fruits, liver, animal blood, milk (especially when mixed with animal blood), red beans and their soup, meat, porridge made of finger millet flour, red soil or red stones and some traditional herbs.

When your blood is less, it will only help you to get a baby, thereafter; you will bleed until your body dries up and you die.

A pregnant woman is also required to be stronger during pregnancy. It is believed that a weak woman will not be able to push the baby out.

If you do not feed well on the pregnancy recommended food, you will not have strength for pushing out the baby during birth. You will be weak, you can even faint. They will demand an operation in order to remove the baby. With the operation you might die.

It is therefore recommended for her to eat "strong" energy-giving food during the pregnancy and minimise "less" energy food. *Ugali* and porridge were the commonly reported foods believed to be rich in energy. Others were milk, rice, sweet potatoes, Irish potatoes and herbs. However, rice and Irish potatoes are regarded as 'less energy-giving food' that should be eaten only once in a while.

Use of preventive herbs during pregnancy was reported by the majority of the respondents, mainly to prevent mother-to-child transmission. A TBA presented 10 different herbal medicines that are boiled together for pregnant women to drink, whether sick or not. Hence, a pregnant woman will be held responsible for any miscarriage if she refuses to take these preventive herbs.

Natural causes

Some aspects of the natural environment were also believed to cause pregnancy complications, though not reported by as many respondents as other aspects of Helman's model. The aspects of natural causes that emerged in this study were mainly infectious and hereditary diseases. Severe pre-pregnancy menstrual cramps (*chepsaliat*), as reported by 19%, are believed to cause miscarriage or pre-term contractions during the first months of pregnancy. Therefore, it is thought that girls who experience severe pre-pregnancy menstrual cramps are likely to abort within 4 months of conception if they do not seek herbal treatment before conceiving.

I had a miscarriage at two and a half months in my previous pregnancy, my grandmother told me it was caused by cramps. When I was a girl, I used to have severe menstrual cramps.

Severe menstrual cramps, as explained by the herbalist, are inherited and are extended to pregnancy and are believed to pierce the capillaries supplying blood to the uterus resulting in "blood leakage" that supposedly causes spontaneous abortion mostly within the fourth month of pregnancy.

To avoid the chances of early miscarriage, girls who experience pre-pregnancy *chepsaliat* are highly recommended to seek herbal treatment before conception. However, if the woman notices unusual contractions or spots of blood and seeks immediate herbal attention, "the capillaries can be sealed" (spontaneous abortion can be controlled) as explained by a TBA/herbalist:

....If someone ignores the herbs and instead opts for hospital treatment before taking the herbs, she cannot control the bleeding even if I give her the herbs. That one is beyond repair, the herbs cannot help her. Whoever ignores these herbs aborts. (Herbalist 2)

If a pregnant woman falls sick, her illness is also believed to be transferable to the foetus causing foetal death (miscarriage or perinatal death). The reported diseases were malaria and yellow fever. As a result, maternal sickness or the possibility of mother-to-child transmission should be prevented by periodically drinking herbs or be treated using mild herbal medicine. Hospital medicines are acceptable but believed to be 'too strong' and may cause spontaneous abortion, hence herbs were preferred.

When I miscarried my previous pregnancy, the TBA told me a different causal reason from my grand mum.... The cause she told me was yellow fever. When I conceived this second pregnancy, she gave me preventive herbs. I started taking from the time my pregnancy was 1 month old. I used to take them daily for 5 days per month until I finished 3 months then she terminated the dose.

Other natural causes were associated with the foetus itself. For instance, the sex of the foetus and its amount of hair were considered a determining factor of the mother's feelings and physical status during pregnancy. Female foetuses are believed to give the mother nausea, lack of appetite, feeling sickly and make her thin and moody, whereas male foetuses are believed to make the mother crave certain types of food, increased appetite, look healthy, strong and jovial. Abundant foetal hair is associated with heartburn to the mother. It is believed that the long hair stretches to the throat causing the irritation.

Numbness of one leg, which complicates movement during pregnancy, is thought to be caused by the abnormal presentation of the foetus and this is believed to cause complicated delivery. TBAs are believed to have inherited skills to massage the uterus and correctly reposition the foetus, hence relieving discomfort to the mother and making birth easier.

Social causes

The social-based explanations that emerged strongly from the study, as reported by 24% of the respondents, is that a pregnant woman should not contact "dangerous people".

Pregnancy complications were believed to be contagious. For instance, a woman who had ever had an abortion or whose child died recently is considered to be contagious, and if she is in contact with a pregnant woman or her shadow falls on the body of a pregnant woman, it is believed to cause miscarriage, stillbirth, and perinatal death or make the woman sick. Other women believed to be dangerous and who should be avoided included those who had a breech or traverse presentation during birth or a multiple birth, or who experience severe menstrual cramps. This can cause pre-term contractions that might cause spontaneous abortion.

I was told not to meet someone whose child died or to get near her or the one who encountered an abortion. If she gets close to you, your baby might also come out [abortion] *or you can even fall sick.*

Some people are known to have evil eyes that can cause a miscarriage if they meet a pregnant woman. Therefore, a pregnant woman should stay away from such people. Some of these "dangerous" people are known, while others are not. Hence, the main way to reduce the chances of meeting them is to restrict movement outside the homestead, avoid walking along public roads, and going to crowded places such as market centres or other social gatherings.

I was just told when someone is pregnant like me now; I should avoid going where there are a lot of people.

Women are not allowed to visit to places when pregnant. They can meet evil people that can cause problems to the foetus. (Herbalist 1)

As a remedy, herbs are available in a roasted powder form, called *bosarok*, which is to be licked every morning. Pig oil can also be applied on the pregnant woman's face and tummy, especially when she is going on a journey, to counter evil eyes. Such herbs were commonly reported by respondents during the study.

When you wake up in the morning, the first thing you should do even before you wash your face is to lick the 'bosarok' [herbs]. *The timings and location of these women is not known. She might come to your house early in the morning to borrow tea leaves for breakfast. These herbs keep the baby safe in the stomach* [womb]. *If you use them as reserved, these spirits cannot attack the baby.*

Social relations
A pregnant woman should not exchange utterances or abusive words with anyone. This is because the opponent might "abuse her badly". The feared abuse mostly reported was "you will give birth but you will not hold that baby", referring to a stillbirth. If a pregnant woman is abused with these words, it is believed that this woman will have a stillbirth, or her baby will die shortly after birth. Moreover, the husband of a pregnant woman or any other close person should not do anything or utter words that might annoy or make her cry or emotionally stressed.

When pregnant, you should not quarrel or exchange words with anybody even if you find a person red handed backbiting you or doing something wrong to you. You simply stay silent and assume that nothing is wrong. If you start exchanging words, the person might abuse you badly and at the end you will give birth and your baby dies.

It is not good for a pregnant woman to cry. This is like moaning for her death or that of her unborn child. She might die or give birth to a dead baby.

Therefore, to avoid complications that may lead to a stillbirth or perinatal death, it is recommended to maintain peaceful relationships by avoiding quarrels. Similarly, a pregnant woman should not be abused or offended even if she transgresses anyone. Should she be abused or offended accidentally, the offending person should apologise immediately. If a pregnant woman had a dispute with someone, and this was not resolved, and she develops a complicated labour, the person concerned or who caused her stress will be sought to come and confess, in order to ease labour and facilitate birth. The offender will be held accountable for any calamity and this will cause the person emotions of shame and guilt. Therefore, a pregnant woman is expected to be respected by members of the community.

Supernatural causes
In this category, explanations of pregnancy complications were ascribed to supernatural causes, mostly spirits and to some extent ancestral spirits and gods.

Evil spirit of the dead
A pregnant woman is not supposed to eat meat of an animal carcass, as reported by 38% of the respondents. Such meat was believed to possess evil spirits that are transferable when eaten. The meat commonly reported to be avoided is an animal that was slaughtered because it suffered and died from pregnancy-related complications, such as placental retention, haemorrhage, an abortion or stillbirth. If eaten, it is believed that the "bad blood" that caused such complications is transferred, causing very similar complications to a pregnant woman who consumed it. Similarly, an animal that was slaughtered because it was sick, for unknown reasons, struck by lightning or by strangling itself with its umbilical cord, should not be consumed. The former is believed to cause maternal death whereas the latter will make the umbilical cord coil around the baby's neck resulting in stillbirth. Thus, a pregnant woman should be aware of the meat she eats. However, if she eats it without knowing its provenance, cleansing rituals must be performed to clear off the spirits of the bad blood.

In case there was a goat which died with kids in the stomach, that meat should not be eaten. Or a cow that died during labour, for example the calf came out but placenta retained she should not eat its meat. If she eats it, the placenta will also be retained during birth or she will die just like that animal.

On the other hand, as reported by 29% of the respondents, a pregnant woman or her husband should not kill any animal (wild nor domestic) or insects. Instead, they should get someone from the neighbourhood to do it for them. Otherwise it is believed that she will give birth to a baby with similar features of that animal. Unless they conduct rituals that involve giving the baby the name of that animal, the baby will retain those features to maturity, some of which are dangerous. The commonly mentioned animals were snakes, cats, dogs and chicken, and the killing was believed to cause disabilities such as blindness, lameness or even death.

I was told not to kill a snake; my baby will look like a snake... will have red eyes that look away from each other and unstable neck, just like a snake. They will call the baby 'Kiberen' continuously until the features disappear. The baby will also cry like a cat if you killed a cat or walk using toes like dog with a funny head if you killed a dog. (TBA 3)

Similarly, 26% of the respondents further reported that a pregnant woman is not allowed to view a dead body. The commonly reported forbidden act is viewing the body while inside the coffin or inside the grave. Traditionally, they were not allowed to even attend the funeral as reported by a key informant. If a person dies in the homestead, she moves away until the burial rituals are completed. The husband of a pregnant woman is not allowed to take part in digging the grave and burying of the dead. Many respondents could not understand why it is prohibited, yet they obeyed the custom. However, some respondents reported that a funeral is emotional and it worsens when viewing the body or burying the corpse. These emotions can make one faint and collapse which can cause damage to the uterus resulting in miscarriage e, stillbirth or maternal death.

Gods
Foetal deformity, as reported by 19% of the respondents, could arise if the pregnant woman makes fun of a person with a physical or mental disability. It is believed that this could result in God afflicting the infant with a similar disability.

Other beliefs ascribed to supernatural causes that emerged in the study were based on ancestral spirits, especially if a close relative of the pregnant woman's husband

committed an evil act to a deceased member of the family and did not reconcile before he/she died. In this case, therefore, when a pregnant woman undergoes prolonged labour, male elders will be called to conduct reconciliation rituals at the graveyard of the deceased.

Discussion
This study examined the lay meanings ascribed to adverse pregnancy outcomes and the adopted treatment and remedies among the Kalenjin in rural Uasin-Gishu County in Kenya. A healthy pregnancy is perceived as a process that pregnant women are able to manipulate by observing behaviours, and taking remedies against natural, social and supernatural forces during pregnancy. The explanatory models of these local meanings are deliberate attempts to reduce and prevent pregnancy complications but are in many cases based on an understanding of disease transmission that differs from biomedical explanations. Some remedies are beneficial, others make no sense at all, while others to some extent can even be detrimental to maternal health as indicated below.

Restricting geographical mobility
In this study, pregnancy complications are attributed to evil people, so pregnant women are confined to the homestead to avoid contracting evil people and are encouraged to apply medicinal herbs to counter evil. Restrictions on geographical mobility reduce vulnerability to contracting infectious diseases. Pregnant women are at a higher risk and more susceptible to or more severely affected by infectious diseases because of the unique "immunological" condition caused by pregnancy. Infections contracted during pregnancy are in most cases associated with maternal death, stillbirth, spontaneous abortion and pre-term birth, hence this is a good practice that should be enhanced. However, the fears of meeting evil people can result in disruptive or non-use of public health facilities by avoiding going outside. Beliefs in witchcraft, poisoning or spiritual attacks are a major component of African cultures' explanatory model of pregnancy complications and illness and have been established as a major barrier to accessing health facilities for care [18, 19].

Use of herbal medicine
Preventive herbs are believed to protect pregnant woman from getting sick and from transmitting sickness to the foetus. Naturally, pregnancy is a state of immunological weakness, and therefore of increased susceptibility to infectious diseases. Improving the immune system is one of the most important ways of protecting the mother against the environmental infections and preventing damage to the foetus. Malaria In Pregnancy (MIP) is a major public health problem in areas of sub-Saharan Africa, including

parts of Kenya, where malaria is endemic, and has important consequences for the birth outcome. Similarly, the risk of pre-term delivery and of miscarriage was found to be high in mothers with HIV and with MIP occurring within 2 weeks of delivery [20]. Use of minerals, plants, and animal products as medicines during pregnancy is a common practice in Kenya, especially among the Kalenjin, to treat pregnancy-related complications and symptoms [10, 21, 22]. Some herbal plants have been confirmed to have antibacterial, anti-inflammatory, antimicrobial and antimalarial properties [23]. However, the safety and efficacy of many of these medicinal herbs, especially during pregnancy, when the human body is vulnerable, still needs to be established.

Avoid sexual intercourse during pregnancy

Ante-natal sexual taboos, which prohibit couples from having sexual intercourse from the second trimester of pregnancy, were also established in the study. In African societies, abstinence from sexual intercourse during pregnancy and for some period after childbirth is a common phenomenon, and is believed to be associated with contamination that might be harmful to the unborn baby or the husband and that the mother is considered to be too fragile to have sex [19, 24, 25]. These women may not justify sexual abstinence during pregnancy in biomedical terms, but scientifically the latent function of this custom is to prevent the transmission of sexually transmitted infections (STIs) to a pregnant woman. STIs, including HIV/AIDS, among pregnant women are common in Kenya [26–28] and have been associated with a number of adverse pregnancy outcomes, such as spontaneous abortion, ectopic pregnancy, pre-term delivery, low birthweight, stillbirth, postpartum sepsis, and congenital infection [28], thus justifying the custom. However, encouraging sexual abstinence during pregnancy might result in men seeking extra-marital sex and might thereby increase the spread of STIs. Some pregnant women in this study opt to use condoms during sexual intercourse to overcome the complications, a practice that needs to be encouraged.

Minimise emotional stress

The belief that a pregnant woman is not supposed to experience emotional stress was also established in this study. Morris [24], in his study in south-eastern Madagascar, also established that prolonged labour and other delivery complications were viewed as resulting from an unsettled feud with someone, especially one's parents or partner, and this can be prevented by resolving feuds or obtaining benediction before or during delivery in order to prevent or resolve complications. A belief that quarrelling, fighting and emotional stress during pregnancy could lead to adverse pregnancy outcomes was also established in some communities

in Ghana and Zambia [24, 27]. This is an adoptive practice that is supported by scientific explanations. It not only enhances social cohesion and harmony, but is also beneficial to the wellbeing of the mother and unborn baby. Studies have confirmed that gastritis, hypertensive disorders, pre-term labour, prematurity birth, low birthweight and perinatal death are significantly more frequent among emotionally stressed women [29, 30].

Avoid heavy duties and risky activities but do not stay idle

A number of activities were considered taboo during pregnancy because of their potentially harmful effect on pregnancy and the foetus. Heavy duties such as collecting water from an open well, splitting firewood, digging and bending for long hours as well as running and standing at the doorway are highly discouraged during pregnancy. Some of these activities endanger the pregnancy and others can cause physical injuries, in the case of a fall. Activity during pregnancy is recommended, but heavy duties should be avoided, and enough rest periods assured, especially in late pregnancy and among women with a high-risk profile [31]. Strenuous work, especially involving long hours of standing and walking, seem to have a negative influence on the growth of the foetus and increase the risk of pre-term delivery [31].

On the other hand, physical activities during pregnancy are encouraged. A pregnant woman is recommended to stay active by engaging in light duties. Bed rest during pregnancy decreases the risk of developing severe hypertension [32] and can improve foetal growth [32]. A belief in maintaining light duties during pregnancy was also established in Zambia [33] and Ghana [34]. Hence this belief and practice of avoiding heavy duties and engaging in light physical activities to exercise the body should be encouraged with scientific explanations.

Observing an appropriate diet

Pregnancy food precautions as a concern for a healthy pregnancy and birth outcome were established in this study. Pregnant women are restricted from consuming protein-rich food such as eggs, meat, and fresh milk for fear of CS arising from big babies. More than half of the respondents in this study reported that they were small-scale farmers and the reported farm produce were vegetables, milk and chicken. This means that eggs, milk and meat are the major sources of protein that are readily available and accessible in their environment are restricted. Protein deficiency is often associated with spontaneous abortion [35] hence there is need for health practitioners to raise awareness against this belief for the benefit of the pregnant women and their children. However, in case of cultural sensitivity against this practice, culturally acceptable high-protein foods should be encouraged. Pregnancy food taboos as a way of restricting the foetus from growing too big in order to facilitate an easy birth as found in this study was also established among other communities in Kenya, Ghana, Ethiopia and south-east Nigeria [36–41].

Consumption of the meat of an animal carcass is a taboo that is highly condemned as reported by 38% of the respondents. This is a good practice that needs to be encouraged because studies have confirmed that bacteria in animal carcasses can lead to human illness if consumed [42].

On the other hand, pregnant women were encouraged to eat certain foods that were believed to be important in increasing blood volume and facilitating easy labour and birth. Food believed to increase blood volume include traditional green leafy vegetables, liver, animal blood, fruits, milk, beans, and fish. Iron deficiency anaemia during pregnancy has long been implicated in miscarriage [43] and is the major contributor to post-partum haemorrhage (PPH), which is the single leading cause of maternal mortality and morbidity in low-income countries [44]. More than half of all maternal deaths occur within 24 h of delivery, mostly from excessive bleeding, thus, women's belief is justified and the foods believed to increase the "volume" of blood are truly rich in iron, hence the practice needs to be encouraged. A belief in the importance of iron-rich food in a successful pregnancy outcome was also established in Ghana [45] and Kenya [37, 38].

Pregnant women were also encouraged to consume foods believed to make a pregnant woman strong, because energy is associated with easy birth. Food believed to make a woman strong include *ugali* and porridge made from finger millet mixed with sorghum, and traditional vegetables, milk, traditional herbs and meat. Some of these foods are indeed energy-rich and studies have confirmed that the risk of spontaneous pre-term birth and low birthweight increases in women with limited weight gain [46], hence this practice needs to be encouraged. The importance of acquiring strength during pregnancy was also established in Ghana [45].

Remedies against supernatural attacks

In this study, pregnant women are restricted from killing any animal. The commonly reported animals that should not be killed because of supernatural reasons include dogs, cats, snakes, chicken and insects. These animals if agitated may produce chemical toxins through a bite or sting, which can kill as a defence against the attacker; hence it is a good practice to avoid them. According to Huntingford [47], among the Nandi, it is believed that the spirits of dead ancestors or relatives return to this world to visit their people and they normally travel in the bodies of snakes, moles, or rats, which they use as vehicles to carry them to and from the houses of the living. If a snake or these animals go to people's houses especially at night or to the pregnant woman's bed or house, they may not be killed, as it is believed that they personify the spirit of a deceased ancestor or relative, and that have been sent to indicate to the woman that her next child will be born safely. Instead milk is poured on the ground for it to drink, and then it is allowed to leave the house. If the animal is killed, it will be unable to get back to spirit-land without great difficulty and will be very angry with the offender, resulting in punishment from the spirit. Usually this punishment takes the form of death or illness in man or beast.

In the event that such animals are killed, a pregnant woman is expected to undergo cleansing rituals to end any calamity that is likely to follow her after exposure. The belief that killing of animals will lead into birth of visually impaired child was also established by Ogechi and Ruto among the Gusii and Nandi of Kenya and these were corrected by conducting a ritual [48]. Scientifically, it has been established that maintaining health through spiritual harmony and spiritual healing reduces anxiety, tension and stress associated with (or causing) illness if the patient has faith in the healer, thus increasing the chance for the prescribed therapy to be effective [49]. However, these spiritual healings may coexist or compete with biomedical treatment, thus negatively affecting access and use of health facilities.

Limitations and strengths of the study

This study focused only on pregnancy-related beliefs up to the point of birth. Post-pregnancy beliefs were beyond the scope of this study and hence need follow-up research. Further exploration of views is necessary to explain some of the Kalenjin perceptions and practices. We are also aware that the respondents who were interviewed were those who had sought care at health facilities. They might have different views from those who do not seek such care. Similarly, respondents were selected from rural Uasin Gishu County health facilities, and we do not know the extent to which respondents attending urban facilities might have different perceptions. However, this being an exploratory qualitative study provides a deeper understanding of the phenomenon on question.

Conclusion

This study aimed to gain insight into the socio-cultural perceptions of maternal morbidity, mortality and other complications associated with pregnancy and childbirth and to establish how these perceptions influence maternal health and care-seeking behaviours. This study has shown that traditional beliefs of health and illness continue to shape reproductive and maternal health practices among the Kalenjin women of Kenya. This is shown by the fact that many respondents attribute maternal health complications to taboos of pregnancy and childbirth, such as acceptable foods to eat, places women can and cannot go, activities in which women should or should not engage during pregnancy and the spirits of dead animals and ancestors. Participants also reported using traditional herbal medicine as a healing and preventive remedy during pregnancy and after birth. These cultural taboos and beliefs allow Kalenjin women to make sense of their maternal experiences, and to care for their health, hence shaping their care-seeking behaviours. Some of the cultural remedies adopted to prevent morbidity and mortality during pregnancy are cultural adaptive mechanisms that indirectly control the transmission of disease and improve maternal health and thus should not be considered to be exclusively folk or primitive. Such activities include: condemning the consumption of meat from a dead animal, avoiding heavy duties and going to crowded areas, maintaining good social relations and avoiding emotional events such as funerals. However, other cultural remedies such as restricting diet and geographical mobility, may pose risks to the pregnant woman's health and access to health facilities. The delay in deciding to seek maternal care is a result of women's failure to recognise symptoms and maternal health problems as potentially needing hospital care, and this failure stems from culturally informed perceptions of symptoms of maternal morbidity and pregnancy complications that differ significantly from biomedical implications.

Abbreviations
ANC: Antenatal care; ASALI: A sustainable approach to livelihood improvement; CHWs: Community health workers; CIS: Centre for International Studies; CS: Caesarean section; FGM: Female genital mutilation; KII: Key informant interviews; MCH: Maternal and child healthcare; MIP: Malaria in pregnancy; MMR: Maternal mortality rate; NACOSTI: National Commission for Science, Technology and Innovation; PNC: Post natal care; SEKU: South Eastern Kenya University; STD: Sexually transmitted diseases; STI: Sexually transmitted infection; TB: Tuberculosis; TBAs: Traditional birth attendants; VU: Vrije Universiteit Amsterdam

Acknowledgements
The authors wish to acknowledge the Uasin Gishu County Director of Health and the Health Officers in charge of the health facilities we visited, who were always willing to collaborate or assist us during field research. We also thank the key informants and the women, who willingly shared their childbirth practices, encounters and beliefs with the research team. I would also like to acknowledge Professor Jos van Roosmalen whose contributions enriched the content of this work.

Funding
The authors acknowledge the financial support from A Sustainable Approach to Livelihood Improvement (ASALI) Project. The Project is coordinated by Dr. Denyse Snelder of the Centre for International Students (CIS) at the VU University Amsterdam. ASALI is a joint collaboration project of Moi University Kenya, South Eastern Kenya University (SEKU) and VU University (Vrije Universteit) Amsterdam that is being implemented in Kenya. This financial support proved fundamental to the design of the study, the collection and analysis of data, and the writing of this manuscript.

Authors' contributions
RMR, a doctoral candidate, is the main author. She contributed to the conception, study design, planning, data collection, analysis and interpretation and prepared a first draft of the paper. JEWB is the promoter and AKN the co-promoter of RR's PhD program. They both contributed to the study design and interpretation of results. All the authors critically revised the paper and approved the final manuscript for submission.

Authors' information
Roselyter Riang'a is an Assistant Lecturer in the Department of Sociology and Psychology, School of Arts and Social Sciences, Moi University, Kenya. She is also a PhD candidate of Maternal Nutrition and Health at Athena Institute for Research on Innovation and Communication, in the Faculty Science, at the VU University Amsterdam, Prof. Anne Nangulu is the director of quality assurance at the Commission for University Education (CUE) in Kenya and also a professor of economic history at Moi University, Kenya. Prof. Dr. Jacqueline Broerse is Professor of Innovation and Communication at the VU University, Amsterdam in the Health and Life Sciences. She is also the Research Director of the Faculty of Sciences, VU University, Amsterdam.

Competing interests
The authors declare that they have no financial or personal relationship(s) that may have inappropriately influenced them in writing this article. The financial grant for this study was only meant for the design of the study, the collection and analysis of data, and the writing of this manuscript.

Author details
[1]School of Arts and Social Sciences, Moi University, P.O. Box 3900-30100, Eldoret, Kenya. [2]Athena Institute, Faculty of Science, Vrije Universiteit Amsterdam, De Boelelaan 1085, 1081 HV Amsterdam, The Netherlands. [3]Commission for University Education, Red Hill Road, off Limuru Road, Gigiri, PO Box 54999 – 00200, Nairobi, Kenya.

References
1. Adegoke AA, Van Den Broek N. Skilled birth attendance-lessons learnt. BJOG Int J Obstet Gynaecol. 2009;116:33–40.
2. Cheptum JJ, Oyore JP. Poor pregnancy outcomes in public health facilities in Kenya. Afr J Midwifery Womens. Health. 2012;6:185–90.
3. World Health Organization. Trends in maternal mortality: 1990 to 2015. Geneva: WHO Press; 2015.
4. Jebet J, Oyore JP. Poor pregnancy outcomes in public health facilities in Kenya; 2015. p. 4–10.
5. Magadi M, Diamond IAN, Madise N. Analysis of factors associated with maternal mortality in Kenyan hospitals. J Biosoc Sci. 2001;33:375–89.

6.   World Health Organization. WHO Global Health Observatory (GHO) data global on maternal health indicators, 2017 update [internet]. Genever: World Health Organization; 2017. Available from: http://www.who.int/gho/maternal_health/en/

7.   Kenya National Bureau of Statistics, ICF Macro. Kenya Demographic and Health Survey 2014. Rockville: ICF International; 2014.

8.   Wanjira C, Mwangi M, Mathenge E, Mbugua G, Ng'ang'a Z. Delivery practices and associated factors among mothers seeking child welfare Services in Selected Health Facilities in Nyandarua South District, Kenya. BMC Public Health. 2011;11:360 Available from: http://www.biomedcentral.com/1471-2458/11/360.

9.   van Eijk AM, Bles HM, Odhiambo F, Ayisi JG, Blokland IE, Rosen DH, et al. Use of antenatal services and delivery care among women in rural western Kenya: a community based survey. Reprod Health. 2006;3:2.

10.   Kaingu CK, Oduma JA, Kanui TI. Practices of traditional birth attendants in Machakos District, Kenya. J Ethnopharmacol. 2011;137:495–502 Available from: http://ac.els-cdn.com/S0378874111004090/1-s2.0-S0378874111004090-main.pdf?_tid=41a99bf2-f8a7-11e4-b07d-00000aacb361&acdnat=1431435977_24d6321d00c99d0e264a9f6cda97caaa.

11.   Kenya National Bureau of Statistics (KNBS); ORC Macro. Kenya Demographic and Health Survey 2008-09. Maryland: Calverton; 2010.

12.   County Government of Uasin Gishu Department of Health Services. County health strategic and investment plan 2013-2018. Nairobi; 2013.

13.   Miller E. Maternal health and knowledge and infant health outcomes in the Ariaal people of northern Kenya. Soc Sci Med. 2011;73:1266–1274. Available from: https://doi.org/10.1016/J.SOCSCIMED.2011.07.009

14.   Montesanti SR. Cultural Perceptions of Maternal Illness among Khmer Women in Krong Kep, Cambodia. vis-à-vis Explor Anthropol. 2011;11:90–106 Available from: http://vav.library.utoronto.ca/index.php/vav/article/view/12664.

15.   Helman CG. Cuture health and Illiness. 5th. Purdy JK and S, editor. London: Hodder Arnold; 2007.

16.   Kothari CR. Research methodology: methods and techniques. New Delhi: New Age International (P) Limited; 2004.

17.   Grinnel RM, Unrau YA. Social work research and evaluation: foundations of evidence based-evaluations. 8th ed. New York: Open University Press; 2007.

18.   Mathole T, Lindmark G, Majoko F, Lecturer S, Ahlberg BM. A qualitative study of women's perspectives of antenatal care in a rural area of Zimbabwe; 2004. p. 122–32.

19.   Ngomane S, Mulaudzi FM. Indigenous beliefs and practices that influence the delayed attendance of antenatal clinics by women in the Bohlabelo district in Limpopo, South Africa. Midwifery. 2012;28:30–8 Available from: http://www.sciencedirect.com/science/article/pii/S0266613810001816.

20.   de Beaudrap P, Turyakira E, White LJ, Nabasumba C, Tumwebaze B, Muehlenbachs A, et al. Impact of malaria during pregnancy on pregnancy outcomes in a Ugandan prospective cohort with intensive malaria screening and prompt treatment; 2013. p. 1–11.

21.   Hillary NC. Utilization of herbal medicine during pregnancy, labour and post-partum period among women at Embu provincial general hospital: Nairobi University, College of Humanities and Social Sciences, Sociology; 2013.

22.   Mothupi MC. Use of herbal medicine during pregnancy among women with access to public healthcare in Nairobi, Kenya: a cross-sectional survey. BMC Complement Altern Med. 2014. Article Number 432. Date Publ. Novemb. 04, 2014. 2014;1–8.

23.   Towns AM, Van Andel T. Wild plants, pregnancy, and the food-medicine continuum in the southern regions of Ghana and Benin. J Ethnopharmacol. 2016;179:375–82.

24.   Morris JL, Short S, Robson L, Andriatsihosena MS. Maternal health practices, beliefs and traditions in Southeast Madagascar. Afr J Reprod Health. 2014;18:101–17.

25.   Maimbolwa MC, Yamba B, Diwan V, Ransjö-Arvidson AB. Cultural childbirth practices and beliefs in Zambia. J Adv Nurs. 2003;43:263–74.

26.   Fonck K, Kidula N, Jaoko W, Estambale B, Claeys P, Kirui P, et al. Validity of the vaginal discharge algorithm among pregnant and non-pregnant women in Nairobi, Kenya; 2000. p. 33–8.

27.   Masha SC, Wahome E, Vaneechoutte M, Cools P, Crucitti T, Sanders EJ. High prevalence of curable sexually transmitted infections among pregnant women in a rural county hospital in Kilifi, Kenya. 2017;1–16. Available from: doi: https://doi.org/10.1371/journal.pone.0175166

28.   Mullick S, Beksinska M, Mabey D. Sexually transmitted infections in pregnancy: prevalence, impact on pregnancy outcomes, and approach to treatment in developing countries. Trop Med. 2005;81:294–302.

29.   Lukasse M, Helbig A, Eberhard-gran M. Antenatal Maternal Emotional Distress and Duration of Pregnancy; 2014. p. 9.

30.   Tandu-umba B, Dedetemo DK, Mananga GL. Maternal stress and pregnancy outcomes *. Open J Obstet Gynecol. 2014;4:361–70.

31.   Ahlborg JG. Physical work load and pregnancy outcome. J Occup Environ Med. 1995;37:941–4.

32.   Crowther CA, Bouwmeester AM, Ashurst HM. Does admission to hospital for bed rest prevent disease progression or improve fetal outcome in pregnancy complicated by non-proteinuric hypertension? Obstet Gynaecol. 1992;99:13–7.

33.   M'soka NC, Mabuza LH, Pretorius D. Cultural and health beliefs of pregnant women in Zambia regarding pregnancy and child birth. Curationis. 2015;38:1–7 Available from: http://www.curationis.org.za/index.php/curationis/article/view/1232.

34.   Dako-Gyeke P, Aikins M, Aryeetey R, McCough L, Adongo PB. The influence of socio-cultural interpretations of pregnancy threats on health-seeking behavior among pregnant women in urban Accra, Ghana. BMC Pregnancy Childbirth. 2013;13:211.

35.   Ebina Y, Ieko M, Naito S, Kobashi G, Deguchi M, Minakami H, Tatsuya Atsumi HY. O127. Low levels of plasma protein S, protein C and coagulation factor XII during early pregnancy and adverse pregnancy outcome. Pregnancy Hypertens An Int J Women's Cardiovasc Heal. 2015;5:239–40.

36.   Ekwochi U, Osuorah CDI, Ndu IK, Ifediora C, Asinobi IN, Eke CB. Food taboos and myths in south eastern Nigeria: the belief and practice of mothers in the region. J Ethnobiol Ethnomed. 2016;12:17 Available from: http://www.ethnobiomed.com/content/12/1/7.

37.   Riang'a RM, Broerse J, Nangulu AK. Food beliefs and practices among the Kalenjin pregnant women in rural Uasin Gishu County , Kenya. J Ethnobiol Ethnomed. 2017;13:29.

38.   Riang'a RM, Nangulu AK, Broerse JEW. "When a woman is pregnant, her grave is open": health beliefs concerning dietary practices among pregnant Kalenjin women in rural Uasin Gishu County, Kenya. J Health Popul Nutr. 2017;36:53 Available from: https://jhpn.biomedcentral.com/articles/10.1186/s41043-017-0130-0.

39.   Zepro NB. Food taboos and misconceptions among pregnant women of Shashemene District, Ethiopia, 2012. Sicnence J Public Heal. 2015;3:410–6.

40.   Arzoaquoi SK, Essuman EE, Gbagbo FY, Tenkorang EY, Soyiri I, Laar AK. Motivations for food prohibitions during pregnancy and their enforcement mechanisms in a rural Ghanaian district. J Ethnobiol Ethnomed. 2015;11:59 Available from: http://www.ethnobiomed.com/content/11/1/59.

41.   Demissie T, Muroki N, Kogi-makau W. Food taboos among pregnant women in Hadiya zone. Ethiop J Heal Dev [Internet]. 1998;12:2–7 Available from: http://www.ethiopianreview.com/1995/Tsegaye_Demissie_Nelson_Muroki_Wamboi_Kogi_Makau_1995.pdf.

42.   Crump JA, Griffin PM, Angulo FJ. Bacterial contamination of animal feed and its relationship to human foodborne illness. Clin Infect Dis. 2002;35:859–65.

43.   Nair M, Choudhury MK, Choudhury SS, Kakoty SD, Sarma UC, Webster P, et al. Association between maternal anaemia and pregnancy outcomes: a cohort study in Assam, India. BMJ Glob Heal. 2016;1:e000026 Available from: http://gh.bmj.com/lookup/doi/10.1136/bmjgh-2015-000026.

44.   Khan KS, Wojdyla D, Say L, Gulmezoglu AM, Van Look PF. WHO analysis of causes of maternal death: a systematic review. Lancet. 2006;367:1066–74.

45.   Aikins A. Food beliefs and practices during pregnancy in Ghana: implications for maternal health interventions. Health Care Women Int. 2014;9332:954–72.

46.   Lumbanraja S, Lutan D, Usman I. Maternal weight gain and correlation with
      birth weight infants. Procedia Soc Behav Sci. 2013;103:647–56 Available
      from: http://www.sciencedirect.com/science/article/pii/S1877042813038287.
47.   Huntingford GWB. The Nandi of Kenya: tribal control in pastoral socirty. First.
      London: Routledge and Kegan Paul Ltd; 1953.
48.   Ogechi NO, Ruto SJ. Portrayal of disability through personal names and
      proverbs in Kenya: evidence from Ekegusii and Nandi. Stichproben Wiener
      Zeitschrift für Krit Afrikastudien. 2002;3:63–82.
49.   Stark L. Cleansing the wounds of war: an examination of traditional
      healing, psychosocial health and reintegration in Sierra Leone.
      Intervention. 2006;4:206–18.

3

Parents' knowledge, awareness and attitudes of cord blood donation and banking options: an integrative review

Lisa Peberdy[1]* ⓘD, Jeanine Young[1], Debbie Louise Massey[1] and Lauren Kearney[1,2]

Abstract

Background: For over 25 years cord blood has been used as an alternative to bone marrow for therapeutic use in conditions of the blood, immune system and metabolic disorders. Parents can decide if they would like to privately store their infant's cord blood for later use if needed or to publicly donate it. Parents need to be aware of the options that exist for their infant's cord blood and have access to the relevant information to inform their choice. The aim of this paper is to identify parent's knowledge and awareness of cord blood donation, private banking options and stem cell use, and parent sources and preferred sources of this information.

Methods: An integrative review was conducted using several electronic databases to identify papers on parents' knowledge, attitudes and attitudes towards umbilical cord blood donation and banking. The CASP tool was used to determine validity and quality of the studies included in the review.

Results: The search of the international literature identified 25 papers which met review inclusion criteria. This integrative review identified parents' knowledge of cord banking and/or donation as low, with awareness of cord blood banking options greater than knowledge. Parents were found to have positive attitudes towards cord blood donation including awareness of the value of cord blood and its uses, with the option considered to be an ethical and altruistic choice. Knowledge on cord blood use were mixed; many studies' participants did not correctly identify uses. Information sources for parents on cord blood was found to be varied, fragmented and inconsistent. Health professionals were identified as the preferred source of information on cord blood banking for parents.

Conclusions: This integrative review has identified that further research should focus on identifying information that expectant parents require to assist them to make informed choices around cord blood banking; and identifying barriers present for health professionals providing evidence based information on cord blood use and banking options.

Keywords: Cord blood banking, Cord blood donation, Cord blood stem cells, Women's knowledge, Expectant parents' knowledge, Information sources

Background

For over 25 years cord blood has been used as an alternative to bone marrow for therapeutic use in conditions of the blood, immune system and metabolic disorders [1]. Cord blood is now one of the main haematopoietic stem cell sources [2]. Umbilical cord blood banking is the process of collecting and storing umbilical cord blood, in the immediate period after the birth of a baby. Cord blood can be collected and stored either publicly or privately.

Public cord blood banks operate in all developed countries, and within most developing countries. By 2014, the international cord blood banking network comprised over 160 public cord blood banks in 36 countries, with over 731,000 umbilical cord blood units stored [3]. Public cord blood banks collect, transport, process, test and store cord blood units which have been altruistically donated for allogeneic use, at no financial cost to the donating parents [4–9]. The donated cord blood unit is not reserved for the use of the donating

---
* Correspondence: Lisa.Peberdy@research.usc.edu.au
[1]School of Nursing, Midwifery and Paramedicine, University of the Sunshine Coast, Locked Bag 4, Maroochydore DC, QLD 4558, Australia
Full list of author information is available at the end of the article

family, who relinquish their rights of ownership of the blood to the banking facility [10].

Private cord blood banks charge parents a fee for the collection, processing and storage of their infant's cord blood for exclusive autologous or family use [4, 8, 9, 11, 12]. Some private cord blood banks now also store cord tissue.

Parents can decide if they would like to privately store their infant's cord blood for later use if needed, publicly donate it, defer cord clamping to allow their infant to receive optimal volumes of cord blood at birth or to discard the remaining cord blood with the placenta after birth. Parents need to be aware of the options that exist for their infant's cord blood and have access to the relevant information to inform their choice. Parents' knowledge and understanding of cord blood banking and donation has been reported to be low and little is known about their source of information on this topic and the quality of the information provided [13–15]. Thus, accuracy of information is difficult to assess and there is limited understanding of how parents use this information to inform their decision making about cord blood banking and donation.

Methods
Aim
In this integrative review, we aimed to identify a) parent's knowledge and awareness relating to cord blood donation, private banking options and stem cell use; b) sources of information received, and c) parents' perceptions of appropriate sources and personnel to provide this information. The rationale for the integrative review was to identify gaps in knowledge and to provide direction for the development of antenatal education frameworks for parents in this important and evolving field of cord blood banking and cord blood use.

Methodology
The integrative method chosen for this review allowed for rigorous evaluation of the strength of the evidence from a combination of diverse methodologies (Whittmore and Knafi 2005), and identification of gaps in the literature and areas for further research [16]. The five stages model [17] of problem identification, literature search, data evaluation, data analysis, and presentation [16], was used as a framework to guide this integrative review.

Literature search
Databases searched included PubMed, Scopus, MIDIRS, CINAHL and Google Scholar using search terms: cord blood banking, cord blood donation, cord blood stem cells, women's knowledge, expectant parents' knowledge, parent/parental knowledge, sources. Publication date limits were set between 1991 and July 2017. Cord blood

banking was reported to have commenced in 1991 [18]; no papers were found on this topic prior to 1998.

Inclusion and exclusion criteria
Inclusion criteria for the review consisted of original research studies that investigated and reported parents' knowledge, awareness and attitudes of cord blood donation and banking options, written in the English language. The initial search was conducted by the first author who identified the potential studies for inclusion based on title and abstract, with all papers for inclusion discussed and agreed upon by co-authors.

Exclusion criteria included papers not available in the English language, discussion papers, papers reporting on knowledge and awareness of embryonic stem cells, and papers which reported only on women's choices and reasons for choice.

Figure 1 details the structured search conducted, including the search strategy and inclusion process applied to the peer reviewed literature which was included in this integrative review.

Data evaluation
Each article was read and summarised to identify the key points and common themes. Following the identification of these, the similarities and differences between studies were compared. Critical Appraisal Skills Programme (CASP) tools appropriate for the study designs were used to determine the quality of the studies [19]. Quantitative studies were assessed using the CASP Cohort Study Checklist (see Additional file 1). Qualitative and mixed methods studies were assessed using the CASP Qualitative Checklist (see Additional file 2). No papers were excluded because of their validity or quality.

Data analysis
A total of 31 articles were retrieved that provided description relating to parents', expectant parents' or pregnant women's knowledge and awareness of cord blood banking and donation. Only one paper retrieved also explored pregnant women's and/or expectant parents' knowledge and awareness of cord tissue banking [20]. Six papers were excluded because they did not meet the inclusion criteria, or aims of this integrative review [11, 21–25].

Thematic analysis [26] was used to identify emerging domains and themes in the literature, with three common domains identified: cord blood banking options, cord blood uses, and information sources.

Findings
This search of the international literature identified 25 papers of parents, pregnant women's and expectant parents' knowledge and awareness of cord blood banking and donation which met the review inclusion criteria

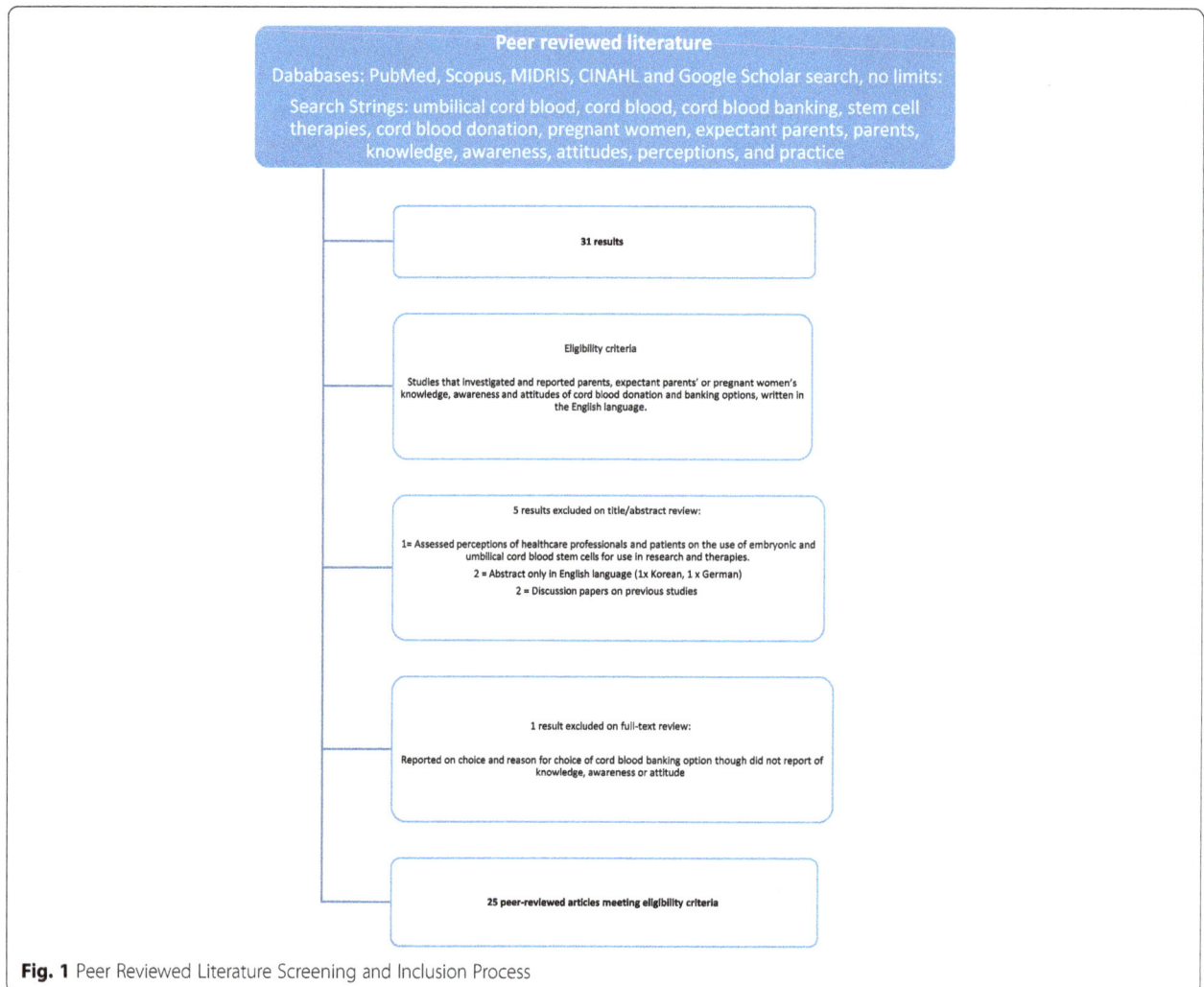

Fig. 1 Peer Reviewed Literature Screening and Inclusion Process

[13–15, 18, 20, 27–46]. Studies selected for inclusion in the review included empirical studies using qualitative (*n* = 5), quantitative (*n* = 18) and mixed methodologies (*n* = 2).

Overall, papers exploring pregnant women's and expectant parents' knowledge and awareness of cord blood donation and banking, were conducted in 15 countries: North America and Canada [13, 15, 18, 27, 28, 31], Europe and the United Kingdom [14, 29, 30, 32, 34, 36, 41, 42, 46], Australia [40], Asia and the Middle East [33, 35, 37, 43–45], Africa [38, 39] and one international study involving countries in Europe, Asia, Australasia, the Americas and Africa [20].

This integrative review included descriptive quantitative studies predominantly using survey designs [13–15, 20, 22, 30, 33–36, 39–43, 46]; qualitative studies predominantly comprising focus groups and interviews [18, 27–29, 31, 37]; or mixed method approaches using a survey design with interviews and focus groups [32, 38] to describe knowledge, awareness and attitudes of cord blood donation and banking options. Table 1 summarises the papers included in this review.

Three domains pertaining to pregnant parents' knowledge, awareness and attitudes were identified: a) cord blood banking and donation; b) cord blood use; and c) cord blood information sources and preferred information sources. Cord blood banking and donation options encapsulated three themes: knowledge, awareness and attitudes. The second domain, cord blood use, comprised two themes: knowledge and awareness. The final domain, information sources, was also divided into two themes: actual sources and preferred sources of information on cord blood banking and donation.

Cord blood banking and donation

Seven papers investigated and reported on cord blood banking awareness [13, 15, 31, 39–41, 46]. Four studies reported a high level of awareness, with around 70% of participants reporting awareness of the topic [15, 40, 41, 46]. Women of lower education levels, age 25 years or less, or of an ethnic minority background were factors associated with less awareness of banking and donation [15, 40].

Table 1 Overview of papers included in the review (Knowledge, awareness, attitude, information source, public donation, private banking)

No.	Author/Year	Country Setting	Sample Inclusion	Design	Findings	Limitations
1	Mathevic & Erjavec (2016)	Croatia 2 Maternity OPD	960 women 96% response rate	Quantitative Questionnaire	*Overall:* Preference of voluntary donation. One-third opted for private donation. 50% pregnant women who were not planning on CCB this pregnancy most often stated insufficient knowledge and too much paperwork *Knowledge and awareness:* Increases with age, education level and pregnancy duration. Majority unaware of practical information. *Information sources:* Media main source; 6% from Obs; nil from other HPs	Strength: Large sample size in two hospitals partly representative of city population. Weakness: Participant demographics representative of urban not general population, although UCB mainly performed in urban populations Validation of tool not disclosed
				To investigate awareness, level of knowledge, attitudes and information sources of pregnant women and hospital maternity staff about cord blood banking.		
2	Matsumoto et al. (2016)	Jordon 6 Maternity Hospitals (4 Private, 2 Public) Maternity OPD	899 women 100% return rate Convenience sample	Quantitative Questionnaire: multi choice, Likert-scale, and coded short answer format. Tool developed and administered by authors.	*Overall:* Positive public opinion about CBB. Most wanted more information on CBB, especially from Obs. *Knowledge & awareness* *69% reported low knowledge of CBB & transplant *77% reported low knowledge of CBD *Higher education & household income = more likely to hear/discuss CBB with Obs. *Only 7% heard about CBB from Obs *Attitudes and opinions* *CBD supported more than CBB; Higher likelihood of CBB if presented with future potential or recommended by Obs *Women with prior knowledge about CB transplants found it ethical /more willing to do CDB *Preference and information* *66% want more CBB information *71% Obs preferred information source	Refusal rate not recorded Not all questions answered fully
		To investigate public opinion and knowledge about cord blood banking in Jordon.				
3	Kim et al. (2015)	Korea 3 metropolitan maternity hospitals	320 early post-partum women who had stored (n = 109), donated	Quantitative 2 Questionnaires, yes/no answer format for knowledge assessment; 4 point scale for attitude format. Tools adapted from 2 previous studies	Overall: CBD decided earlier than CBB. Mass media most influential factor for CBD *Reasons for CBB/CBD* *93% CBB - as insurance for baby. *73% CBD - due to unlimited	Lacked thorough examination on delivery of CB education Some participants believed they
				To assess the knowledge & attitude of early post-partum women in Korea with regard to storage,		

Table 1 Overview of papers included in the review (Knowledge, awareness, attitude, information source, public donation, private banking) (Continued)

No.	Author/Year	Aim	Country Setting	Sample Inclusion	Design	Findings	Limitations
		donation & disposal of CB, & to identify factors influencing CB donation.		(n = 34), discarded (n = 177) their cord blood. Convenience Sample	Kim et al. (2009) and Lee (2006)	uses of CB. *Knowledge and Attitude of CB use* *Higher knowledge and positive attitude towards CBB & CBD increased likelihood of CBD. *CB Education* *Women who used CBD were encouraged by media *44.2% who CBB and 12% who CBD were educated HP	were educated on CBB by HP but they were CBB employees working in the hospitals
4	Bioinformant (2014)	To determine the factors involved in expectant parents' decision to privately store, publicly donate or discard their infant's cord blood.	International: Australia, NZ, Asia, Europe, USA, Canada, Middle East, Sth America, Mexico, Central America, Caribbean, Africa	603 Expectant parents and recent parents (within 3 years) Sample method unsure	Quantitative Survey Questionnaire Branched survey. Specific questions asked of different respondent populations.	Overall: Most study participants had not been informed of CBB options by their antenatal health care professional. *Source of CB banking information:* Obs (35%), Family & friends (35%), ANC (14%). 45%: Information from CBB was influential in their decision. 30%: Obs significantly influential in parent decision. 77%: did not CBB as unaware of option. 62%: Obs did not mention CBB. 63%: ANC did not mention cord blood banking.	Analytical strategy was not described
5	Jordens et al. (2014)	To explore awareness and understanding of cord blood banking among Australian women, and the effect of education of planned choices on the disposal of cord blood.	Australia, NSW 14 public and private antenatal clinics and classes in maternity hospitals in metropolitan (n = 8), regional (n = 4) and rural (n = 2) [included 3 hospitals that facilitate CB donation]	1873 Pregnant women (> 24 wks gestation, low risk) Target n = 2050 Response rate = 87% Purposive Sampling	Quantitative Self-administered Questionnaire: multi-choice format. (modified version of Fernandez et al., 2003)	Overall: Most women wanted information from ANC provider. Many respondents were aware of CBB. CBB education increased intention to CBB / CBD. *Awareness* *71% indicated awareness of CBB; more likely to know of CBB vs CBD. *Source of CB banking information* *Hospital print information (43%); print media (22%); ANC (21%); TV / radio (19%), family/relatives (17%) *Decisions about CBB*	Only 1 State of Australia sampled; not representative of national population. Awareness knowledge was reported

Table 1 Overview of papers included in the review (Knowledge, awareness, attitude, information source, public donation, private banking) (Continued)

No.	Author/Year	Aim	Country Setting	Sample Inclusion	Design	Findings	Limitations
						*After receiving CBB basic information, proportion who indicated they would CBB or CBD increased from 30 to 68%. *CBB preferences and beliefs* *Only 13% had been asked about CBB or CBD prior to commencing survey. *93%: CBB and CBD information during pregnancy should be given by ANC giver.	
6	Alexander et al. (2014)	To determine awareness of CB donation and banking among pregnant women.	Nigeria 1 tertiary university teaching hospital, ANC	302 Pregnant women Convenience sampling	Quantitative Structured Questionnaires	Overall: Awareness of CBD and CBB among pregnant women is low, with media the main source of information. *Awareness* *Only 19% aware of CB due to the absence of CBB and CBD in Nigeria. *Information sources* *Hospitals (30%); Media (39%), Friends (24%), Internet (7%)	CBB and CBD not available in the Country so may contribute to low awareness.
7	Karagiorgou et al. (2014)	To analyse the attitudes and knowledge of Greek citizens with high reproductive capacity (aged 18–24 years) about cord blood banking and therapies.	Greece 5 Greek cities, 2 Greek island communities.	1019 Public citizens; 292 parents Response rate = 100% of approached target population Random Sampling	Quantitative Standard anonymous multi-choice questionnaires	Findings from parents only reported here Overall: High CBB awareness level, with almost half informed by a HP *Knowledge and attitudes about CBB* *80% knew of CBB; 83% aware of CB uses; 87% positive about CBB *Information quality* *48% stated main source of CBB information, 43% of CB use information came from HP. *Future attitudes* *53% preferred CBD vs 47% preferred CBB for future use.	Focused on general population of childbearing age. Did not clearly represent pregnant women or expectant couples. Awareness not knowledge reported.
8	Vijayalakshmi, (2013)	To assess antenatal mothers' knowledge	India 1 regional hospital's ANC	100 Antenatal mothers Non-probability	Quantitative Questionnaires	Overall: 95% had poor knowledge of CBB and collection.	Minimal information on knowledge questions asked

Table 1 Overview of papers included in the review (Knowledge, awareness, attitude, information source, public donation, private banking) (Continued)

No.	Author/Year	Aim	Country Setting	Sample Inclusion	Design	Findings	Limitations
		regarding cord blood collection and storage. To find an association between knowledge and demographics on cord blood collection and storage.		Purposive sampling		*Significant association between knowledge scores and demographics (live birth, abortion, death, place of residence, type of family and membership to any organization) was found *Age, religion, gravida, para, education, occupation, income, newspaper and magazine subscription showed no correlation with knowledge score	Minimal analysis of findings presented Survey tool not validated
9	Meissner-Roloff & Pepper (2013)	To assess the extent of public support for the establishment of a public cord blood bank.	South Africa 1 urban university hospital, ANC	217 Mothers Convenience sampling	Mixed methods Qualitative Interview and education Quantitative Anonymous Questionnaires Survey tools validated	Overall: Study revealed positive support for a public CB bank in South Africa *Willingness to donate placenta and CB *80% supported placental donation, while 2.5% unwilling to donate placenta would do CBD *78% supported a public bank; 78% willing to have HIV testing for CBD process *Knowledge of CB stem cells *70% unaware of stem cells prior to education session; 94% opinion that stem cells could treat blood disorders *Influence of Age *Younger women more willing to donate placentas than older women (84% v 77%), more likely support CBD (92% v 82%)	Centre specialized in high risk pregnancies; participants may have had better access to, and received more, information than rest of population attending other clinics
10	Padmavathi (2013)	To assess stem cell and CB banking knowledge among antenatal mothers before and after a structured teaching program. To assess the effectiveness of structured teaching	India 1 district maternity hospital, ANC	30 Antenatal mothers Purposive sampling	Qualitative Structured interviews pre and post education Post education interviews attended 7 days following education	Overall: Results suggest a structured teaching program was effective and increased ANC mothers' knowledge on stem cells and CB. Pre-test Knowledge *57% had poor knowledge; 43% had average knowledge.	Unclear of education content in teaching session and how knowledge was assessed Unclear if same interview questions used pre and post education.

Table 1 Overview of papers included in the review (Knowledge, awareness, attitude, information source, public donation, private banking) (Continued)

No.	Author/Year	Aim	Country Setting	Sample Inclusion	Design	Findings	Limitations
		program on cord blood banking and stem cell knowledge among antenatal mothers.				*Post-test knowledge* *70% had good knowledge; 30% had average knowledge. *Mean post-test knowledge higher (21.9%) then pre-test knowledge (10.2%).	
11	Screnci et al. (2012)	To explore knowledge about CB stem cells, and preferences for donation or private banking and the motivation behind the decision.	Italy University of Rome, ANC	239 pregnant women before CB education given Surveys distributed n = 300 Response rate = 80% [298 female blood donors] Convenience Sampling 100 mothers who had donated CB (for verification of donation motivation)	Quantitative Anonymous Questionnaires	Findings reported for pregnant women only. Overall: Large support for CBD suggests CBB is not an obstacle to expansion of CBD. HP and institutions should provide CBB information. *Knowledge of CB* *93% general knowledge; 42% probability of clinical use; 31% therapeutic uses; 58% difference CBD Vs CBB; 71% donation criteria *CBD awareness* *95% aware of CBD *Information source* *42% Obs; 25% internet CB choice (n = 215) *61% would CBD, 56% had altruistic and other reasons; *7% would CBB, 73% would do so to safeguard future *32% would discard CB, logistics (28%), lack of interest (28%)	Sample from one Institution only so may not be generalised Survey tool not validated
12	Shin et al. (2011)	To investigate the knowledge of CB and attitudes towards CB banking among well educated, high-potential donors.	Korea 1 Maternity hospital	863 pregnant women attending antenatal classes which did not consist of CB banking education component Convenience sampling Surveys distributed = 1430 Response = 60.3%	Quantitative Questionnaires Questionnaire adapted and enhanced from 3 previous studies (Fernandez et al. 2003,Perlow et al. 2006, Fox et al. 2007)	Overall: Minimal level of knowledge was recorded. Obs have insignificant role in disseminating knowledge *Knowledge* 57% correctly answered CB current use and limitations *CB collection reason* *CBD: Altruism most common reason (94%) *Safeguard for	Only highly educated, urban women who received antenatal care and education were included. Results may not be generalized. Survey Tool not validated.

Table 1 Overview of papers included in the review (Knowledge, awareness, attitude, information source, public donation, private banking) (Continued)

No.	Author/Year	Aim	Country Setting	Sample Inclusion	Design	Findings	Limitations
						future was most common reason for CBB (75%) *Most common reason for no CB collection was inconvenience of consent and medical questionnaire *CB Donation motivation* *54% of CBD were blood donors *Source of Information* *88% received CBD information; most common sources CBD of information was media/internet (37%) and brochures (31%). * 2% and 4% learnt about CBD and CBB respectively from Obs. *97% received CBB information; most common CBB information source was advertisements (38%) and media/internet (36%).	
13	Manegold et al. (2011)	To explore the attitudes of donating parents towards public and private CB banking.	Switzerland Public CB bank	300 Recent Swiss, western and eastern European public CB donors. Purposive Sampling Surveys distributed = 621 Response rate = 48.3%	Quantitative Standardised anonymous questionnaire 20 multi-choice and open ended questions	Overall: Motivation for private or hybrid CB banking is low in this population. *Source of CBD information* *54% from HP *22% from more than 1 source: family, friends and media *34% actively sought CBD information *CBD vs CBB Options* *2% would CBB for next infant *27% did not know of CBB *69% opted for CBD due to altruism and cost of CBB	84% of the open questions were unanswered Only donors whose CB was accepted for storage were included in study May not be generalized to the entire donor population Survey tool not validated
14	Katz et al. (2011) Europe	To explore pregnant women's awareness of CB stem cells and their	5 European countries: France, Germany, Italy, Spain, United Kingdom.	1620 Pregnant women who had not previously	Quantitative Anonymous self-directed	Overall: Study revealed strong preference for CBD. Attitudes were not an	Ethnic breakdown was not reported. Data collection differed

Table 1 Overview of papers included in the review (Knowledge, awareness, attitude, information source, public donation, private banking) (Continued)

No.	Author/Year	Aim	Country Setting	Sample Inclusion	Design	Findings	Limitations
		attitude towards banking.	6 urban maternity hospital antenatal clinics with over 1000 births per annum (Germany = 2 antenatal classes in lieu of clinic)	enrolled in a CB banking program. France n = 318 UK n = 290 Germany n = 313 Spain n = 323 Italy n = 376 Purposive Sampling	multi-choice questionnaire	obstacle to CBB. *CB Information and knowledge* *79.4% declared poor CBB knowledge. *59.6% received information via mass media and internet. *20% received information from HP. *91.6% believed they should be systematically informed. *CB banking choices* *89% would collect CB; 11% would discard CB; 77% would CBD; 12% would CBB; 12% would store in hybrid bank *Choice for CBD* *59% said altruism; 30% believe a duty to donate *24% would change birth hospital in order to be able to CBD *Choice for CBB* *12% would CBB; 51% of these women would do so due to possible future medical research therapies *16% would do so for insurance reasons	across sites: German questionnaires conducted in antenatal classes not clinics as in other 4 countries CBB not available in 3 countries at time of study (France, Italy and Spain) Knowledge not awareness reported. Survey tool validated
15	Suen et al. (2011)	To assess knowledge of private cord blood banking among pregnant women	Hong Kong 2 large public maternity units	1866 Pregnant women accessing antenatal clinic. Surveys distributed = 2000 Response rate = 93.3% Convenience Sampling	Quantitative Cross-sectional self-administered questionnaire Survey validated	Overall: Study revealed inadequate knowledge on CBB and use. *Understanding* *78.2% reported no understanding of likelihood CBB use *Awareness* *Only 58.5% were aware of CB use for childhood leukemia *Knowledge* *20.3% knew of CB availability from public CB banks	Sampling limited to public patients who did not have the option of CBB unless indicated for medical reasons.

Table 1 Overview of papers included in the review (Knowledge, awareness, attitude, information source, public donation, private banking) *(Continued)*

No.	Author/Year	Aim	Country Setting	Sample Inclusion	Design	Findings	Limitations
						Preferred source of CBB information *44% stated Dr.; 32% stated CBB staff *22% stated unsure who to receive information from; 7% stated N/MWs Government involvement * 89% wanted more promotion and education on CBB	
16	Salvaterra et al. (2010)	To analyze knowledge, comprehension, opinions, attitudes and choices related to cord blood donation of pregnant women, future parents, donors, midwives, obstetricians/ gynaecologists. To compare preferences of public versus private banking.	Italy Hospital, community & academic sector participation	Pregnant women, future parents and donors (n = 30) 32 antenatal health care providers consisting of: 10 community midwives 12 hospital midwives 10 obstetricians (public and private) Multiple sampling methods	Mixed methods using participatory approach with establishment of a taskforce and public multidisciplinary round table Focus groups; (max. n = 10 participants, led by 2 psychologists) Self-administered questionnaires at completion of focus groups (n = 20)	Findings reported from pregnant women, future parents and donor perspectives: Overall: *CBD considered a gift of moral and social value; Participants would CBD for altruistic purposes. *CBB was associated with egoism and fraud. *100% wanted more information and clear procedures on CBB. *100% stated HP should be educated on CBB/CBD and inform future parents during pregnancy *70% (14/20) reported poor knowledge of CBD	Included only those in an urban setting and didn't include any minority groups. Few knowledge questions; most opinion based. Small sample sizes allowed for limited between group comparisons Researchers developed own assessment tool Knowledge not reported
17	Rucinski et al. (2010)	To explore the knowledge, attitudes, beliefs and practices regarding cord blood donation among Hispanic and non-Hispanic black women.	United States of America 1 Community Health Centre and 1 Community Hospital in Chicago, Illinois	41 Hispanic and non-Hispanic pregnant black women, or who had given birth in the last 12 months, > 18 yrs, had received antenatal care by the 2nd trimester; did not have any religious objections to donation. Purposive sampling.	Qualitative 5 Focus groups: 1 Hispanic (English) n = 5 1 Hispanic (Spanish) n = 9 3 non-Hispanic n = 8/9/10	Overall: Most not aware of, what it involved, or the value of, CBD for treatment and research. Participants believed that Drs provide CBD information Initial analysis did not reveal strong ethnic difference in knowledge or attitudes towards CBD. *Knowledge/Awareness* *Participants who reported awareness of saving CB, was in reference to CBB not CBD. *Participants reported confusion between CBD and CBB options. *Information needs and sources* *Those who had birthed	Very specific inclusion criteria so results could not be generalized to the wider population.

Table 1 Overview of papers included in the review (Knowledge, awareness, attitude, information source, public donation, private banking) *(Continued)*

No.	Author/Year	Aim	Country Setting	Sample Inclusion	Design	Findings	Limitations
						expressed concern that they had't been informed by HP on CBD option *Many wanted CBD info from their Dr. due to trust/respect in Dr. being source of factual information and perceived ability to answer questions on topic. *Some parents reported Dr. indifference on topic and Dr. failure to spend time providing health related answers to questions which reduced faith that Drs were reliable source of information.	
18	Patten & Dudenhausen (2010)	To evaluate the correlation between German-speaking women's knowledge of cord blood banking and their level of education.	Germany (Perlow, 2006) 1 obstetric hospital in Berlin, 3 ANC	300 Pregnant women over the age of 18 years in their 3rd trimester Surveys distributed = 313 Response rate = 96% Quota Sampling: to gain comparative number to Fox et al. (2007) study	Quantitative Multi-choice response Questionnaire	Overall: Women were poorly educated about CB storage usefulness, costs and methods. *Education* *35% well educated (University degree). *Women with higher education level had read more CBB information *Knowledge* * 50-65% were unaware of CB treatable illnesses *Source of CB information* *74%: reading material and commercials. *59%: material by private CBB. *26%: public CBD banks. *CB discussion with obstetrician* *5% discussed it with Obs; 1% had it raised by Obs	Language interpreted tool used by Fox et al. (2007), although cultural and health system differences make comparisons of findings difficult. Awareness not knowledge reported.
19	Dinc & Sahin (2009)	To determine pregnant women's knowledge and attitudes towards stem cells and cord blood banking in Instanbul.	Turkey 2 Antenata clinics: 1 in a University Medical Centre, 1 in a Family Planning Centre.	334 Pregnant women accessing antenatal clinic in Instanbul. Convenience Sampling	Qualitative Exploratory descriptive study of Interviews: yes/no and open ended questions	Overall: Women with a higher education had higher levels of knowledge about CB and stem cells. Most had a lack of knowledge on the topics and wanted more information from HP.	Select sample of women in 2 antenatal clinics in 1 location so may not be generalized to the rest of the population.

Table 1 Overview of papers included in the review (Knowledge, awareness, attitude, information source, public donation, private banking) (Continued)

No.	Author/Year	Aim	Country Setting	Sample Inclusion	Design	Findings	Limitations
						Knowledge *Only 26.9% aware of CB and stem cells. *Source of CB information* *72% stated media; 28% stated Obs *Preferred source of information* *79% stated Obs; 21% stated N/MW *Main reasons for CBB* *48.9% stated possible future need *22% it is beneficial; 10% future regret *8% insurance for child *Main reasons against CBB* *68.7% not necessary; 21% limited information	Awareness not knowledge reported.
20	Fox et al. (2007)	To evaluate patient understanding of cord blood banking.	United States of America 1 large Obstetric Hospital, New York with access to public and private CB banking, ANC	325 pregnant women Quota sampling Surveys distributed =724 Response rate = 44.9%	Quantitative Anonymous multi-choice questionnaire	*Overall:* Women had very poor understanding of CB uses and banking. *Education status* 94% completed undergraduate degree 58% completed post graduate degree. *Awareness* *54.4% unaware of medical conditions treatable with CB. *Main CB Information source* *86.5%: private CBB literature *29.2%: Public CBD banks literature *36.9%: Discussion with Obs though not stated who initiated the conversation. *Reasons for private CBB* *83%: protect infant in future	Survey conducted in early pregnancy. Only 45% of surveys completed so may indicate a bias of results. Study did not examine the extent of the women's knowledge of CBB.
21	Perlow (2006)	To determine patients' knowledge of cord	United States of America	425 Pregnant women attending for antenatal	Quantitative Convenience Sampling	*Overall:* Patients poorly informed	Addressed private CBB only.

Table 1 Overview of papers included in the review (Knowledge, awareness, attitude, information source, public donation, private banking) *(Continued)*

No.	Author/Year	Aim	Country Setting	Sample Inclusion	Design	Findings	Limitations
		blood banking.	1 Obstetric Medical Centre Phoenix, Arizona.	consultation, or ultrasound. Convenience Sampling	2. part questionnaire: 1. Awareness 157 (37%) unaware of CB banking. Completed part 1 only. 2. Knowledge 268 (63%) completed part 1&2.	about CBB (74%, 315/425). Few receive CB education from HP. Lack of knowledge and expense CBB barriers. *Awareness of CBB* *63% were aware. Remainder excluded from part 2 of study. *Women with lower education less likely to be aware than women with a University degree (22% v 78%). * Women under age 25 less likely to be aware (53% v 68%). *Ethnic women had less awareness then Caucasian women. *Knowledge of CBB* *74% stated minimally informed. *3% stated extremely knowledgeable on the subject. *Source of CBB information* *53% informed by media; 17.5% informed by Dr; 8.2% informed by other HP. *Barriers to CBB* *Cost (30%); low knowledge (31%), misinformation on who could use CB (50%).	Conducted in one location only so may not be representative of the general population. Lack of cultural diversity, small numbers of Native and African Americans in the survey. Last two questions of the survey were not completed by all participants.
22	Danzer et al. (2003)	To evaluate the attitudes of mothers towards cord blood donation for therapeutic use 6 months post donation.	Switzerland 1 University Hospital with a CB collection centre	78 Women 6 months post-partum who donated cord blood Purposive Sampling Response rate = 59.5% (Total surveys distributed = 131)	Quantitative Survey Standardized anonymous questionnaires Multi-choice format, with 1 open ended question.	Overall: A High degree of satisfaction with CBD. *Responses regarding CBD* 100% believed CBD was ethical *96.1% would CBD again *74.8% emotionally satisfied about CBD *Original source of CBD information*	Women from one Institution only were surveyed. A total of 131 were sent surveys however, 40.5% did not respond.

Table 1 Overview of papers included in the review (Knowledge, awareness, attitude, information source, public donation, private banking) (*Continued*)

No.	Author/Year	Aim	Country Setting	Sample Inclusion	Design	Findings	Limitations
						*81.3% from their Dr; 18.7% from media and friends. *No significant association between information source and decision to donate again. Open ended question comments *8 women supported importance of CB collection centres; 5 expressed concern for improper use, 2 expressed concern donated CB may not be available for own child.	
23	Fernandez et al. (2003)	To examine pregnant women's knowledge and attitudes regarding CB banking, which maybe used in the development of policies and procedures for public and private CB banking?	Canada 1 Regional Women's Hospital	443 English speaking pregnant women attending antenatal clinic. Response rate = 68% (Total surveys distributed = 650) Convenience Sampling	Quantitative Questionnaires developed by Authors	Overall: Most women were supportive of CBD for transplantation and research. *Knowledge* *72% reported poor or very poor CBB knowledge ($n = 310$) 25% overestimated risk of a child requiring a stem cell transplant *Preferred CB education source* *66% HP; 68% Dr; 70% ANC. *CB Banking option* *14% would choose CBB due to a good investment. *86% would choose to CBD due to altruism.	High proportion of participants were university or college educated. Little ethnic diversity in group. No established public or private CB banks in the area at the time the study was conducted.
24	Sugarman et al. (2002)	To evaluate the informed consent process for cord blood donation.	United States of America 2 CB Collection centres associated with a Public CB Bank.	170 Pregnant women in the 3rd trimester who had consented to cord blood donation Convenience Sampling	Qualitative Telephone interviews	Overall: Women were satisfied with consent process (96.9%), most (98.8%) would donate again, though did not seem to know about alternatives to CBD. *Other responses to CBD process* *Only 32.9% understood they had the option not to have CB collected.	Sample limited to those who had consented to CBD at 1 public bank. Understanding of CBD and uses may differ in women who chose not to CBD and where CBB is

Table 1 Overview of papers included in the review (Knowledge, awareness, attitude, information source, public donation, private banking) *(Continued)*

No.	Author/Year	Aim	Country Setting	Sample Inclusion	Design	Findings	Limitations
						*Only 55.3% understood the option of CBB. 78.8% incorrectly thought they could donate CB to a specific recipient. Incorrect endorsement of CBD *Diagnosis of genetic disease of infant (92.9%) and mother (88.2%) * Diagnosis of infectious disease of infant (88.2%) and mother (87.1%) *Protection for infant (48.8%)	an option. Interviews were conducted 1 month post-partum so information previously conveyed and understood may have been forgotten.
25	Sugarman et al. (1998).	To learn about pregnant women's concerns regarding CB collection and banking in order to establish a comprehensive recruitment and informed consent process for donation.	United States of America 3 antenatal clinics (1 private, 2 public) affiliated with CB collection centres.	19 Pregnant women in their 2nd & 3rd trimester Purposive sampling	Qualitative Focus group discussions	Overall: 100% indicated they lacked sufficient or substantial prior knowledge of CB technology. Desire for more information about collection, storage and use of CB, especially difference between CBB and CBD was identified. *CB education* *100% believed in importance of CBB education including collection, storage and use. *Earlier the education was provided promoted a feeling of choice. *CB education should be in various formats: clinic pamphlets/posters, parenting magazines, information hotlines, television advertisements & reports, ANC. *Safety of mother and infant* *Important to inform women that CB collection does not alter the birth process. *Reasons for CBD* *Altruism was main reason *Influence of others may give cause for more likely CBD.	Findings context specific, not able to be generalized to broader population.

Three papers reported low awareness of cord blood banking and donation [13, 31, 39]. Participants who had heard about cord blood banking expressed considerable confusion between public and private banking options [31], with cord blood donation having the least awareness reported in North America [13, 31].

Thirteen studies reported on cord blood banking and donation knowledge [14, 15, 18, 27, 28, 32–34, 37, 41, 43–46], with most studies assessing knowledge by participant self-report, as opposed to knowledge being measured by assessment of associated facts. Ten studies identified parent-reported suboptimal knowledge about collection and storage options for cord blood [15, 18, 27, 28, 32–34, 37, 43, 44], and of parents being minimally informed about cord blood banking and donation options [15, 28, 32–34, 37, 44, 45].

Exceptions to these low knowledge findings were reported by four studies, with more than 70% of participants of three studies reported to be knowledgeable about cord blood banking and donation [14, 41, 46]. Findings from early postpartum women (n = 320) surveyed by Kim et al. (2015) on their knowledge and attitudes of storage, donation and disposal of cord blood suggested that a high level of knowledge about cord blood was associated with women opting for cord blood donation.

Ten papers investigated parents' attitudes towards cord blood banking and donation with samples including pregnant women, expectant parents and new parents [14, 28, 29, 32, 34, 35, 41, 42, 44, 46]. Overall, the findings from these studies indicated that parents were more inclined to support donation than private cord blood banking [14, 28, 32, 34, 35, 42, 45]. Key themes of parent attitudes towards donation and storage of cord blood included altruism, ethical practice, duty to society and insurance for the baby. Only one paper reported low regard for altruism or public benefit surrounding cord blood donation, however this may be attributed to lack of awareness of cord blood donation as public cord blood banking was not available at the time of this study's data collection [45].

Several papers found parents to be positive towards cord blood banking [29, 41, 44, 45]. Reasons given for private cord blood banking included insurance for their baby [44], the cord blood may be needed in the future and they may have future regret of not storing their baby's cord blood [29].

Cord blood use

Five papers reported on cord blood use awareness [13, 31, 38, 41, 46], with only one paper reporting high awareness, which included participants who were already parents [41]. Three studies used mixed methods and reported that considerable proportions of the parent population had relatively low awareness relating to uses of cord blood [13, 31, 38].

Nine papers reported knowledge of cord blood use [13, 27–30, 33, 35, 36, 46] and knowledge deficits were identified. Treatment of blood cancers was the most commonly known use of cord blood [13, 29, 30, 35], with over 50% of participants correct in their responses in studies by Fox and colleagues (n = 70%) [14] and Palten and Dudenhausen (50–65%) [26]. Limited knowledge was reported for other uses [13, 30, 36], including the likelihood of use of cord blood stem cells [28, 33]. Matijevic and Erjavec (2016) reported 95% of participants in their study self-reported knowledge of cord blood treatments as either insufficient or basic [46].

Cord blood information
Source of information

Source of cord blood banking information was investigated by 16 of the reviewed papers [13–15, 20, 28, 30, 31, 34–36, 39, 40, 42, 44–46]. The main sources of parent information were hospitals; health professionals, including antenatal classes; media and magazines; cord blood banks; and family and friends. Table 2 summaries the sources of information reported in the studies reviewed.

Six authors reported health professionals and/or antenatal classes were the main source of information on cord blood banking [14, 20, 36, 41, 42, 44], with a further two authors reporting these were the second most common sources [39, 40]. Health professionals, particularly doctors, were identified as important informers of cord blood banking options [20, 36, 42, 45]. Receiving this information from a health professional significantly influenced the parental decision to store cord blood [20].

Four authors reported low numbers of participants had received cord blood information from health professionals [15, 34, 35, 45, 46], and a further study found that participants had to actively enquire in order to receive information on cord blood donation [14].

Print and electronic (including internet) media and advertising were the main information source of cord blood banking reported in six studies [15, 30, 34, 35, 39, 46], and was the second most common source in two further papers [36, 40] after health professionals [36] and private cord blood banks [40].

Four studies listed cord blood banks as a source of cord blood banking information [13, 20, 30, 40], with Jordens and colleagues [36] reporting this was the main source for their participants. Private banking information was reported as a more common source of information compared to public banks [13, 30]; one study reported that almost half of their sample indicating that information from private cord blood banks was influential in their decision to store cord blood [20].

Six reports noted family and friends to be a source of information [14, 20, 36, 39, 42, 47], though only one paper stated this was their main source [20]. Three studies combined 'family, friends and media' as a single information source category [15, 28, 32]. These studies reported similar findings with approximately 20% of participants identifying this category as a source of cord blood banking information and an influence in their decision-making [15, 32, 38].

Preferred source of information
Five papers reported on participants preferred source of information on cord blood banking and donation [28, 29, 31, 33, 40, 45]. Four studies listed antenatal health professionals, including antenatal classes, as the most important and preferred source [29, 31, 33, 40, 45]. Only one paper reported cord blood banks as a preferred source of information [33]. Table 2 displays the preferred information sources reported by participants of studies included in this review.

Discussion
Cord blood banking and donation has been an option for parents for the past quarter century, yet an understanding of knowledge and awareness of these options, and consistency of information provided to parents, remains low. This is the first integrative review to explore parents' knowledge, awareness and attitudes towards cord blood banking and donation, and parent sources, and preferred source, of information on this topic.

This integrative review identified parents' knowledge of cord banking and/or donation as generally low [18, 27, 28, 32–34, 37, 44–46]. Higher knowledge levels were identified where participants had previously donated cord blood and where participants had been provided with information on these options by their antenatal health care provider or in antenatal classes [14, 41, 44]. This finding highlighted the importance of providing parents with this information as part of routine antenatal education. Overall, awareness of cord blood banking options was found to be higher than knowledge in this integrative review [15, 41, 47]. Like knowledge findings, this may be attributed to the availability of information provided at birthing facilities, and the level of education of participants [15, 40, 41].

Positive attitudes towards cord blood donation among parents were found, with the option considered to be an ethical [42] and altruistic choice for parents [14, 28, 34, 35, 41]. This could be indicative that cord blood donation has a moral association, and this finding may be important when health professionals discuss this option with parents as they may feel pressure or an obligation to choose this option. Positive attitudes towards private cord blood banking were also found, with only one study reporting negative findings [32]. Participants who chose to privately store their infant's cord blood did so because they viewed this option as an investment for future use, insurance or protection for their child or family [28, 29, 34, 35, 44]. The desire of parents to do the best for their children and provide for their future may influence their interpretation of the importance of the scientific benefit on storing cord blood stems cells for future health protection, and illustrates the emotional element frequently attached to this option.

Knowledge on cord blood use among study participants was mixed. Over 50% of participants in many of the studies could not correctly identify uses of cord blood [13, 18, 27, 29, 30, 33, 36, 46]. This lack of knowledge emphasises the uncertainty about the source and the quality of the information being provided. When knowledge was self-reported by participants, general uses for cord blood was higher than specific uses [29, 30, 36], with treatment of blood cancers the highest correct response reported [14, 26].

Awareness among parents of the value of cord blood and cord blood uses was found to be less than knowledge levels of cord blood value and use. We identified that the provision of information by health professionals greatly influenced awareness of the value of cord blood and its' potential uses. This finding again emphasises the need for information to be provided as part of routine antenatal care.

In this integrative review, we found that there was inconsistency in information provided to parents about cord blood banking and cord blood use. This inconsistency created awareness and knowledge deficits and arguably prevents parents from making informed choices. This is an important finding; in Australia, the Health and Safety commission have identified involving consumers in health care choices is associated with better client experience and promotes client centered care [48].

Information sources for parents on cord blood was found to be varied, fragmented and inconsistent [14, 20, 35, 40]. This inconsistency of information is concerning because for parents to make informed choices about cord blood banking or donation they need appropriate, relevant, objective information that is accurate, valid, regulated and based on the latest evidence in a variety of consumer-friendly formats through trustworthy sources [49].

Health professions were identified as the preferred source of information on cord blood banking for parents [28, 29, 31, 33, 40, 45]. The views of clients are among many factors that influence change to health services [50] and it is imperative that information on cord blood banking and donation is considered as part of routine antenatal education for parents.

Strengths and limitations of this study
The integrative approach chosen for this review of parent knowledge and awareness of cord blood banking, donation and cord blood banking, including sources and preferred sources of information, allowed for the

inclusion of a diverse range of qualitative, quantitative and mixed methods studies with participant samples from nations representing most world continents. Despite the literature review being extensive, inclusive of published studies meeting eligibility criteria since cord blood banking became available in 1991, this integrative review was limited to studies published in the English language only. Different terminology and sampling descriptions (pregnant women and / or parent / couples' knowledge) used across studies, and a lack of clarity and consistency within studies relating to study aims and methods reported, limited interpretation of some study results.

The papers included in this review varied significantly in sample size ($n = 30$ to 1873), but this may have been driven by the research approach chosen [18, 31, 32, 37]. Survey tools to measure knowledge, awareness and attitudes were poorly described or not validated in some studies [14, 32, 35–37, 43, 46], with only two studies using the same (or modified version) tool [13, 30].

Several papers reported on awareness, not knowledge, as indicated in their title or abstract [29, 30, 32, 40, 41] or on knowledge, when awareness was indicated [34]. The findings of some studies were context specific and may not be generalised [14, 18, 31, 35–37], or participants did not have access to both cord blood banking and donation which may have influenced study findings [15, 27, 28, 33, 34, 39].

Implications for practice, education and research

In this integrative review, inconsistencies, and uncertainty in knowledge and awareness that parents have regarding cord blood use and banking options have been highlighted. These findings are indicative of the need for expectant parents to be informed of the cord blood banking options available to them by their antenatal care providers and/or at their birthing facility so that they can make an informed decision about what option is appropriate for their family circumstances. Maternity care policy and practice evolve with the emergence of new research evidence [49]; health services therefore need to be responsive to client and consumer input and needs [48] and involve clients in health care and informed decision making.

Research

Parent knowledge of cord blood banking options and cord blood use has been identified as poor. This integrative review identified that parents have a lack of knowledge about the options of cord blood banking and donation, and the uses of cord blood. There is lack of clarity and consistency in the information provided for parents on cord blood banking, donation and cord blood use. Future research is needed to explore health professionals' knowledge of, and attitudes towards, cord blood banking, donation and cord

blood use and how this impacts on the information that they provide to expectant parents in their care. The option of cord blood banking and donation has been available to parents for over 25 years so it is timely to investigate where the gaps in health professionals' knowledge lie.

Practice

Information on cord blood banking and cord blood use is not a standard element of antenatal education and this is concerning because parents require this information to make a fully informed choice of their options regarding their infant's cord blood following birth. We argue that there is a need for health professionals to provide accurate and evidence-based information to parents. This integrative review has demonstrated that information provision to expectant parents by health professionals on the topic of cord blood banking and donation is not a consistent part of antenatal education. Research is needed to identify and understand barriers to the information provision to parents on cord blood banking and donation, and why this important topic is not yet a standardised part of antenatal education.

Education

Health professionals are the parent preferred source of cord blood banking information. It is vital that health professionals are educated and informed of all aspects and elements of cord blood banking to enable them to provide appropriate information to parents. We argue that cord blood banking should be incorporated into health professional curricula and antenatal education.

Conclusion

Cord blood banking is complex and often poorly understood by parents and health professionals. This integrative review makes an important contribution to the body of knowledge in this field by identifying knowledge, highlighting gaps and suggesting direction for future research, practice and education in relation to cord blood banking and donation and cord blood use.

Significant gaps in parents' knowledge and awareness of cord blood banking have been identified in this review of current evidence. This is an important topic and one that requires parents to make informed and rationale choices. For this to occur, information provided needs to be accurate, objective valid, timely and appropriate, and supplied by parent preferred sources. As identified in this integrative review, currently this is not the case.

This integrative review has identified that further research should focus on identifying the information expectant parents would like to receive to assist them to make an informed choice around cord blood banking and to identifying the barriers to health professionals providing this evidence-based information on cord blood use and banking options.

Parents' knowledge, awareness and attitudes of cord blood donation and banking...

45

Authors' contributions

All authors conceptualized the review and selected the review methodology. LP conducted the literature search, identified articles for inclusion and analysis, and drafted the initial manuscript. JY, DM and LK checked the search strategy, reviewed included articles, and contributed to the contributed to critical revisions of the manuscript. All named authors contributed sections of the text and approved the final manuscript.

Competing interests

The authors declare that they have no competing interests.

Author details

[1]School of Nursing, Midwifery and Paramedicine, University of the Sunshine Coast, Locked Bag 4, Maroochydore DC, QLD 4558, Australia. [2]Sunshine Coast Hospital and Health Service, Maroochydore DC, Queensland, Australia.

References

1. Navarrete C, Contreras M. Cord blood banking: a historical perspective. Br J Haematol. 2009;147(2):236–45.
2. Gluckman E. Milestones in umbilical cord blood transplantation. Blood Rev. 2011;25:255–9.
3. Ballen KK, Verter F, Kurtzberg J. Umbilical cord blood donation: public or private? Bone Marrow Transplant. 2015:1–8.
4. Yoder MC. Cord blood banking and transplantation: advances and controversies. Pediatrics. 2014;26(2).
5. Waller-Wise R. Umbilical cord blood: information for childbirth educators. J Perinat Educ. 2011;20(1):50–60.
6. Guilcher G, Fernandez CV, Joffe S. Are hybrid umbilical cord blood banks really the best of both worlds? J Med Ethics. 2013;41:272–5.
7. Han MX, Craig ME. Research using autologous cord blood - time for a policy change. Med J Aust. 2013;199(4):288–90.
8. Mayani H. Umbilical cord blood: lessons learned and lingering challenges after more than 20 years of basic and clinical research. Arch Med Res. 2011; 42:645–51.
9. Petrini C. Ethical issues in umbilical cord blood banking: a comparative analysis of documents from national and international institutions. Transfusion. 2013;53:902–10.
10. Skabla P, McGadney-Douglas B, Hampton J. Educating patients about the value of umbilical cord blood donation. Journal of American Academy of Physician Assistants. 2010;23(11) 33–34, 39–40.
11. Plant M, Knoppers BM. Umbilical cord blood banking in Canada: socio-ethical and legal issues. Health Law Journal. 2005;13:187–212.
12. Samuel G, Kerridge IH, O'Brien TA. Umbilical cord blood banking: public good or private benefit? Med J Aust. 2008;188(9):533–5.
13. Fox NS, Stevens C, Ciubotariu R, Rubinstein P, McCullough LB, Chervenak FA. Umbilical cord blood collection: do patients really understand? J Perinat Med. 2007;35(4):314–21.
14. Manegold G, Meyer-Monard S, Tichelli A, Granado C, Hosli I, Troeger C. Controversies in hybrid banking: attitudes of Swiss public umbilical cord donors towards private and public banking. Arch Gynecology Obstetrics. 2011;284:99–104.
15. Perlow JH. Patients' knowledge of umbilical cord blood banking. J Reprod Med. 2006;51(8):642–8.
16. Kornhaber RA, McLean LM, Baber RJ. Ongoing ethical issues concerning authorship in biomedical journals: an integrative review. Int J Nanomedicine. 2015;10:4837–46.
17. Whittmore R, Knafi K. The integrative review: updated methodology. J Adv Nurs. 2005;52(5):546–53.
18. Sugarman J, Cogswell B, Olson J. Pregnant Women's Perceptives on umbilical cord blood banking. J Women's Health. 1998;7(6):747–57.
19. CASP: Making sense of evidence.
20. Bioinformant Worldwide LLC. Cord blood banking survey 600+ recent and expectant parents; Geography Worldwide. *WwwBioInformantcom* 2014. 2014:1–51.
21. Surbrek D, Islebe A, Schonfeld B, Tichelli A, Holgreve W. Umbilical cord blood transplantation: acceptance of umbilical cord blood donation by pregnant patients. Schweiz Med Wochenschr. 1998;128(18):689–95.
22. Kim MO, Yoo JS, Park CG, Ahn HM. Knowledge and attitude to cord blood of early postpartum women after donating cord blood or storing cord blood. Korean Journal of Womens Health Nursing. 2009;15(1):13–23.
23. Dunbar NM. Between the trash can and the freezer: donor education and the fate of cord blood. Transfusion (Philadelphia, Pa). 2011;51:234–6.
24. Wagner AM. Use of human embryonic stem cells and umbilical cord blood stem cells for research and therapy: a prospective survey among health care professionals and patients in Switzerland stem cell survey in Switzerland. Transfusion (Philadelphia, Pa). 2013;53(11):2681–9.
25. Parco S, Vascotto F, Visconti P. Public banking of umbilical cord blood or storage in a private bank:testing social and ethical policy in northeastern Italy. Journal of Blood Medicine. 2013;4:23–9.
26. Braun V, Clarke V. Using thematics analysis in psychology. Qual Res Psychol. 2006;3:77–101.
27. Sugarman J, Kurtzberg J, Box TI, Horner RD. Optimization of informed consent for umbilical cord blood banking. American Journal of Obstetrics and Gynaecology. 2002;187(6):1642–6.
28. Fernandez CV, Gordon K, Van den Hof M, Taweel S, Baylis F. Knowledge and attitudes of pregnant women with regard to collection, testing and banking of cord blood stem cells. CMAJ. 2003:695–8.
29. Dinc H, Sahin NH. Pregnant Women's knowledge and attitudes about stem cells and cord banking. Int Nurs Rev. 2009;56(2):250–6.
30. Palten PE, Dudenhausen JW. A great lack of knowledge regarding umbilical cord blood banking among pregnant women in Berlin, Germany. J Perinat Med. 2010;38(6):651–8.
31. Rucinski D, Jones R, Reyes B, Tidwell L, Phillips R, Delves D. Exploring opinions and beliefs about cord blood donation among Hispanic and non-Hispanic black women. Transfusion. 2010;50:1057–63.
32. Salvaterra E, Casati S, Bottardi S, Brizzolara A, Calistri D, Cofano R, Folliero E, Lalatta F, Maffioletti C, Negri M, et al. An analysis of decision making in cord blood donation through a participatory approach. Transfus Apher Sci. 2010; 42(3):299–305.
33. Suen SSH, Lao TT, Chan OK, et al. Maternal understanding of commercial cord blood storage for their offspring - a survey among pregnant women in Hong Kong. Acta Obstet Gynecol Scand. 2011;90(9):1005–9.
34. Katz G, Mills A, Garcia J, Hooper K, McGuckin C, Platz A, Rebulla P, Salvaterra E, Schmidt AH, Torrabadella M. Banking cord blood stem cells: attitudes and knowledge of pregnant women in five European countries. Transfusion. 2011;51:578–86.
35. Shin S, Yoon JH, Lee HR, Kim BJ, Roh EY. Perspectives of potential donors on cord blood and cord blood crypreservation: a survey of highly educated, pregnant Korean women receiving active prenatal care. Transfusion. 2011;51:277–82.
36. Screnci M, Murgi E, Pirre G, Valente E, Gesuiti P, Corona F, Girelli G. Donating umbilical cord blood to a public bank or storing it in a private bank: knowledge and preference of blood donors and of pregnant women. Blood Transfus. 2012;10:331–7.
37. Padmavathi P. Effects of Structured Teaching Programme regarding Stem Cells and Umbilical Cord Blood Banking on Knowledge among Antenatal Mothers. Nurs J India. 2013;CIV(4):30–2.
38. Meissner-Roloff MP, M. Establishing a public umbilical cord blood stem cell Bank for South Africa: an enquiry into public acceptability. Stem Cell Review and Reproduction. 2013;9:752–63.

39. Alexander NI, Olayinka AO, Terrumun S, Felix EA. Umbilical cord blood donation and banking: awareness among pregnant women in Makurdi, Nigeria. Journal of dental and Medical Sciences. 2014;13(1):16–9.

40. Jordens CF, Kerridge IH, Stewart CL, O'Brien TA, Samuel G, Porter M, O'Connor MA, Nassar N. Knowledge, beliefs, and decisions of pregnant Australian women concerning donation and storage of umbilical cord blood: a population-based survey. Birth. 2014;41(4):360–6.

41. Karagiorgou LZ, Pantazopoulou MP, Mainas NC, Beloukas AI, Kriebardis AG. Knowledge about umbilical cord blood banking and Greek citizens. Blood Transfus. 2014:353–60.

42. Danzer E, Holzgreve W, Troeger C, Kostka U, Steimann S, Bitzer J, Gratwohl A, Tichelli A, Seelmann K, Surbek DV. Attitudes of Swiss mothers towards unrelated umbilical cord blood banking 6 months after donation. Transfusion. 2003;43:604–8.

43. Vijayalakshmi S: Knowledge on collection and storage of cord blood banking. Singhad e Journal of Nursing 2013, 111(1):14–17.

44. Kim M, Han S, Shin M. Influencing factors on the cord blood donation of post-partum women. Nursing and Health Science. 2015;17:269–75.

45. Matsumoto M, Dajani R, Khader Y, Matthews K. Assessing women's knowledge and attitudes towards cord blood banking: policy and ethical implications for Jordan. Transfusion. 2016;56:2052–60.

46. Matijevic R, Erjavec K. Knowledge and attitudes among pregnant women and maternity staff about umbilical cord blood banking. Transfus Med. 2016;26(6):462–6.

47. Jordens CF, O'Connor MA, Kerridge IH, Stewart CL, Cameron A, Keown D, Lawrence RJ, McGarrity A, Abdulaziz S, Tobin B. Religious perspectives on umbilical cord blood banking. J Law Med. 2012;19:497–511.

48. Australian Commission on Safety and Quality in Health Care: National Safety and Quality Health Service Standards. In., vol. September. Sydney: Commonwealth of Australia; 2012.

49. Cook Carter M, Correy M, Delbanco S, Foster CS, Friedland R, Gabel R, Gipson T, Rima Jolivet R, Main E, Sakala C, et al. 2020 vision for a high-quality, high-value maternity care system. Womens Health Issues. 2010;20:7–17.

50. Crawford M, Rutter D, Manley C, Weaver TKB, Fulop N, Tyrer P. Systematic review of involving patients in the planning and development of health care. British Medical Journal. 2002;325.

4

Is anemia an independent risk factor for postpartum depression in women who have a cesarean section? - A prospective observational study

Nirmala Chandrasekaran[1]*[iD], Leanne R De Souza[1], Marcelo L Urquia[2], Beverley Young[3], Anne Mcleod[4], Rory Windrim[5] and Howard Berger[1]

Abstract

Background: The symptoms of anemia and depression are very similar suggesting that there may be an association between the two entities. The aim of this study is to assess whether postpartum anemia (PPA) is an independent risk factor for de novo postpartum depression (PPD)in women undergoing elective cesarean section.

Methods: Women after an uncomplicated term cesarean section were recruited and their hemoglobin and iron status were measured on day 3–5 post section and again at 6 weeks. Postpartum depression was screened using the Edinburgh Postnatal Depression Scale (EPDS) and functional capacity was assessed with the RAND 12-item Health survey.

Results: One hundred and three women completed the study. The incidence of probable postpartum depression (PPD) as defined by EPDS score ≥ 10 was 17% at 6 weeks. There was no difference in hemoglobin or iron status in women who had PPD compared to those without (OR-0.69; 95% CI-0.15-2.49). Similarly, there was no significant association between low hemoglobin and maternal functional status (OR -1.03; 95% CI-0.34 - 2.94).

Conclusions: Neither anemia or low iron stores were found to be an independent risk factors for postpartum depression or decreased postpartum functional capacity in women who undergo an elective cesarean section.

Keywords: Anemia, Iron stores, Cesarean section, Postpartum depression, Functional status

Background

Postpartum anemia (PPA) is a serious health condition affecting approximately 27% of North American women during the early postpartum period (puerperium). Among women with PPA, an estimated 50% are also iron deficient, wherein iron stores are depleted while hemoglobin could be normal or low [1–3]. Maternal consequences of anemia are well known and include cardiovascular symptoms like palpitations and dizziness, fatigue, reduced physical and mental performance, reduced immune function, reduced peripartum blood reserves and increased risk of blood transfusion [4].

Postpartum depression (PPD) is one of the most common conditions in the postnatal period affecting between 10 and 15% of women [5]. The causes of postpartum depression remain unclear and risk factors include a family or personal history of depression before pregnancy, low income, poor social support, poor interfamilial relationships, low self-esteem, parental stress, unwanted or unplanned pregnancy and recent stressful life events in a woman's life [6, 7]. Up to 50% of women with PPD will go on to develop PPD in subsequent pregnancies, and their offspring are at increased risk of impaired psychological and intellectual development [8, 9]. The classic symptoms associated with PPD are depressed mood, anxiety, anhedonia, appetite and sleep disturbances, physical agitation, fatigue, feelings of worthlessness and

* Correspondence: chandrasekan@smh.ca
[1]Department of Maternal and Fetal Medicine, St Michaels Hospital, 30 Bond street, Toronto, ON M5B 1W8, Canada
Full list of author information is available at the end of the article

excessive guilt, decreased concentration and recurrent thoughts of death or suicidal ideation [10].

Symptoms of PPD are common to those found in women with PPA. Whether a causal pathway relates PPD and PPA, is unknown, however identifying a physiological link between these two conditions may help identify women at increased risk of PPD. Such an association has been suggested in the literature but there are few studies that specifically address the association between postpartum anemia and postpartum depression [11–13]. Furthermore the association between PPA and maternal functional status, defined by an individual's ability to perform normal daily activities required to meet basic needs, fulfill usual roles, and maintain health and well-being has not been previously studied in the context of developing PPD.

Moreover, some studies show that women who undergo cesarean delivery could potentially be at increased risk of developing PPD possibly due to perceived pain and immobility of recovery, stress response to surgery and perceived failure to undergo vaginal birth as potential reasons for the association. A meta-analysis of the effects of cesarean delivery on the risk of PPD concluded that although the risk of PPD was higher with both elective and emergency Cesarean sections compared to vaginal delivery, no statistically significant association was identified for elective section and PPD [14].

We aimed to determine whether anemia and iron deficiency, or the combination of these, are independent risk factors for newly diagnosed postpartum depression and decreased functional capacity in women who deliver by elective cesarean section.

Methods

The study was approved by the Research and Ethics board (REB) of St Michaels Hospital (REB #08–155). Informed written consent was obtained from all the women that agreed to participate in the study.

All women 18 years of age or older, with a full term, singleton pregnancy (37–41 weeks' gestation), undergoing elective Caesarean section were eligible to enroll in the study. Emergency Caesarean sections were excluded to avoid potential obstetric confounders associated with adverse labor and delivery experiences. Women were excluded from the study if they had symptomatic anemia necessitating blood transfusion, significant fetal anomalies, preexisting severe chronic maternal illness (e.g. cardiac disease with functional class >II, chronic renal failure), preexisting maternal depression or other psychiatric illness, preexisting hemoglobinopathy (e.g. thalassemia, sickle cell disease) or confounding social factors (e.g. single parent or no fixed address).

The primary outcome for our study was the incidence of probable postpartum depression determined by the Edinburgh postpartum depression scale (EPDS). The secondary outcomes were the association of PPD with measures of iron stores, measured by hemoglobin and soluble transferrin receptor and functional status measured by the RAND test.

Eligible women were approached within 24 h of delivery and followed prospectively for 6 weeks. Baseline demographic (age, ethnicity, gestational age) and clinical data (use of prenatal vitamins or iron supplements and any medical comorbidities) were collected, followed by venous blood collection for hemoglobin (gm/dl), ferritin (ng/ml) and soluble transferrin receptor (mg/L) levels. The intention to breastfeed was documented. Anemia was defined as hemoglobin < 110 g/l as described by the World Health Organization (WHO, 2007) [15]. A venous blood draw was repeated at 3 weeks postpartum to assess hemoglobin and ferritin levels. Women identified with anemia were prescribed iron supplements, with compliance monitored using a pill counter. At 6 weeks postpartum, a thyroid function test was administered to exclude postpartum thyroiditis as a potential confounder.

Functional status was assessed by administering the RAND 36-item health survey (SF-36). The RAND is a validated questionnaire that evaluates 8 health concept sub scales that include physical functioning, bodily pain, role limitations due to physical health problems, role limitations due to personal or emotional problems, emotional well-being, social functioning, energy/fatigue, and general health perceptions that may affect quality of life [16, 17]. From these 8 individual subscales, 2 overall scores were generated: physical health component (PCS) and mental health component (MCS). The scoring for the 8 domains and the 2 overall components are based on a 0–100 General Health Rating index scale, with a higher value corresponding to a higher quality of life [16].

The EPDS was administered at enrollment, 24 h after elective Cesarean section and again at 3 and 6 weeks postpartum. A score of ≥ 10 on the EPDS was considered positive for postpartum depression, as this has previously been shown to be highly sensitive for the detection of minor depression. Despite its intended use as a screening tool, the EPDS is widely accepted as a validated method to detect postpartum depression and the cut off threshold score of 10, readily identifies all cases of major depression with a negative predictive value of 99.7% [18–21]. Patients with a score ≥ 10 in the EPDS or > 2 in question 10 (thoughts of self-harm), were referred to a staff psychiatrist for the administration of the gold standard diagnostic tool - the Structured Clinical Interview for DSM-III-R (SCID, nonpoint version) and treatment if deemed necessary.

A lactation consultant contacted each woman at 2, 4 and 6 weeks postpartum to inquire about the frequency of breastfeeding or bottle-feeding and supplementation with formula among women who were breastfeeding. Women who reported rare supplementation with formula were coded as predominantly breastfeeding. Among those who reported exclusive bottle feeding, the number of weeks of any breastfeeding was recorded.

Statistical analysis

Previous studies indicate approximately 13% of women are diagnosed with major or minor PPD [5]. Using a 13% incidence of PPD among non-anemic patients, a sample size of 100 women would detect a 2.8-fold increase in PPD (37%) or higher in the defined anemic group (hemoglobin < 110), with a statistical power of 80% and alpha 0.05. This magnitude of increased risk is similar to the risk observed for other accepted risk factors for PPD [e.g. History of psychiatric disease OR 3.1 (2.3–4.2; Social isolation OR 3.6 (1.9–7.0)] [22] and would thus be a clinically significant effect size. This sample size also offers 80% power to detect a 50% increase in mean EPDS score.

Fisher's exact test was used to test the association between categorical variables and PPD and a T-test assessed continuous variables. We also used exact logistic regression to obtain odds ratios with 95% confidence intervals. Linear regression was used for the comparison of means between groups.

Given the lower than expected incidence of anemia in the study cohort, data were stratified according to the lowest quartiles to enable a comprehensive description of the effects of hemoglobin and iron status on functional capacity and postpartum depression. In multivariable analyses, we controlled for maternal age at delivery, parity, prenatal intake of vitamins and continuation of breastfeeding, each collected at 6 weeks postpartum. Data was analyzed with SAS 9.4 (SAS Institute Inc., Cary, NC).

Results

A total of 248 women were recruited for the study, with 145 lost to follow-up (Fig. 1). The excluded women were not demographically different from the study group (data not shown). Demographic characteristics of the 103 women are as listed in Table 1. There were no statistical differences in the baseline characteristics of women who screened positive for PPD and those who did not have any indication of PPD (Table 1).

The incidence of probable postpartum depression in our study population was 17% at 6 weeks postpartum. There were 14 women (13%) who were anemic prior to the Cesarean section. There were no cases of anemia identified at the 6-week follow-up visit. Patients who

scored > 10 on EPDS and > 2 on question 10 (self-harm) were referred to a psychiatrist. Not all patients accepted the referral. The 3 patients who accepted the referral had the diagnosis confirmed and were commenced on SSRIs.

Anemia indices and PPD

The incidence of postpartum depression was not different in anemic vs. non-anemic mothers (Table 2).

There was no statistical difference in hemoglobin, ferritin and soluble transferrin receptor levels between women who had a positive screen for PPD and those who did not have PPD according to EPDS scores.

To assess a possible effect of acute blood loss on PPD, we calculated the change in pre-operative hemoglobin values to those at 6 weeks' post-partum (ΔHb). There was no significant association between ΔHb and the presence of PPD (Table 2). There were also no significant differences in the thyroid stimulating hormone levels between the women with and without a positive screen for post-partum depression.

Functional capacity as assessed by the RAND score did not significantly differ between the two groups (Table 2) and, scores on the RAND showed no relation to the scores on the EPDS.

Anemia indices and postpartum functional capacity

There is no established cut off threshold values for RAND scores. Therefore, we compared the lowest RAND score quartile to the upper three quartiles. As indicated in Table 3, there was no correlation between either the hemoglobin or the iron store indices with measures of functional status.

Exact binary logistic regression analysis showed that neither anemia nor iron status independent predictor of postpartum depression or post-partum functional status (Table 2).

Discussion

We found that neither anemia nor iron stores measured postpartum are associated with postpartum depression or functional status postpartum.

The biological association between PPD and PPA could be attributed to iron deficiency rather than decreased hemoglobin levels. Iron is critical for adequate myelination, neurotransmitter metabolism and function, and neuronal cellular and oxidative processes and through these processes, may contribute to the development of clinical depression [23]. The association between anemia and poor functional status is well established in the non-pregnant population and has been attributed to poor muscle oxygenation and reduced exercise tolerance. To date, there have been no studies that evaluated this association in the pregnant population.

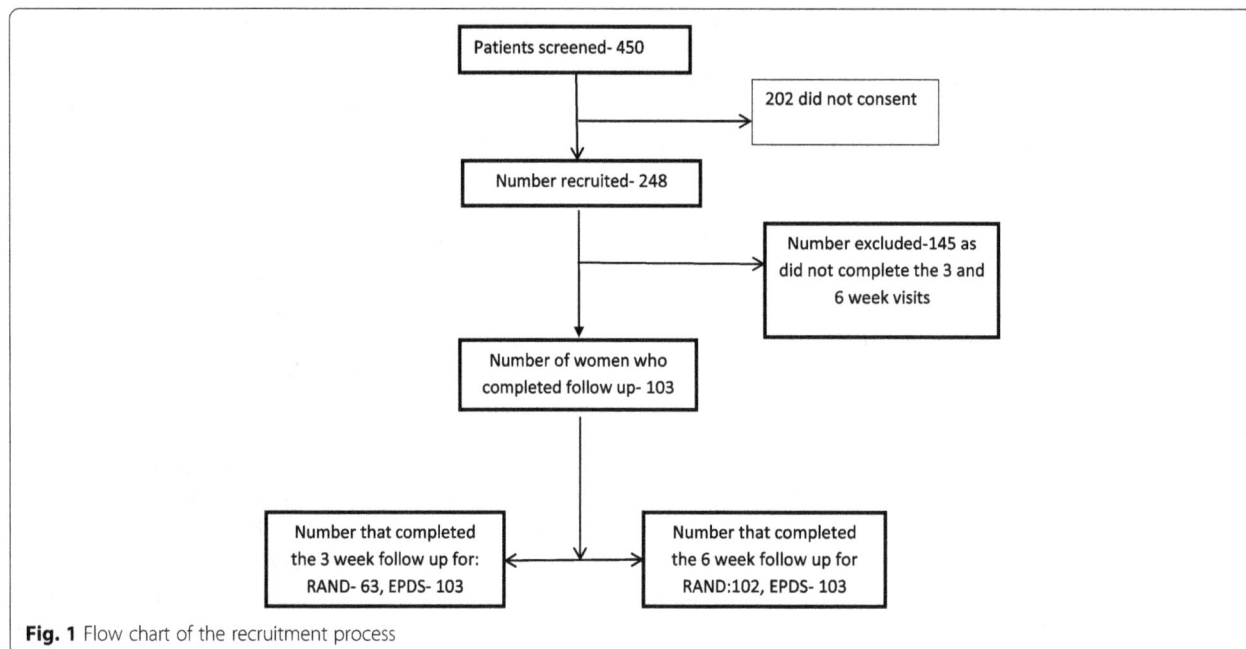

Fig. 1 Flow chart of the recruitment process

While iron deficiency and anemia have been related to poor cognition, depression and reduced functional capacity in the non-pregnant population, there have been conflicting results in studies examining pregnant populations. In one study [11], the authors used the Center for Epidemiological Studies-Depressive Symptomatology Scale (CES-D) to screen for symptoms of depression on day 28 postpartum and reported that hemoglobin concentration on day 7 to be negatively correlated with self-reported depressive symptoms on day 28, however this study had a relatively small sample size and did not measure iron status or thyroid function. In contrast, other research reported no correlation between low hemoglobin levels and high Edinburgh test for post-partum depression (EPDS) scale [12]. Possible cohort effects may impede extrapolation of study findings as those with low hemoglobin were also more likely to have had an abnormal delivery and a consequent propensity for

Table 1 Characteristics of the study population

Maternal characteristics	EPDS ≥10 at any visit (PPD = yes)	EPDS < 10 at any visit (PPD = no)	p-value**
N (%)	18(17.5%)	85 (82.5%)	
Age: mean (SD)	34.1 (4.1)	34.9 (4.3)	0.46
Nulliparous (%)	2/18 (11%)	31/85 (36%)	0.17
Number of previous livebirths or stillbirths: mean (SD)	0.7 (0.8)	0.9 (0.8)	0.36
Gestation weeks at delivery: mean (SD)	38.9 (0.6)	38.8 (0.9)	0.72
Less than 13 years of education, N (%)	3 (16.7)	4 (4.7)	0.11
Ethnicity (non-White) *N = 102	10 (55.6)	36 (42.9)	0.44
Pregnancy complications (GDM, PIH, IUGR and Preeclampsia)	6 (33.3)	23 (27.1)	0.58
Smoking during pregnancy *N = 102	0 (0.00)	1 (1.19)	1.00
alcohol use during pregnancy *N = 102	5 (27.8)	9 (10.7)	0.07
Illegal Drug use during pregnancy*N = 102	0 (0.00)	1 (1.19)	1.00
Birth weight: N, mean (SD)	3334 (401)	3370 (470)	0.76
BMI: N; mean (SD)	25.9 (6.9)	25.6 (5.5)	0.84
Prenatal Vitamins (%)	12 (66.7)	60 (70.6)	0.78
Breastfeeding (%)	15 (83.3)	76 (89.4)	0.44

*Indicates total N, excluding missing/unknown values for row characteristics (1 subject in the PPD = yes group)
**Fisher's test for proportions, 2-sided

Table 2 Associations between anemia indicators, functional status and postpartum depression

Maternal characteristics	N	EPDS >= 10 at any visit (PPD = yes N = 18)	EPDS < 10 at any visit (PPD = no N = 85)	Odds Ratio[a] (q1 vs. rest) or mean differences (95% CI)	Adjusted Odds Ratio[b] (q1 vs. rest) or mean differences (95% CI)
Anemia indicators					
HGB quartile 1 at pre-c/section), N (%)	103	3 (16.67)	27 (31.76)	0.43[a] (0.07 to 1.72)	0.44[b] (0.08 to 1.74)
HGB quartile 1 at visit 1 N (%)	101	3 (16.67)	24 (28.92)	0. 50[a] (0.08 to 1.98)	0.53[b] (0.09 to 2.12)
Mean HGB at pre-c/ section (SD)	103	124.0 (9.9)	119.2 (9.2)	4.8 (−0.4 to 10.0)	4.6 (−0.2 to 9.5)
Mean HGB at visit 1 (SD)	101	109.4 (9.6)	105.2 (9.7)	4.2 (−0.4 to 10.0)	3.8 (−1.3 to 8.8)
HGB quartile 1 at visit 3, N (%)	103	4 (22.22)	25 (29.41)	0.69[a] (0.15 to 2.49)	0.73[b] (0.15 to 2.82)
Mean HGB at visit 3 (SD)	103	133.4 (8.1)	129.0 (8.1)	4.4 (0.2 to 8.5)*	4.2 (0.1 to 8.2)*
Delta Hgb_visit 1 - Hgb_presection (note 1)	101	− 13.9 (9.0)	−14.0 (8.3)	−0.1 (− 6.7 to 6.5)	− 1.1 (− 6.9 to 4.7)
Delta Hgb_visit 3 - Hgb_presection (note 2)	103	8.1 (9.8)	10.0 (8.9)	1.9 (−3.6 to 7.4)	−1.0 (− 7.2 to 5.3)
Delta Hgb_visit 3-Hgb visit 1 (note 2)	101	22.7 (11.09)	24.1 (9.2)	1.4 (−4.4 to 7.2)	− 0.2 (− 6.8 to 6.3)
Ferritin quartile 1 at visit 1, N (%)	103	6 (33.33)	20 (23.53)	1.62[a] (0.44 to 5.42)	1.80[b] (0.46 to 6.60)
Mean ferritin at visit 1 (SD)	103	48.8 (27.7)	46.7 (25.4)	2.12 (−11.2 to 15.4)	0.9 (− 12.7 to 14.4)
Ferritin quartile 1 at visit 3, N (%)	103	3 (16.67)	23 (27.06)	0.54[a] (0.09 to 2.18)	0.52[b] (0.09 to 2.20)
Mean ferritin at visit 3 (SD)	103	54.9 (41.0)	42.7 (29.6)	12.3 (−4.1 to 28.7)	13.1 (−3.5 to 29.7)
Soluble transferrin receptor quartile 1 at visit 1, n (%)	103	3 (16.67)	24 (28.24)	0.51[a] (0.09 to 2.05)	0.46[b] (0.08 to 1.87)
Mean Soluble transferrin receptor at visit 1 (SD)	103	1.21 (0.33)	1.14 (0.43)	0.1 (−0.1 to 0.3)	0.1 (− 0.1 to 0.3)
Rand, quartile 1 at visit 3, n (%)	102	8 (44.44)	19 (22.35)	2.75[a] (0.82 to 9.04)	3.24[b] (0.92 to 11.70)
Exclusive Breastfeeding at visit 3, n (%)	103	10 (55.56)	59 (69.41)	0.55 (0.17 to 1.82)	0.39*
Rand mean score at visit 3 (SD)	102	83.7449 15.1247	89.1667 13.1908	−5.4 (−12.4 to 1.6)	−5.8 (−12.7 to 1.1)

*P-value < 0.05; [a]Unadjusted Odds ratio; [b]Odds ratio adjusted for age, parity, prenatal vitamins, breastfeeding at week 6

PPD regardless of degree of anemia. A randomized control trial demonstrated an improvement in emotional and cognitive measures at 9 months postpartum in iron treated anemic women but not in placebo controls [13]. A study examining risk factors for postpartum psychosis demonstrated anemia in 51.4% of cases with postpartum psychosis. However, there is no information about the incidence of anemia in a control group of women without postpartum psychosis. These results are most likely not applicable to the postpartum population in developed countries and cannot be extrapolated to patients with PPD.

Another study illustrates no relation between maternal iron stores and postpartum depression [24]. The incidence of postpartum depression in this population was significantly higher (> 20%) and again the authors did not control for hemoglobin. Some authors have suggested that anemia, but not iron deficiency is associated with a higher incidence of postnatal depression [25]. But this study was limited by a small sample size. Also, the incidence of PPD was significantly lower (5.5%) compared to what is quoted in the literature. A similar finding was reported in a recent study from Saudi Arabia by Alharbi et al. [26].They found that anemia but not iron deficiency is a significant risk factor for postpartum depression, but this study had a higher than normal incidence of PPD (33%) and the investigators did not control for confounders like traumatic delivery or history of preexisting depression.

In a recent nested cohort study, the authors demonstrate a positive association between anemia at

Table 3 Associations between anemia indicators and postpartum functional status

Maternal characteristics	N	RAND Quartile 1 at visit 3 (n = 27)	RAND Quartiles 2, 3 and 4 at visit 3 (N = 76)	Odds Ratio[a] (q1 vs. rest) or mean differences (95% CI)	Adjusted Odds Ratio[b] (q1 vs. rest) or mean differences (95% CI)
Anemia indicators					
HGB quartile 1 at pre-csection, N (%)	103	8 (29.63)	22 (28.95)	1.03[a] (0.34 to 2.94)	1.13[b] (0.37 to 3.28)
Mean HGB (pre-csection) (SD)	103	120.3 (11.16)	119.9 (8.84)	0.4 (−4.6 to 3.9)	0.1 (−4.2 to 4.4)
HGB quartile 1 at visit 1, N (%)	101	7 (25.93)	20 (27.03)	0.95[a] (0.29 to 2.80)	1.01[b] (0.30 to 3.12)
Mean HGB at visit 1 (SD)	101	105.9 (8.88)	105.9 (10.16)	0.01 (−4.4 to 4.4)	0.04 (−4.6 to 4.5)
HGB quartile 1 at visit 3, N (%)	103	10 (37.04)	19 (25.00)	1.75[a] (0.61 to 4.92)	2.44[b] (0.76 to 8.00)
Mean HGB at visit 3 (SD)	103	129.2 (9.20)	130.0 (7.89)	−0.8 (−2.9 to 4.5)	−1.8 (−5.4 to 1.7)
Delta Hgb_visit 1 - Hgb_presection (note 1)	101	−14.4 (7.9)	−13.9 (8.6)	−0.5 (−4.3 to 3.2)	− 0.3 (− 4.2 to 3.5)
Delta Hgb_visit 3 - Hgb_presection (note 2)	103	8.9 (11.2)	10.1 (8.1)	−1.2 (−5.2 to 2.8)	− 1.9 (−6.0 to 2.2)
Delta Hgb_visit 3-Hgb visit 1 (note 2)	101	23.3 (7.9)	24.2 (10.0)	−0.9 (−5.2 to 3.3)	−1.9 (− 6.2 to 2.4)
Ferritin quartile 1 at visit 1, N (%)	103	5 (18.52)	21 (27.63)	0.60[a] (0.16 to 1.91)	0.77[b] (0.19 to 2.70)
Mean ferritin at visit 1 (SD)	103	50.4 (26.1)	45.9 (25.7)	4.5 (−6.9 to 16.0)	5.0 (−6.9 to 16.8)
Ferritin quartile 1 at visit 3, N (%)	103	5 (18.52)	21 (27.63)	0.60[a] (0.16 to 1.91)	0.71[b] (0.18 to 2.39)
Mean ferritin at visit 3 (SD)	103	50.5 (35.2)	42.8 (30.8)	7.7 (−6.5 to 21.9)	5.5 (−9.2 to 20.2)
Soluble transferrin receptor quartile 1 at visit 1, n (%)	103	8 (29.63)	19 (25.00)	1.26[a] (0.41 to 3.65)	1.26[b] (0.41 to 3.65)
Mean Soluble transferrin receptor at visit 1 (SD)	103	1.1 (0.3)	1.2 (0.5)	−0.1 (−0.3 to 0.1)	−0.1 (−0.2 to 0.1)

[a]Unadjusted Odds ratio; [b]Odds ratio adjusted for age, parity, prenatal vitamins, breastfeeding at week 6

discharge from the maternity ward and the development of PPD symptoms, even after controlling for plausible confounders such as previous psychological contact, experience of delivery, mood during pregnancy and no exclusive breastfeeding at 6 weeks postpartum (OR = 2.29, 95%CI = 1.15–4.58) [27].

Anemia has been shown to be a possible risk factor for reduced functional status and is well studied in cardiac, elderly and cancer patients but there are no studies addressing this issue in pregnant patients.

The strengths of this study include the use of a prospective study design, limiting the cohort to women who had an elective Caesarean section which eliminated potential obstetric confounders that have known associations with postpartum depression. The exclusion of women with preexisting depression was a strength as this is a known risk factor and permitted the determination of de novo postpartum depression in a cohort of low risk women. We also controlled for the continuation of breast feeding as there is evidence that there is reduced risk of PPD in women who continue to breast feed [28]. In addition, we controlled for thyroid function - a well-known confounder for postpartum depression. The use of soluble transferrin receptor levels allowed us

to more accurately define true iron deficiency. This is first study to our knowledge that explored the effects of anemia and iron status on functional scores in Obstetric population.

Our limitations include a potential selection bias as only 103 out of the 248 women recruited completed the planned follow up. The incidence of anemia and iron deficiency in our population was lower than expected, thereby limiting the variability in the exposure and an ability to detect significant effects, if they exist. We attempted to overcome this by analyzing hemoglobin using the lowest quartile values. There is the possibility of an association between maternal anemia (or iron deficiency) and the risk of developing PPD, but this association will manifest only at certain threshold values. Given that all anemic women post Cesarean section were treated with iron supplements, there were no anemic patients at the 6 weeks visit when the second EPDS was administered. The results reported herein are applicable only to women undergoing elective Cesarean sections and it is possible that there would be different results in women having CS in labour or vaginal delivery which need to be explored further. Finally, there is also a possibility that the women who did not complete the 3 and 6 weeks follow up might have been affected by postpartum depression that the study did not capture.

Conclusion

We did not find any evidence of an association between postpartum anemia and postpartum depression, despite this association occurring in the non-pregnant population. Further research is needed to ascertain why iron status relates to these symptoms in some contexts but not in others.

Abbreviations
EPDS: Edinburgh Postnatal Depression Scale; PPA: Postpartum anemia; PPD: Postpartum depression

Acknowledgements
We thank all the women that agreed to participate in the study.

Funding
This study was funded by Canadian Foundation for Women's Health (The Garfied Weston award grant received by Dr. Berger).

Authors' contributions
NC was involved in data collection and writing the manuscript, LD was involved in recruitment and revising the manuscript critically, MU was involved in statistical support. Authors BY, AM, RW were involved in conceiving the idea and initiation of the proposal. Author HB was the principle investigator of the study that was involved in conception, design and approval of the final manuscript. All authors participated in the editing of manuscript and have given their final approval for publication.

Competing interests
HB is a member of the editorial board (section editor) of the journal.

Author details
[1]Department of Maternal and Fetal Medicine, St Michaels Hospital, 30 Bond street, Toronto, ON M5B 1W8, Canada. [2]Li Ka Shing Knowledge Institute, St Michael's Hospital, Toronto, Canada. [3]Perinatal Mental Health Program, Mount Sinai Hospital, Toronto, Canada. [4]Sunnybrook Health Sciences, Toronto, Canada. [5]Mt Sinai Hospital, Toronto, Canada.

References
1. Recommendations to prevent and control iron deficiency in the United States. Centers for Disease Control and Prevention. MMWR Recomm Rep. 1998;47(RR-3):1–29.
2. Bodnar LM, Siega-Riz AM, Miller WC, et al. Who should be screened for postpartum anemia? An evaluation of current recommendations. Am J Epidemiol. 2002;156(10):903–12.
3. Bodnar LM, Scanlon KS, Freedman DS, et al. High prevalence of postpartum anemia among low-income women in the United States. Am J Obstet Gynecol. 2001;185(2):438–43.
4. Breymann C. Iron deficiency and anaemia in pregnancy: modern aspects of diagnosis and therapy. Blood Cells Mol Dis. 2002;29(3):506–16.
5. O'Hara MW, Swain AM. Rates and risk of postpartum depression - a meta-analysis. International Review of Psychiatry. 1996;8(1):37–54.
6. Evagorou O, et al. Cross cultural approach of postpartum depression: manifestation, practices applied, risk factors and therapeutic interventions. Psychiatr Q. 2016;87:129–54.
7. Nielsen FD, Videbech P, Hedegaard M, et al. Postpartum depression: identification of women at risk. BJOG. 2000;107(10):1210–7.
8. Caplan HL, Cogill SR, Alexandra H, et al. Maternal depression and the emotional development of the child. Br J Psychiatry. 1989 Jun;154:818–22.
9. Cogill SR, Caplan HL, Alexandra H, et al. Impact of maternal postnatal depression on cognitive development of young children. Br Med J (Clin Res Ed). 1986;292(6529):1165–7.
10. The diagnostic and statistical manual of mental disorders, 4th ed.:DSM-IV. 4th ed. Washington, D.C.: American Psychiatric Association, 1994.
11. Corwin EJ, Murray-Kolb LE, Beard JL. Low hemoglobin level is a risk factor for postpartum depression. J Nutr. 2003;133(12):4139–42.
12. Paterson JA, Davis J, Gregory M, et al. A study on the effects of low haemoglobin on postnatal women. Midwifery. 1994;10(2):77–86.
13. Beard JL, Hendricks MK, Perez EM, et al. Maternal iron deficiency anemia affects postpartum emotions and cognition. J Nutr. 2005;135(2):267–72.
14. Hui X, Ding Y, Ma Y, Xin X, Zhang D. Cesarean section and risk of postpartum depression: a meta-analysis. J Psychosom Res. 2017;97:118–26 https://doi.org/10.1016/j.jpsychores.2017.04.016.
15. Candio F, Hofmeyr GJ. Treatments for iron deficiency anemia in pregnancy. RHL commentary. The WHO reproductive health library. Geneva: WHO; 2007.
16. Ware JE Jr, Gandek B. Overview of the SF-36 health survey and the international quality of life assessment (IQOLA) project. J Clin Epidemiol. 1998;51(11):903–12.
17. Stewart AL, Hays RD, Ware JE Jr. The MOS short-form general health survey. Reliability and validity in a patient population. Med Care. 1988;26(7):724–35.
18. Navarro, P., Ascaso, C., Garcia-Esteve, et al 2007. Postnatal psychiatric morbidity: a validation study of the GHQ-12 and the EPDS as screening tools. Gen. Hosp. Psychiatry 29, 1–7.
19. Boyd RC, Le HN, Somberg R. Review of screening instruments for postpartum depression. [review] [92 refs]. Archives of Women's. Mental Health. 2005;8(3):141–53.
20. Cox JL, Holden JM, Sagovsky R. Detection of postnatal depression. Development of the 10-item Edinburgh postnatal depression scale. Br J Psychiatry. 1987;150:782–6.
21. Harris B, Huckle P, Thomas R, et al. The use of rating scales to identify post-natal depression. Br J Psychiatry. 1989;154:813–7.
22. Murray L, Carothers AD. The validation of the Edinburgh post-natal depression scale on a community sample. Br J Psychiatry. 1990;157:288–90.
23. Beard JL, Connor JR. Iron status and neural functioning. Annu Rev Nutr. 2003;23:41–58.
24. Armony-Sivan R, Shao J, Li M, et al. No relationship between maternal Iron status and postpartum depression in two samples in China. J Pregnancy. 2012;2012:521431.
25. Goshtasebi A, Alizadeh M, Gandevani SB. Association between maternal anaemia and postpartum depression in an urban sample of pregnant women in Iran. J Health Popul Nutr. 2013;31(3):398–402.
26. Alharbi AA, Abdulghani H. Risk factors associated with postpartum depression in the Saudi population. Neuropsychiatr Dis Treat. 2014;10:311–31.
27. Eckerdal P, Kollia N, Löfblad J, et al. Delineating the association between heavy postpartum Haemorrhage and postpartum depression. PLoS One. 2016;11(1):e0144274. https://doi.org/10.1371/journal.pone.0144274.
28. Nam JY, et al. The synergistic effect of breastfeeding discontinuation and cesarean section delivery on postpartum depression: a nationwide population-based cohort study in Korea. J Affect Disord. 2017;218:53–8 https://doi.org/10.1016/j.jad.2017.04.048.

5

Preeclampsia by maternal reasons for immigration: a population-based study

Roy M Nilsen[1*], Eline S Vik[1], Svein A Rasmussen[2], Rhonda Small[3,4], Dag Moster[5,6], Erica Schytt[4,7] and Vigdis Aasheim[1]

Abstract

Background: To investigate whether the occurrence of preeclampsia varied by maternal reasons for immigration.

Methods: We included 1,287,270 singleton pregnancies (163,508 to immigrant women) in Norway during 1990–2013. Individual data were obtained through record linkage between the Medical Birth Registry of Norway and Statistics Norway. Analyses were performed for preeclampsia overall and in combination with preterm birth < 37 and < 34 weeks of gestation, referred to as preterm and very preterm preeclampsia. Odds ratios (ORs) with 95% confidence intervals (CIs) were estimated using logistic regression with robust standard errors, adjusted for relevant covariates, including maternal income and education.

Results: Preeclampsia was reported in 3.5% of Norwegian women and 2.5% of immigrants. Compared with Norwegian women, the adjusted OR for preeclampsia was lowest in labour immigrants (adjusted OR 0.55 [95% CI 0.49–0.62]), followed by family immigrants (0.62 [0.59–0.65]), immigrant students (0.75 [0.65–0.86]), refugees (0.81 [0.75–0.88]), and immigrants from other Nordic countries (0.87 [0.80–0.94]). Compared with Norwegian women, labour immigrants also had lower adjusted odds of preterm and very preterm preeclampsia, whereas refugees had increased adjusted odds of preterm and very preterm preeclampsia (< 37 weeks: 1.18 [1.02–1.36], and < 34 weeks: 1.41 [1.15–1.72]).

Conclusions: The occurrence of preeclampsia was lower overall in immigrants than in non-immigrants, but associations varied by maternal reasons for immigration. Maternity caregivers should pay increased attention to pregnant women with refugee backgrounds due to their excess odds of preterm preeclampsia.

Keywords: Education, Family, Immigration, Labour, Preeclampsia, Pregnancy, Refugee

Background

People with an immigrant background constitute an increasing proportion of populations in many European countries. In 2017, the Norwegian population comprised 13.8% (~ 725,000) immigrants from 221 countries, with the largest proportions being from Europe, Asia, and Africa [1]. Major reasons for immigrating to Norway include employment, education, family reunion or establishment, as well as seeking refuge due to war and political conflicts [1, 2]. These immigration reasons may not be deterministically linked to countries of origin. Individuals from the same country may have different reasons for leaving, and individuals who arrive from very different countries may share immigration reasons.

Immigrants vary in health and disease compared with individuals born in the receiving countries [3, 4]. In terms of immigration reasons, individuals with a refugee background are considered a particularly vulnerable group and refugee background has been associated with several adverse outcomes in both pregnant and non-pregnant individuals [5, 6]. In particular, refugee women giving birth in receiving countries have been found to have higher risks of preterm birth [7], infant mortality and morbidity [8], and postpartum depression [9]. While these findings suggest the need for closer health monitoring of pregnant refugee women in receiving countries, knowledge of health disparities associated with other reasons such as employment, education, family reunion or establishment is lacking.

* Correspondence: roy.miodini.nilsen@hvl.no
[1]Faculty of Health and Social Sciences, Western Norway University of Applied Sciences, Inndalsveien 28, 5063 Bergen, Norway
Full list of author information is available at the end of the article

Increased knowledge of disparities in preeclampsia among immigrant pregnant women is of particular interest as preeclampsia is a leading cause of maternal and perinatal morbidity and mortality in many countries [10, 11]. Previous studies of preeclampsia in immigrant women in Western countries have shown that the occurrence of preeclampsia varies considerably by maternal birthplace [12–15]. A few studies have also reported that the occurrence of preeclampsia among immigrants increases with increasing length of residence in host countries [15, 16]. However, none of these studies performed analyses according to refugee status or other maternal reasons for immigration.

The main objective of the present study was to investigate whether the occurrence of preeclampsia varied by maternal reasons for immigration to Norway. We also explored whether the occurrence of preeclampsia varied with the length of residence for each immigration reason. Additionally, country-specific occurrences of preeclampsia in women from a number of countries were examined.

Methods

Data sources

Data were obtained through individual record linkage between the Medical Birth Registry of Norway (MBRN) and Statistics Norway. In brief, MBRN is a national health registry in which registration of all births after gestational week 16 has been compulsory in Norway since 1967 [17]. The registry comprises data on the mother's health before and during pregnancy, on birth, and on the infant. Statistics Norway is the Norwegian institution for collection, processing, and dissemination of official statistics in Norway [18]. The collection of data relies on official registries and administrative data, including the National Registry, which contains data on individuals who either are, or have been resident in Norway [2].

Preeclampsia

Preeclampsia for a given pregnancy was recorded once in the MBRN by a check box or open text coded according to the *International Statistical Classification of Diseases and Related Health Problems*, 8th revision for the years 1967–98 and 10th revision since 1999. The diagnostic criteria were defined as maternal blood pressure 140/90 mmHg or higher after gestational week 20 on at least 2 occasions, combined with proteinuria (+ 1 point increase on urinary dipstick) [19]. As an indicator of severity of preeclampsia, preeclampsia was analyzed overall as well as in combination with time point of birth. If a woman was diagnosed with preeclampsia and gave birth before gestational week 34 and 37, we defined her preeclampsia as very preterm preeclampsia and preterm preeclampsia, respectively. A validation study covering the years

1999–2010 showed that preeclampsia in MBRN corresponds well with medical records, although the sensitivity of the diagnosis may be somewhat low [20].

Reasons for immigration

The collection of data regarding reasons for immigration to Norway has been described in detail elsewhere [2]. In brief, the information is obtained from the Norwegian Directorate of Immigration, which is the Norwegian authority for processing applications from foreign nationals who wish to visit or live in Norway. The immigration reason is recorded in connection with the first positive decision on the individual's application for permission to stay in Norway which may or may not concur with the immigrant's original motivation for immigration. Nordic citizens can move freely to Norway and therefore have no data regarding immigration reasons.

We used the variable derived by Statistics Norway, in which immigrants were allocated to one of five main categories of immigration reason: *refuge, family (reunion or establishment), labour, education, and unspecified reasons* [2]. For comparison, we also included immigrants from other Nordic countries (i.e., Sweden, Denmark, Finland, and Iceland) as a separate exposure group. Norwegian women constituted the reference group, and the group of women with unspecified reasons was excluded due to low numbers. Notably, data on immigration reasons were only available from 1990 onwards. Therefore, women who had received permission to stay in Norway before this time, but gave birth from 1990 onwards, were excluded from the study (see details below).

Other variables

From the MBRN, we obtained data on year of birth, maternal age at birth, parity (0, 1, 2, 3, ≥4 previous births), marital status at birth (married/partner, single/widowed/other), chronic hypertension (yes, no) and pre-pregnancy diabetes (yes, no). Prenatal smoking and pre-pregnancy body mass index (kg/m^2) were available from 1999 and 2008 onwards, respectively. From Statistics Norway, we obtained maternal data on country of birth (smaller countries with < 15 preeclampsia cases throughout the study period were grouped), maternal parents' background (Norwegian born, foreign born), income (quartiles calculated for the whole study period) and educational level (no education, primary school, secondary school, university/college). The mother's length of residence in years was calculated as year of childbirth in the MBRN minus the year of official permission to stay in Norway.

Study sample

The study was restricted to include only ethnic Norwegian women (Norwegian-born with two Norwegian-born parents), other Nordic women, and first-generation immigrant women (foreign-born with two foreign-born parents) with a registered reason for immigration. Initially, there was a total 1,439,913 births during the period 1990–2013. We excluded 48,102 births due to multiple pregnancies and 389 pregnancies for which information on country of birth for the woman was missing. We additionally excluded 13,478 pregnancies of women who were born outside Norway but had two Norwegian born parents (including adoptees), 53,532 pregnancies of women who had one Norwegian and one foreign born parent (mixed-ethnic), and 6432 pregnancies of women who were born in Norway but had immigrant parents (second-generation immigrants). We further excluded 30,710 pregnancies for which information on immigration reasons was unavailable (permission to stay before 1990; $n = 28,088$), unspecified ($n = 1886$), or missing ($n = 736$), leaving 1,287,270 singleton pregnancies for analyses.

Statistical analyses

To examine how the occurrence of preeclampsia varied by immigration reason we used binary logistic regression models. Immigration reason was incorporated in the models as a categorical variable with Norwegian women as the reference group. We calculated both crude and adjusted odds ratios (ORs) with 95% confidence intervals (CIs). Adjustment variables were year of birth, maternal age at birth, parity, marital status at birth, chronic hypertension, pre-pregnancy diabetes, maternal income and education. Year of birth and maternal age at birth were included in the regression models as polynomial quadratic terms. To account for dependency among births by the same mother, we used robust standard errors that allowed for within-mother clustering.

We also estimated the incidence of preeclampsia in relation to length of residence for each immigration group. The length of residence was modeled as a continuous exposure using generalized additive logistic regression models, allowing for nonlinear relationships. The predicted incidences are presented in graphical format for primiparous and multiparous women, with adjustment for the same variable as previously. To test if preeclampsia incidence trajectories differed across immigration groups, we performed a likelihood ratio test by comparing the log-likelihood for a model with and without the interaction between length of residence and immigration reasons. Due to limited data within subgroups, estimations were performed only for preeclampsia overall and not for preterm and very preterm preeclampsia.

All statistical analyses were performed by using R 3.4.1 software for Windows [21]. Missing data on maternal income and education (shown in footnotes of Table 1) were assumed to be missing at random and were replaced by using a multiple imputation technique [22].

Five imputed datasets were created using the predictive mean matching algorithm. The imputation model included the same adjustment variables as before, as well as data on immigration reason, maternal country of birth and preeclampsia.

Results

The number of immigrants and non-immigrants giving birth in the current sample was 163,508 (13%) and 1,123,762 (87%), respectively. The number of registered maternal birth countries was 186.

Among immigrant births, 18% ($n = 29,422$) were to women coming as refugees, 55% ($n = 89,523$) to family immigrants, 8% ($n = 13,618$) to labour immigrants, 5% ($n = 8351$) to immigrant students, and 14% ($n = 22,594$) were to Nordic immigrant women. There was a steady increase in the number of immigrants in all groups from 1990 to 2013, although labour immigrants increased more rapidly during the most recent period than did other groups (Table 1). The countries dominating each immigration reason are shown in Additional file 1.

Immigrants differed on several sample characteristics (Table 1). Refugees were younger when giving birth, had a higher parity, and were more often single than others. They also had lower income and lower education than that of others. In contrast, women coming for employment or education had lower parity, lower mean body mass index and higher education and income than others. Refugees and family immigrants had less chronic hypertension than Norwegians. Norwegian and Nordic immigrant women had the highest smoking prevalence (18% and 12%, respectively).

There was considerable variation in the mean length of residence from arrival to childbirth across immigration groups (Table 1). Nordic immigrant women and those coming for education had nearly twice the residence length (mean 7.0 and 6.1 years, respectively) compared to labour and family immigrants (mean 3.2 and 4.1 years, respectively).

Overall, preeclampsia was reported in 3.5% ($n = 39,251$) of non-immigrants and in 2.5% ($n = 4133$) of immigrants. The corresponding incidences in nulliparous women were 5.2% ($n = 24,043$) and 3.5% ($n = 2461$), respectively. The lower incidence of preeclampsia in immigrant women remained constant throughout the study period (Fig. 1). However, there was considerable variation across women's countries of birth with immigrants from several countries having adjusted odds of preeclampsia higher than that seen in Norwegian women (Additional file 2).

Table 2 shows the incidence and the corresponding OR for preeclampsia in relation to immigration reasons. All immigration reasons were associated with lower preeclampsia incidence. Relative to Norwegian women, the adjusted OR for preeclampsia was lowest in labour

Table 1 Sample characteristics by reasons for immigration to Norway, 1990–2013

Characteristics	Norwegian women (non-immigrants)	Nordic immigrant women	Reasons for immigration			
			Refuge	Family	Labour	Education
No. of women	1,123,762	22,594	29,422	89,523	13,618	8351
Period of birth (%)						
1990–1993	18.6	12.5	5.2	3.4	0.4	1.0
1994–1998	22.4	18.1	11.4	11.1	2.2	6.0
1999–2003	20.4	21.9	19.5	20.2	6.6	12.7
2004–2008	19.7	21.9	27.7	28.8	18.0	26.6
2009–2013	18.9	25.6	36.2	36.4	72.8	53.6
Maternal age at birth, years (mean ± SD)	29.0 ± 5.1	30.6 ± 4.8	28.6 ± 5.6	29.1 ± 5.4	30.2 ± 4.7	30.1 ± 4.0
Parity (%)						
Primiparous	41.2	45.6	31.5	41.7	60.8	58.7
Multiparous	58.8	54.4	68.5	58.3	39.2	41.3
Single/widowed/other (%)	8.2	5.0	19.3	5.3	4.0	5.5
Maternal income, NOK per 1000 (quartiles)[a]						
< 125.0	24.7	16.3	37.3	35.3	13.0	24.3
125.0–195.5	25.6	20.7	18.7	20.2	12.5	12.0
195.6–287.4	25.0	28.1	23.0	24.0	28.1	22.0
≥ 287.5	24.7	34.8	21.0	20.5	46.3	41.6
Maternal educational level (%)[b]						
No education	0.0	0.4	7.6	2.8	0.3	0.2
Primary school	21.6	10.6	50.5	36.0	7.6	12.5
Secondary school	38.5	31.2	25.5	26.8	21.9	16.5
University/college	39.9	57.8	16.5	34.3	70.2	70.8
Smoking early in pregnancy (%)[c]	18.3	11.6	7.5	5.7	8.5	2.8
Pre-pregnancy BMI, kg/m^2 (mean ± SD)[d]	24.6 ± 4.9	24.0 ± 4.5	24.7 ± 4.8	23.5 ± 4.4	23.0 ± 4.0	22.8 ± 3.9
Chronic hypertension (%)	0.5	0.6	0.4	0.3	0.6	0.5
Pre-pregnancy diabetes (%)	0.4	0.4	0.6	0.6	0.4	0.4
Length of residence, years (mean ± SD)[e]		7.0 ± 6.1	5.5 ± 5.2	4.1 ± 4.0	3.2 ± 2.7	6.1 ± 3.8
Maternal age at arriving, years (mean ± SD)[e]		23.6 ± 6.6	23.1 ± 6.9	25.0 ± 5.8	27.0 ± 4.3	24.0 ± 3.6

SD standard deviation, *NOK* Norwegian kroner, *BMI* body mass index

[a]Information on income was missing for 94,234 (8.4%) among non-immigrants and 70,977 (43.4%) among immigrants

[b]Information on education was missing for 2229 (0.2%) among non-immigrants and 45,779 (28.0%) among immigrants

[c]Information on smoking (1999–2013) was missing for 96,763 (14.6%) among non-immigrants and 31,306 (22.7%) among immigrants

[d]Information on body mass index (2008–2013) was missing for 137,574 (53.5%) among non-immigrants and 39,014 (53.1%) among immigrants

[e]Excluded were 1303 (0.8%) immigrant women who were registered with births before receiving permission to stay in Norway

immigrants (adjusted OR 0.55 [95% CI 0.49–0.62]), followed by family immigrants (0.62 [0.59–0.65]), immigrant students (0.75 [0.65–0.86]), refugees (0.81 [0.75–0.88]), and Nordic immigrant women (0.87 [0.80–0.94]).

Additional adjustment for maternal prenatal smoking (1999–2013; $n = 673,286$) had essentially no impact on the estimates, compared with the adjusted OR (excluding smoking) in the same period (data not shown).

Women coming for employment also had lower adjusted odds if preeclampsia occurred preterm or very preterm (Table 2). In contrast, refugees had excess adjusted odds of preterm and very preterm preeclampsia

(< 37 weeks: 1.18 [1.02–1.36] and < 34 weeks: 1.41 [1.15–1.72]). For other groups, adjusted ORs for preterm or very preterm preeclampsia were either attenuated (family and education) or remained essentially unchanged (Nordic immigrant women).

Among immigrant women for which information on immigration reasons was unavailable, unspecified or missing, the incidence of preeclampsia was 2.7% (833/30,710).

Figure 2 shows the estimated adjusted incidence of preeclampsia according to length of residence for each immigration group. The adjusted incidence of preeclampsia

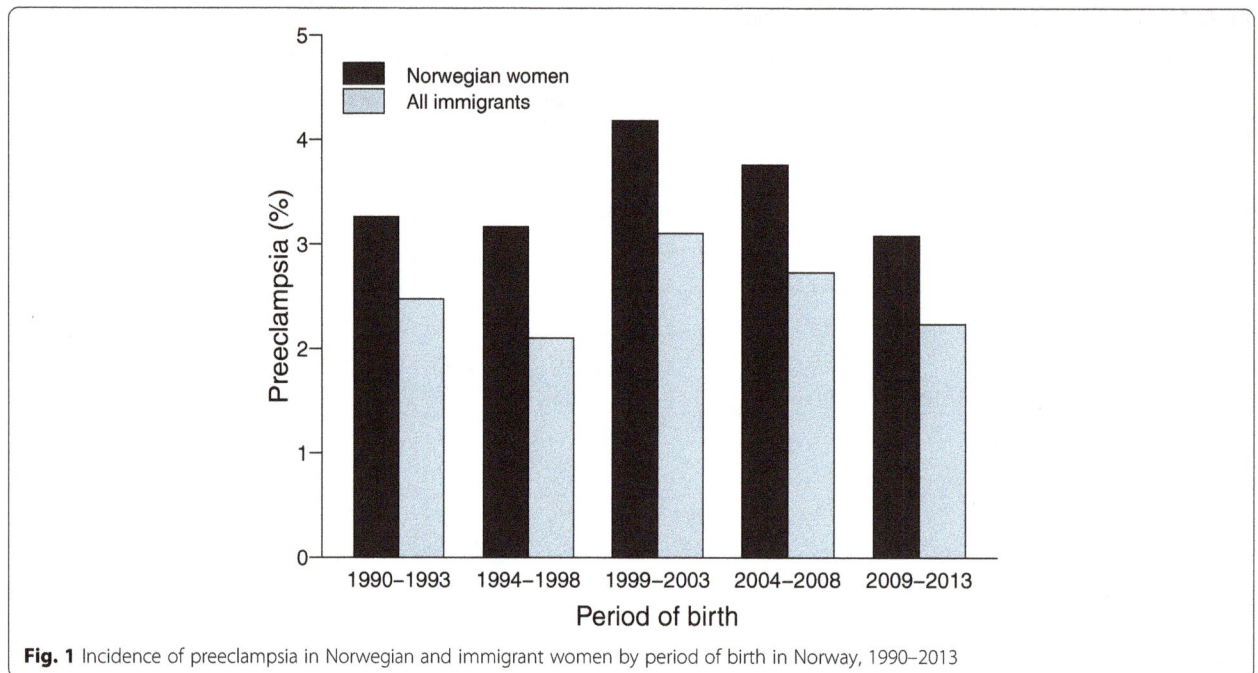

Fig. 1 Incidence of preeclampsia in Norwegian and immigrant women by period of birth in Norway, 1990–2013

Table 2 Odds ratio for preeclampsia by reasons for immigration to Norway, 1990–2013

Reasons for immigration	No. of women	With outcome, No. (%)	Crude OR [95% CI]	Adjusted OR [95% CI][a]	Adjusted OR [95% CI][b]
Preeclampsia (all cases)					
Norwegian women (non-immigrants)[c]	1,123,762	39,251 (3.5)	1	1	1
Nordic immigrant women	22,594	723 (3.2)	0.91 [0.84–0.99]	0.86 [0.79–0.93]	0.87 [0.80–0.94]
Refuge	29,422	800 (2.7)	0.77 [0.71–0.84]	0.87 [0.81–0.95]	0.81 [0.75–0.88]
Family	89,523	2074 (2.3)	0.66 [0.62–0.69]	0.65 [0.62–0.69]	0.62 [0.59–0.65]
Labour	13,618	293 (2.2)	0.61 [0.54–0.68]	0.56 [0.49–0.63]	0.55 [0.49–0.62]
Education	8351	243 (2.9)	0.83 [0.72–0.95]	0.75 [0.66–0.86]	0.75 [0.65–0.86]
Preterm preeclampsia (< 37 weeks)[d]					
Norwegian women (non-immigrants)[c]	1,077,269	8431 (0.8)	1	1	1
Nordic immigrant women	21,948	157 (0.7)	0.91 [0.77–1.08]	0.84 [0.71–1.00]	0.86 [0.72–1.01]
Refuge	28,304	257 (0.9)	1.16 [1.01–1.34]	1.28 [1.11–1.47]	1.18 [1.02–1.36]
Family	87,571	647 (0.7)	0.94 [0.87–1.03]	0.93 [0.85–1.02]	0.88 [0.80–0.96]
Labour	13,513	68 (0.5)	0.64 [0.50–0.81]	0.58 [0.45–0.73]	0.58 [0.45–0.74]
Education	8254	64 (0.8)	0.99 [0.76–1.29]	0.89 [0.68–1.16]	0.89 [0.69–1.16]
Very preterm preeclampsia (< 34 weeks)[d]					
Norwegian women (non-immigrants)[c]	1,077,269	3480 (0.3)	1	1	1
Nordic immigrant women	21,948	57 (0.3)	0.80 [0.61–1.06]	0.73 [0.56–0.97]	0.75 [0.57–0.98]
Refuge	28,304	132 (0.5)	1.45 [1.19–1.75]	1.56 [1.28–1.89]	1.41 [1.15–1.72]
Family	87,571	280 (0.3)	0.99 [0.87–1.13]	0.98 [0.86–1.12]	0.91 [0.80–1.05]
Labour	13,513	32 (0.2)	0.73 [0.52–1.04]	0.64 [0.45–0.92]	0.65 [0.46–0.93]
Education	8254	30 (0.4)	1.13 [0.78–1.63]	0.99 [0.68–1.44]	1.00 [0.69–1.46]

OR odds ratio, *CI* confidence interval

[a]Adjusted for year of birth, maternal age at birth, parity, marital status at birth, chronic hypertension, and pre-pregnancy diabetes

[b]Additional adjustments for maternal income and education

[c]Reference category

[d]Excluded were 50,411 pregnancies (1736 with and 48,675 without preeclampsia) due to missing data on gestational age

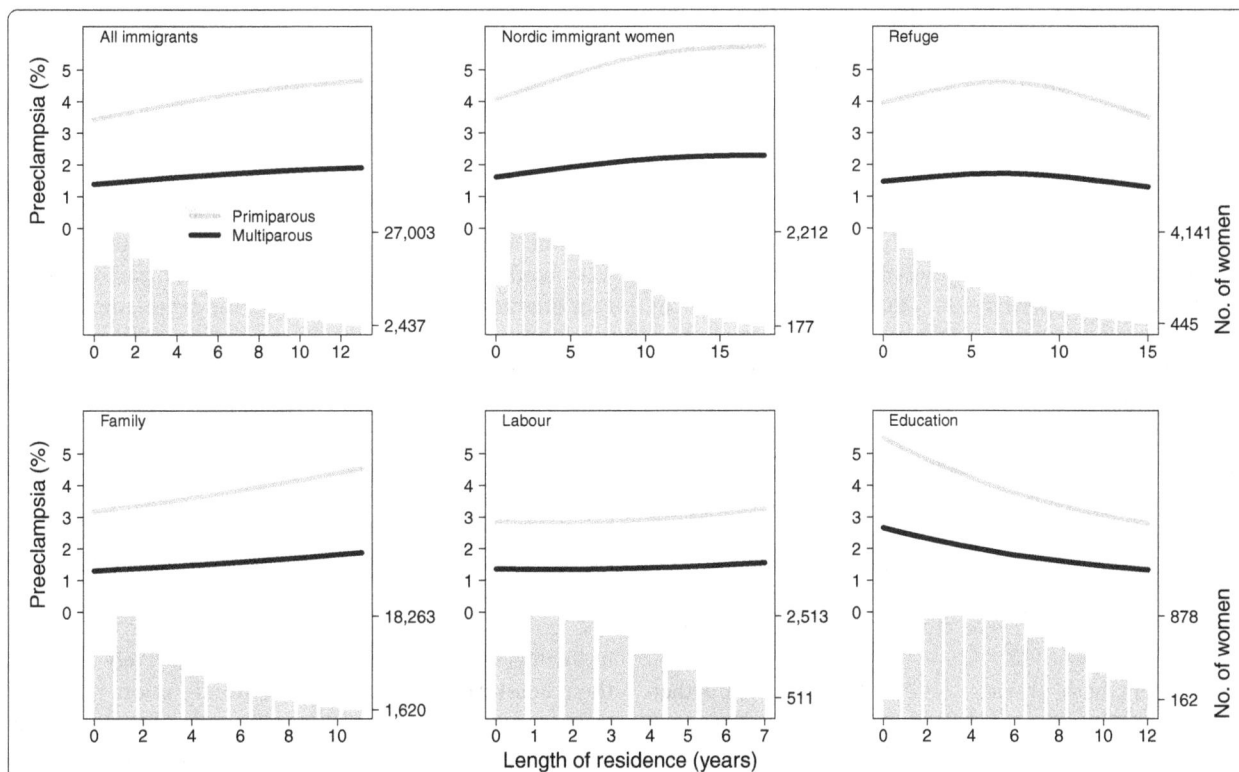

Fig. 2 Estimated adjusted incidence of preeclampsia by length of residence for various immigration reasons in Norway, 1990–2013. The incidences were estimated for primiparous and multiparous immigrant women by using generalized additive logistic regression models, adjusted for year of birth, maternal age at birth, parity, marital status at birth, chronic hypertension, pre-pregnancy diabetes, maternal income and education. The incidence trajectories for each immigration group are shown for secondary school and third income quartile and at the means of the other covariates (see Table 1). Due to small numbers, lengths of residence above the 95th percentile of the distributions were excluded. The distribution of length of residence is shown on the x-axis as frequency bars (highest and lowest frequencies are shown on right vertical axis)

for Nordic immigrant women and family immigrants appeared to increase with increasing length of residence. For labour immigrants and refugees, the adjusted incidence of preeclampsia remained essentially constant over time, while there was a decline in the adjusted incidence for students. The P for interaction across immigration groups was estimated to be < 0.001.

Discussion

We found that the occurrence of preeclampsia was generally lower in immigrants than in non-immigrants, but that the disparity varied by reasons for immigration and severity of preeclampsia. Particularly, labour immigrants had a substantially lower OR for preeclampsia overall as well as for preterm and very preterm preeclampsia. In contrast, refugees had an excess OR for preterm and very preterm preeclampsia. Furthermore, there was an increase in the adjusted incidence of preeclampsia with the length of residence for Nordic immigrant women and family immigrants, but not for the other immigrant groups.

As far as we are aware, this represents the first study investigating how the occurrence of preeclampsia varies

by maternal reasons for immigration. Strengths of our study include the large sample size, the standardized collection of data on both preeclampsia and migrant-related variables and the comprehensive adjustment for covariates in regression analyses.

The results of our study are not generalizable to all women giving birth in Norway. Particularly, we excluded second-generation immigrants, mixed-ethnic mothers, and adoptees, as these were neither ethnic Norwegian women nor non-Nordic immigrants with an immigration reason. Additionally, as the composition of immigrant groups in Norway may differ from that in other countries, our results may not be completely generalizable to other countries. Additional file 2 shows the largest groups dominating each immigration reason in our study (i.e., countries covering at least 50% of each group).

Pre-pregnancy body mass index is associated with both preeclampsia and immigrant background, but was not adjusted for in the analyses due to the variable's limited registration history in the MBRN (registered from 2008). Adjusting for body mass index would probably have attenuated the difference between Norwegian women and labour immigrants and immigrant students, because these immigrant groups were leaner than others. However, the adjustment of several demographic and socioeconomic variables might have compensated for some of this variation as demographic and socioeconomic variables are related to both obesity and preeclampsia.

The estimated incidences of preeclampsia for specific maternal countries of birth in our study were somewhat lower than those estimated in a previous Norwegian study including women from eight birth countries for the period 1986–2005 [15]. Variation in preeclampsia incidences between studies may reflect different study periods, different inclusion criteria (e.g., multiple births vs singletons), or variation in sample characteristics and immigrant groups over the study periods. Nonetheless, we found that Vietnamese and Chinese women had the lowest incidence of preeclampsia while women from Bangladesh and several countries from sub-Saharan Africa had among the highest (see Fig. 2). This partly agrees with the Norwegian study and a recent study from Canada on preterm preeclampsia [12, 15].

Consistent with previous studies [23], we found that immigrants had an overall lower incidence of preeclampsia than non-immigrants. In our sample, results were particularly strong for labour immigrants, but family immigrants, immigrant students, refugees, and immigrants from other Nordic countries also exhibited lower overall incidence of preeclampsia compared with Norwegian women. Our results regarding a lower overall incidence of preeclampsia in refugees agree with two recent studies comparing refugee pregnant women with Turkish and Canadian-born pregnant women [24, 25]. A comparison of results with studies concerning other immigration reasons was difficult due to the scarce literature.

The phenomenon that immigrants exhibit lower disease rates than the host population has been reported for numerous health outcomes. It is usually explained in terms of "the healthy immigrant effect", i.e., people who immigrate are a selected group and on average healthier than the population they move to [26]. Indeed, immigrants tended to be healthy in our study; in addition to having lower incidence of preeclampsia, we found that several immigrant groups were less often smokers, had a lower mean body mass index, and had less chronic hypertension than Norwegian mothers (see Table 1).

We did not find consistent lower incidences for preterm and very preterm preeclampsia among immigrants. Rather, in comparison with Norwegian women, a higher incidence for preterm and very preterm preeclampsia was found for refugees, and no increased or reduced incidence was observed for immigrant students. Our finding that refugee women were more vulnerable to preterm preeclampsia appears to be supported by previous literature. Particularly, refugees suffer more frequently than others from mental health problems, such as posttraumatic stress disorders, depression and schizophrenia [27, 28]. These disorders have been associated with increased risk of both preeclampsia and preterm birth in pregnant women [29–33].

We found an overall increase in the adjusted incidence of preeclampsia with the length of residence (see Fig. 2). This confirms previous findings and may partly be due to a gradual change in risk factors for preeclampsia after immigration [15, 16]. For instance, dietary changes over time may contribute to increased risk of obesity, diabetes, and cardiovascular disease [34]. Notably, in the present analysis, we did not find positive associations between length of residence and preeclampsia among refugees, students and labour immigrants. This may suggest that positive and negative determinants of preeclampsia in these groups were unchanged or cancelled each other out over the study period.

It could be argued that the information about an individual's reason for immigration merely reflects their country of birth, and that immigration reason is therefore superfluous. Although this may be partly true for refugees coming from conflict-laden countries, such an assumption would be problematic for the other immigration reasons, such as labour, family or education, which are less country-specific. Additionally, using country as an indicator for immigration reasons could lead to biased conclusions, as immigration reasons from any one country can, and do, vary between individuals, or, in some instances, change over time depending on a country's economic and political situation. In light of this, we believe that immigration reasons attributed individually to immigrant woman are likely to be a valuable indicator for investigating perinatal health among immigrants.

Conclusions

In this large population-based study, we used immigration reason as a health indicator for identifying immigrant women with high and low occurrence of preeclampsia in Norway. Our study suggests that maternity caregivers should pay increased attention to pregnant women of refugee background due to their higher odds of preterm preeclampsia. Among Nordic immigrant women and family immigrants, the aim should be to support the maintenance of healthy behaviors in these women to keep the occurrence low after immigration. Labour immigrants and immigrant students appear to be the least vulnerable groups, as the occurrence of preeclampsia in these groups was unchanged or decreased over time. However, from a public health perspective continued monitoring of all groups is necessary to detect potential variation in preeclampsia over time.

Abbreviations
CI: Confidence interval; MBRN: Medical Birth Registry of Norway; OR: Odds ratio

Authors' contributions
ES and VA have made substantial contributions to conception, design and planning of the study; RMN, ES and VA made substantial contributions to drafting the first version of the manuscript and revising the manuscript critically for important intellectual content; RMN and ESV have made substantial contributions to data management, statistical analysis and interpretation of data; SAR, RS, and DM made their contribution in drafting and revising the manuscript. All authors read and approved the final manuscript.

Competing interests
The authors declare that they have no competing interests.

Author details
[1]Faculty of Health and Social Sciences, Western Norway University of Applied Sciences, Inndalsveien 28, 5063 Bergen, Norway. [2]Department of Clinical Science, University of Bergen, Bergen, Norway. [3]Judith Lumley Centre, School of Nursing & Midwifery, La Trobe University, Melbourne, Australia. [4]Reproductive Health, Department of Women's and Children's Health, Karolinska Institute, Stockholm, Sweden. [5]Department of Paediatrics, Haukeland University Hospital, Bergen, Norway. [6]Department of Global Public Health and Primary Care, University of Bergen, Bergen, Norway. [7]Centre for Clinical Research Dalarna, Uppsala University, Falun, Sweden.

References
1. Sandnes T. Statistical analyses. Immigrants to Norway 2017. Oslo-Kongsvinger: Statistics Norway; 2017.
2. Dzamarija MT. Statistics on reasons for immigration 1990-2011, what do we know and how can we best use this information? Oslo-Kongsvinger: Statistics Norway; 2013.
3. Malmusi D. Immigrants' health and health inequality by type of integration policies in European countries. Eur J Pub Health. 2015;25(2):293–9.
4. Gagnon AJ, Zimbeck M, Zeitlin J, Collaboration R, Alexander S, Blondel B, Buitendijk S, Desmeules M, Di Lallo D, Gagnon A, et al. Migration to western industrialised countries and perinatal health: a systematic review. Soc Sci Med. 2009;69(6):934–46.
5. Malebranche M, Nerenberg K, Metcalfe A, Fabreau GE. Addressing vulnerability of pregnant refugees. Bull World Health Organ. 2017;95(9):611–A.
6. Gerritsen AA, Bramsen I, Deville W, van Willigen LH, Hovens JE, van der Ploeg HM. Physical and mental health of afghan, Iranian and Somali asylum seekers and refugees living in the Netherlands. Soc Psychiatry Psychiatr Epidemiol. 2006;41(1):18–26.
7. Liu C, Urquia M, Cnattingius S, Hjern A. Migration and preterm birth in war refugees: a Swedish cohort study. Eur J Epidemiol. 2014;29(2):141–3.
8. Carolan M. Pregnancy health status of sub-Saharan refugee women who have resettled in developed countries: a review of the literature. Midwifery. 2010;26(4):407–14.
9. Stewart DE, Gagnon A, Saucier JF, Wahoush O, Dougherty G. Postpartum depression symptoms in newcomers. Can J Psychiatr. 2008;53(2):121–4.
10. Duley L. The global impact of pre-eclampsia and eclampsia. Semin Perinatol. 2009;33(3):130–7.
11. Sibai B, Dekker G, Kupferminc M. Pre-eclampsia. Lancet. 2005;365(9461):785–99.
12. Ray JG, Wanigaratne S, Park AL, Bartsch E, Dzakpasu S, Urquia ML. Preterm preeclampsia in relation to country of birth. J Perinatol. 2016;36(9):718–22.
13. Urquia ML, Glazier RH, Gagnon AJ, Mortensen LH, Nybo Andersen AM, Janevic T, Guendelman S, Thornton D, Bolumar F, Rio Sanchez I, et al. Disparities in pre-eclampsia and eclampsia among immigrant women giving birth in six industrialised countries. BJOG. 2014;121(12):1492–500.
14. Urquia ML, Ying I, Glazier RH, Berger H, De Souza LR, Ray JG. Serious preeclampsia among different immigrant groups. J Obstet Gynaecol Can. 2012;34(4):348–52.
15. Naimy Z, Grytten J, Monkerud L, Eskild A. The prevalence of pre-eclampsia in migrant relative to native Norwegian women: a population-based study. BJOG. 2015;122(6):859–65.
16. Ray JG, Vermeulen MJ, Schull MJ, Singh G, Shah R, Redelmeier DA. Results of the recent immigrant pregnancy and perinatal long-term evaluation study (RIPPLES). CMAJ. 2007;176(10):1419–26.
17. Irgens LM. The medical birth registry of Norway. Epidemiological research and surveillance throughout 30 years. Acta Obstet Gynecol Scand. 2000;79(6):435–9.
18. Statistics Norway: About Statistics Norway. http://www.ssb.no/en (2018). Accessed 19 Jan 2018.
19. Haugen M, Brantsaeter AL, Trogstad L, Alexander J, Roth C, Magnus P, Meltzer HM. Vitamin D supplementation and reduced risk of preeclampsia in nulliparous women. Epidemiology. 2009;20(5):720–6.
20. Klungsoyr K, Harmon QE, Skard LB, Simonsen I, Austvoll ET, Alsaker ER, Starling A, Trogstad L, Magnus P, Engel SM. Validity of pre-eclampsia registration in the medical birth registry of Norway for women participating in the norwegian mother and child cohort study, 1999-2010. Paediatr Perinat Epidemiol. 2014;28(5):362–71.
21. R Core Team: R: A language and environment for statistical computing. R Foundation for Statistical Computing, Vienna, Austria. http://www.R-project.org (2017). Accessed 19 Jan 2018.
22. Harrell Jr FE: rms: Regression Modeling Strategies. R package version 5.1-1. http://CRAN.R-project.org/package=rms (2017). Accessed 16 August 2017.
23. Mogos MF, Salinas-Miranda AA, Salemi JL, Medina IM, Salihu HM. Pregnancy-related hypertensive disorders and immigrant status: a systematic review and meta-analysis of epidemiological studies. J Immigr Minor Health. 2017;19(6):1488–97.
24. Demirci H, Yildirim Topak N, Ocakoglu G, Karakulak Gomleksiz M, Ustunyurt E, Ulku Turker A. Birth characteristics of Syrian refugees and Turkish citizens in Turkey in 2015. Int J Gynaecol Obstet. 2017;137(1):63–6.
25. Khan S, Yao Z, Shah BR. Gestational diabetes care and outcomes for refugee women: a population-based cohort study. Diabet Med. 2017;34(11):1608–14.
26. Kennedy S, Kidd MP, McDonald JT, Biddle N. The healthy immigrant effect: patterns and evidence from four countries. J Int Migr Integr. 2015;16(2):317–32.
27. Hollander AC, Dal H, Lewis G, Magnusson C, Kirkbride JB, Dalman C. Refugee migration and risk of schizophrenia and other non-affective psychoses: cohort study of 1.3 million people in Sweden. BMJ. 2016;352:i1030.
28. Fazel M, Wheeler J, Danesh J. Prevalence of serious mental disorder in 7000 refugees resettled in western countries: a systematic review. Lancet. 2005;365(9467):1309–14.

29. Vigod SN, Kurdyak PA, Dennis CL, Gruneir A, Newman A, Seeman MV, Rochon PA, Anderson GM, Grigoriadis S, Ray JG. Maternal and newborn outcomes among women with schizophrenia: a retrospective population-based cohort study. BJOG. 2014;121(5):566–74.

30. Palmsten K, Setoguchi S, Margulis AV, Patrick AR, Hernandez-Diaz S. Elevated risk of preeclampsia in pregnant women with depression: depression or antidepressants? Am J Epidemiol. 2012;175(10):988–97.

31. Liu C, Cnattingius S, Bergstrom M, Ostberg V, Hjern A. Prenatal parental depression and preterm birth: a national cohort study. BJOG. 2016;123(12):1973–82.

32. Shaw JG, Asch SM, Katon JG, Shaw KA, Kimerling R, Frayne SM, Phibbs CS. Post-traumatic stress disorder and antepartum complications: a novel risk factor for gestational diabetes and preeclampsia. Paediatr Perinat Epidemiol. 2017;31(3):185–94.

33. Shaw JG, Asch SM, Kimerling R, Frayne SM, Shaw KA, Phibbs CS. Posttraumatic stress disorder and risk of spontaneous preterm birth. Obstet Gynecol. 2014;124(6):1111–9.

34. Holmboe-Ottesen G, Wandel M. Changes in dietary habits after migration and consequences for health: a focus on south Asians in Europe. Food Nutr Res. 2012. https://doi.org/10.3402/fnr.v56i0.18891.

6

Cost analysis of implementing mHealth intervention for maternal, newborn & child health care through community health workers: assessment of ReMIND program in Uttar Pradesh, India

Shankar Prinja[*], Aditi Gupta, Pankaj Bahuguna and Ruby Nimesh

Abstract

Background: The main intervention under ReMIND program consisted of a mobile health application which was used by community health volunteers, called ASHAs, for counselling pregnant women and nursing mothers. This program was implemented in two rural blocks in Uttar Pradesh state of India with an overall aim to increase quality of health care, thereby increasing utilization of maternal & child health services. The aim of the study was to assess annual & unit cost of ReMIND program and its scale up in UP state.

Method and materials: Economic costing was done from the health system and patient's perspectives. All resources used during designing & planning phase i.e., development of application; and implementation of the intervention, were quantified and valued. Capital costs were annualised, after assessing their average number of years for which a product could be used and accounting for its depreciation. Shared or joint costs were apportioned for the time value a resource was utilized under intervention. Annual cost of implementing ReMIND in two blocks of UP along and unit cost per pregnant woman were estimated. Scale-up cost for implementing the intervention in entire state was calculated under two scenarios – first, if no extra human resource were employed; and second, if the state government adopted the same pattern of human resource as employed under this program.

Results: The annual cost for rolling out ReMIND in two blocks of district Kaushambi was INR 12.1 million (US $ 191,894). The annualised start-up cost constituted 9% of overall cost while rest of cost was attributed to implementation of the intervention. The health system program costs in ReMIND were estimated to be INR 31.4 (US $ 0.49) per capita per year and INR 1294 (US $ 20.5) per registered women. The per capita incremental cost of scale up of intervention in UP state was estimated to be INR 4.39 (US $ 0.07) when no additional supervisory staffs were added.

Conclusion: The cost of scale up of ReMIND in Uttar Pradesh is 6% of annual budget for 'reproductive and child health' line item under state budget, and hence appears to be financially sustainable.

Keywords: mHealth, Health system cost, Costing analysis, Maternal and child health, Community health volunteers

* Correspondence: shankarprinja@gmail.com
School of Public Health, Post Graduate Institute of Medical Education and Research, Sector-12, Chandigarh 160012, India

Background

Despite the rapid improvement in maternal, newborn and child health (MNCH) indicators in India, many districts in the country still face high maternal and infant mortalities [1]. On the basis of a composite health index indicator, Government of India (GOI) identified 184 high priority districts across 29 states for focused integrated planning and monitoring of reproductive, maternal, newborn, child and adolescent health care program (RMNCH+A) [2]. District Kaushambi in Uttar Pradesh (UP) state is a high priority district with high maternal mortality ratio (MMR) of 283 per 100,000 live births and infant mortality rate (IMR) of 82 per 1000 live births [3] which are way above the national and state averages of 178 & 258 MMR and 40 & 68 IMR respectively [3]. Most of these maternal and newborn deaths are preventable if a continuum of care is followed right from pregnancy to newborn care. This includes whole spectrum of services including utilization of antenatal care, institutional delivery, early initiation of breastfeeding, essential newborn care, early recognition and referral of maternal and newborn complications with timely access to quality healthcare [4]. In order to strengthen the service provision, National Rural Health Mission (NRHM) was introduced in 2005 to augment primary health care and build capacity of community health workers (CHW) in remote areas to deliver affordable, equitable and accessible care [5]. With this aim, concept of Accredited Social Health Activist (ASHA) was envisaged. These are local women who serve as first contact between public health system and communities. ASHA as a cadre were included in the health system with intent to fulfil three roles i.e., creating awareness among communities for health issues, facilitating access to healthcare services, and as a provider for a limited range of basic health services. They help in addressing community health needs and generating demand for health service utilisation. This huge human resource of 890,000 ASHAs in the country holds immense potential and perform range of services such as mobilizing community for antenatal services during pregnancy, institutional delivery, identification and referral for maternal & newborn complications, home-based postnatal care, universal immunization, prevention of water-borne & other communicable diseases, and nutrition & sanitation [6]. With a minimal educational qualification of high school, ASHAs are provided on job training in various modules as specified by GOI [7, 8]. Various studies have been conducted to determine the effectiveness and functionality of ASHA workers in India. A study conducted in eight states of India highlighted that 75% pregnant women received services from ASHAs across all the states which included whole range of services from antenatal care, accompanying for institutional delivery, immunization etc. [9]. Findings of

the 10th Common Review Mission also highlighted that coverage of antenatal care, institutional delivery and immunization services have improved in 16 states of India, which were also attributed to the role of ASHA workers [10]. Another study found that ASHA workers were valued, as service providers by rural communities in creating awareness and behaviour change towards maternal and child care [11]. However, many studies highlighted that the quality and pace of trainings provided to ASHA workers after recruitment were inadequate and service provisioning by ASHA was largely limited to health education and referral. Thus, a need for regular and refresher trainings were realised for improving ASHAs' performance [12]. A review of the home-based care highlighted that skill retention and thus quality of care provided by ASHA could be improved by either conducting periodic refresher trainings or by using information technology, or using audio visual teaching aids that are more interactive and engaging [13]. These job aids are likely to improve retention of information and make ASHAs communication effective [13].

Mobile technology based health solutions are increasingly being utilized in health sector in low and middle income countries to strengthen skills of CHWs. Mobile Health (mHealth) as defined by World Health Organization (WHO) is an area of electronic health that provides health services and information via mobile technologies such as mobile phones and personal digital assistants [14]. For instance, mHealth application has been used for improving maternal and child health indicators in Ethiopia [15], as web based mobile applicable modules for treatment and follow up of malaria cases along Thai-Myanmar border and for community case management of malaria in Saraya, Senegal [16, 17], as diagnostic and management tool in diabetes [18] and as a cardiovascular risk assessment tool in Nyanga district of Cape town [19]. Similarly, one mobile based application was implemented as ReMiND (Reducing Maternal and Newborn Deaths) program in routine health care service delivery through ASHA workers in two blocks of district Kaushambi in UP state. The overall aim of this intervention was to increase the quality of counselling provided by ASHAs with the help of mobile application as an audio visual aid, thereby increasing utilization of MCH services.

However, a global survey done by WHO highlighted the lack of cost effectiveness data as one of major barrier in justifying implementation of mHealth services. It reported that only 13 out of the 112 countries have ever evaluated cost effectiveness of their mHealth programs [20]. Also, a recent systematic review from India highlighted the lack of sufficient evidence on cost effectiveness of mHealth interventions [21]. In order to fill this gap in evidence base, we undertook a study to evaluate the impact of ReMiND program on utilization of MNCH services & its cost effectiveness. In this paper, we specifically report the cost of ReMiND program in district Kaushambi.Also, we estimated the scale up cost of this program in Uttar Pradesh state which is relevant from the fiscal planning point of view.

Methods

Study setting & background

The ReMiND program was undertaken in district Kaushambi which is one of the high priority districts of Uttar Pradesh. Ninety two percent of its 1.6 million population resides in rural areas [22]. The female literacy rate of district is 52.7% in contrast to state average of 63.9% [3]. The district MMR of 283 deaths per 100,000 live births, was 25 and 105 points higher than the state and national averages respectively [3]. The coverage of full antenatal care checkups; haemoglobin and ultrasound test during routine ANC of pregnant women were 5%, 11.3% & 10.7% respectively [3]. Nearly 60% women in the district delivered in health facilities, while 46.9% children had full course of primary immunization during infancy [3].

To improve these maternal and child health indicators, a mHealth program named ReMiND was introduced in two community development blocks namely, Manjhanpur and Mooratganj, of district Kaushambi in year 2012. It resulted from collaborative work of two Non- Government Organizations (NGOs) i.e. Catholic Relief Services (CRS) & Vatsalya; and a social technology innovator, Dimagi. The main focus of the program was to improve the counselling skills of ASHA workers with the help of mHealth application. The detailed description of mHealth application under ReMiND program, its study setting, objectives and methodology are available as a published literature [23].

The preplanning phase of the program started with ten ASHA workers who were trained for piloting an early pregnancy checklist in March 2011. Subsequently, 111 ASHAs from Manjhanpur block were trained in August 2012 followed by training of 148 ASHAs of Mooratganj block in March 2013. These 259 ASHAs were provided Java based phones and trained on use of mobile application to register and counsel women for various MNCH services. The application had a built-in algorithm in the form of five modules which were used to advice and counsel registered women on the complete continuum of care; right from registration and antenatal care to, postnatal & newborn care as per individualized needs and requirements [24]. The data entered by ASHAs were received at Dimagi's online cloud server. Commcare is an open source, mobile platform that enables non-technical users to build mobile applications for their frontline programs across numerous sectors

reducing the need for paper based data collection. The data in variety of formats like multiple choice questions, dates, images, videos, global positioning system (GPS) coordinates can be collected through simple mobile interfaces. The data can be collected in offline mode and is sent automatically to the server on regaining internet connectivity. Thus, it can be widely used in rural areas of India which may not have good internet connectivity. Data about pregnant women were restricted and were only accessible to few authenticated users from the program with valid username and password. The data were de-identified before analysis and no reports generated by Dimagi using commcare included information about individual pregnant women. The ASHA supervisors, also called Sector facilitators, used this data to monitor the timeliness and frequency of antenatal and postnatal home care visits by ASHAs to discuss their performance in monthly meetings at block level [24].

Data collection

Economic costing was done from the health system and patient's perspectives to estimate the annual and per-capita cost of implementing the ReMiND program. The cost of resources spent under three time heads were obtained – preplanning phase extending from October 2010 to March 2012, start-up phase from April 2012 to July 2012, and implementation phase from August 2012 to August 2015.

We collected data from all the agencies involved in the program namely, i.e. CRS, Vatsalya, Dimagi and health department of district Kaushambi from May to October, 2015. Cost data was collected from different sources such as financial records, program budget, audit reports, agreements, etc. Data was collected from country office of Dimagi & CRS in New Delhi, state office of CRS in Lucknow and health department in district Kaushambi for health systems costs. Since CRS funded Vatsalya for implementing ReMiND program, the records for latter's expenses were also obtained from CRS. The details about the expenditure on development and maintenance of the software were obtained from Dimagi. Maintenance cost of application included any technical assistance from the designers of the application including assistance on bug fixing and update. Along with this, costs on housing, serving, and maintaining files on the cloud, also called 'hosting service charge', were also obtained from Dimagi. All the cost data were obtained in US dollars, which were converted to Indian Rupees using exchange rates for the respective years. Research costs for two evaluations done during the program namely; baseline study in 2012–13 and mid-term evaluations in 2014 were excluded from the analysis.

Intervention costing methodology

The present analysis determines the cost of ReMiND program from both the health system and patient's perspective separately. The health system costs were stratified based on the agencies which incurred the cost (i.e. developmental partners & government health system) and nature of cost (start-up capital cost and recurrent cost). The recurrent cost in turn is stratified into cost on program implementation by development partners, cost of monitoring & supervision by government officials and the cost of providing services as a result of increased demand in public health system. The scale-up costs were estimated from the health system perspective alone. In addition to the health system cost, we also measured out of pocket expenditures (OOPE) on doctor or nurse fee, medicines, diagnostic tests, medical or surgical procedures, transportation and boarding/lodging which is called as 'cost from patient's perspective'. We measured OOPE incurred by households in seeking health care during pregnancy, delivery and post delivery period from a household survey [14].

Start-up capital cost

We included two cost heads i.e. start-up capital cost and recurrent implementation cost. Start-up costs included all the capital costs incurred during the initial preplanning phase and start-up phase. Technically, any cost whose inputs may last for more than one year was considered as capital cost [25]. This was categorised as costs levied on modules' development and piloting, development and maintenance of software, equipment cost, mobile phones and overhead costs. Apart from these costs; pre-planning meetings, trainings of ASHAs & their supervisors and translation of modules into local dialect were also taken as capital costs because the effect of these inputs were likely to last for the life of the program.

All the capital costs were apportioned in terms of their time value devoted in ReMiND program out of all the programs running simultaneously by the implementing agencies. The program was piloted in two blocks but it was designed such that it could be launched in 821 blocks of Uttar Pradesh. Accordingly, we apportioned the entire start up expenditure for the two blocks of district Kaushambi where intervention was actually piloted. After obtaining the apportioned value, costs in dollars were converted to Indian National Rupee (INR) by applying the dollar conversion rates given by the US Internal Revenue Service for a particular year of purchase of equipment [26]. The converted rates were then inflated from the year of purchase to the current value of product in 2015 by applying Consumer Price Index in India [27]. These inflated values of capital were then annualized as per the average life of utilization of the product at a discount rate of 3% [28]. The annual

maintenance rates for capital items as given by the implementing agency were used in calculations.

The average life of software was assumed to be 12 years as the cost incurred on software may last either till strategies of the program remained the same; or if there was a change in technology itself. We chose former based on expert consultation as it is unlikely that any drastic paradigm change may happen in the content of the programme for another 12 years. Further, any change in technology would have had only marginal effect on costs if it requires any revision. The hosting charges were annualized for 3 years as these charges would be revised and added again like recurrent cost if the program extends beyond three years. For mobile phones, laptops, furniture and vehicle, the average life were taken as 3.5 years, 5 years, 6 and 10 years respectively as per the policy of the implementing agencies.

Recurrent implementation cost

The implementation costs included recurrent costs which were required to sustain the intervention. All the recurrent costs were categorized as cost on human resource, travel, ASHA data/internet usage charges for mobile application, utilities like office rent, electricity, telephone bills & internet bills and stationary & printing. Other program support expenses at state and national office like the office rent and salaries were also accounted. Shared costs were apportioned as per the time value devoted by that given resource in performing a particular activity. The office rents were spent at three levels i.e. at district, state and country level. At the district level, entire rent were spent on the activities related to ReMiND program only and hence no apportioning was required. However, at the state and national levels, multiple programs were being handled simultaneously. Therefore, office rent was apportioned in proportion of floor area occupied by the staff involved in ReMiND program to the total office staff. The travel costs in form of vehicle or fuel for carrying out planning and supervisory activities during the start-up and implementation phase were dedicated to ReMiND program only as no other program was being implemented concurrently at the block levels.

For the recurrent costs, we converted the expenses levied by the partner agencies over 37 months i.e. from Aug 2012 to August 2015, into average annual expense. For converting US dollars into Indian rupees, the average dollar rate for these three years was taken as 1 US $ = INR 58.84.

Government health system program cost

Apart from costs spent by implementing agencies, additional costs incurred by district health system were also estimated. It included three components – first, health system cost on monitoring and supervision of ASHA activities under ReMiND program. It includes the time value of the personnel involved either in their supervision through household visits, interactions with ASHA workers or indirectly via review meetings; second, incremental cost of service delivery due to increased utilization of MNCH services as the result of given intervention and third, incremental effect of intervention on ASHAs payment in terms of incentives. The direct supervisory costs were calculated considering that supervisors spend 13% of their total time in monitoring and supervisory activities, as mentioned in another study conducted in developing country [29].

For program implementation, the extra cost of monthly meetings at the block levels, quarterly meetings at district level and bi-annual meetings at the state level were calculated by apportioning the time devoted by government officials in meetings for review of ASHAs' performance under the program. The effect of ReMiND program on overall utilization of MNCH services was evaluated using a quasi-experimental design with a difference in difference analysis [14]. The unit costs for these services were obtained from economic evidence available in the Indian context [30–32].

Economic implications of changes in service utilization in the intervention and control blocks in terms of the performance based incentives for ASHA workers were evaluated using data from health management information system (HMIS) and financial records as obtained from the office of Chief Medical Officer of the district for year 2014–15 [23].

Unit costs

For calculation of unit costs, the population under the intervention area (387,030) was used as denominator for per capita calculation. For cost per pregnant woman, the number of women registered under mHealth was used as denominator. A total of 28,169 women have been registered under ReMiND program since its inception (over three years) as per data provided by Management Information System of the implementing agencies, so the annual number of beneficiaries was taken as 9390.

Scale up costs of ReMiND program for Uttar Pradesh state

The intervention was implemented on pilot basis in two blocks of Uttar Pradesh state. Subsequently the estimates on the cost of implementation of ReMiND program in two blocks were used to estimate the scale up cost of this program, if the government of UP state decided to roll out intervention in the entire 821 blocks in the state. The scale up costs of mHealth intervention in entire state included costs on purchase of mobile phones, internet usage, trainings of ASHAs & their supervisors

for use of application and health system costs on review meetings in the entire state. The scale up cost also implicitly included the costs of ASHAs performance based incentives. For scale up, two case scenarios were assumed. First, if current available human resource in the health system could be utilised for monitoring and supervision of this intervention. In UP, Block Community Managers (BCM) and Health Education Officers (HEO) are employed at block and district levels respectively to coordinate and supervise ASHAs' performance. These are regular salaried staff unlike ASHAs whose remunerations were incentive based. In second scenario, a separate supervisory cadre like sector facilitators in ReMiND program were assumed at block level.

At sub-block level also, one ASHA facilitator was employed for monitoring and supervision of 20 ASHAs as guided by the National Health Mission [33], and the same pattern was followed by the implementing agencies. These were promoted ASHAs and did not receive any extra incentives for holding the position. Supervisory training costs of these ASHA facilitators were also included in the scale up cost.

As there was dearth of data on time value spent by different supervisors on various activities in our study and Indian literature [12], we assumed the time apportioned on supervisory and monitoring activities as 13% of total activity time based on findings from a similar study [29]. Though as per directions given by MoHFW, a block ASHA facilitator shall spend 20 days in field in a month [34].

From the perspective of UP state, there would be no requirement to change the content of the software or the built in audio-visual support as the same dialect could be understood in the entire state. Therefore, the start-up capital costs which included the costs on development of software, preplanning meetings, initial translation of modules were not included in scale up cost. Dimagi Inc. developed the software and provided free of cost server support services to first 50 beneficiaries and thereafter charged US$ 1 per year per beneficiary. Therefore, 5 million US$ have to be spent for 5 million (50 lakh) pregnant women in Uttar Pradesh as scale up hosting server charges. Table 1 describes the different types of costs calculated in the study.

Out of pocket expenditures (Patient's perspective)

A patient's perspective is important to consider in costing studies as it includes expenditures borne by households in form of out of pocket expenditures (OOPE) for seeking health care. Aiming patient's perspective helps in adopting policies that intend to provide financial risk protection against OOPE and minimize the losses to households. The data on mean OOP for utilization of

Table 1 Various types of cost with the data sources and methodology

Area	Type of cost	Type of Data collected	Source of data	Method of data collection
At two block levels	Start up/Capital cost	Cost on Module development, translation & piloting. Development of software, Equipment and mobile cost, overheads. Preplanning meetings, ASHA trainings	Official documents of CRS, Vatsalya & Dimagi. Annual budget reports, bills receipts, Personal Interviews	Primary data collection. Time value contributed over the average age of the program
	Implementation cost	Salaries, travel, ASHA internet usage, utilities like office rent, electricity, telephone bills, stationary and printing. Program support cost at state and national office	Official documents like bills, annual budget reports, Personal interview	Primary data collection. Time apportioned as per the time value spent/utilized on the activities related only to ReMiND program
	Health system cost	Health system cost on program implementation. Incremental cost of service delivery due to increased utilization of MNCH services. unit cost for per service utilization) Incremental effect of intervention on ASHA payment.	Financial documents on ASHA incentives from Chief Medical officer's Office, Personal Interviews, Observations during meetings at block, district and state level. Literature review for unit cost per service utilization	Primary data collection. Apportioning of the salaries of the officials as per the time spent on attending meetings at block, district and state level.
	Costs from Patient perspective	Out of pocket expenditure(OOPE) incurred by the households in seeking health care services for various maternal, newborn and child illnesses	OOPE were obtained from the Impact assessment study carried out n two intervention blocks and two control blocks.	Primary data collection
	Annual Program cost	It is sum of startup cost and implementation cost	–	Derived indicator
	Overall annual unit cost per pregnant women	Annual programmatic cost divided by average annual number of women registered under ReMiND	Management information system (MIS) data from CRS on number of registered women	Derived indicator
	Unit health system cost per pregnant women	Annual health system cost divided by average annual number of women registered under ReMiND	MIS data from CRS	Derived indicator
At state level –Uttar Pradesh	Scale up cost	Number of ASHAs in entire state, training cost of ASHA and supervisors, mobile phone cost, hosting service charges, health system cost	NRHM website, Observations, Calculations from available data	Unit costs of pilot at two blocks were expanded to 821 blocks in Uttar Pradesh state.
	Per capita scale up cost	Total scale up cost divided by Total population of state	Census 2011	Derived indicator
	Per pregnant women scale up cost	Total scale up cost in Uttar Pradesh divided by average number of pregnant women in the state in an year	Crude Birth Rate	Derived indictors

ASHA- Accredited Social Health Activist, CRS-Catholic Relief Services, MNCH- Maternal, Newborn and Child Health, OOP- Out of Pocket Expenditure, ReMiND- Reducing Maternal and Newborn Deaths

specific MNCH services was obtained from a household survey undertaken to evaluate impact of ReMiND and its cost effectiveness [14]. The detailed information about the household survey and its methodology are described in details in our protocol paper and impact assessment paper [14, 23]. The household questionnaire included questions to assess any cost borne by patients and their families for treatment, consultation from doctors, purchase of drugs and consumables, travel, lodging & boarding, or any money spent elsewhere. Figure 1 illustrates the conceptual framework of costing process of ReMiND program explaining both health system perspective and patient perspective.

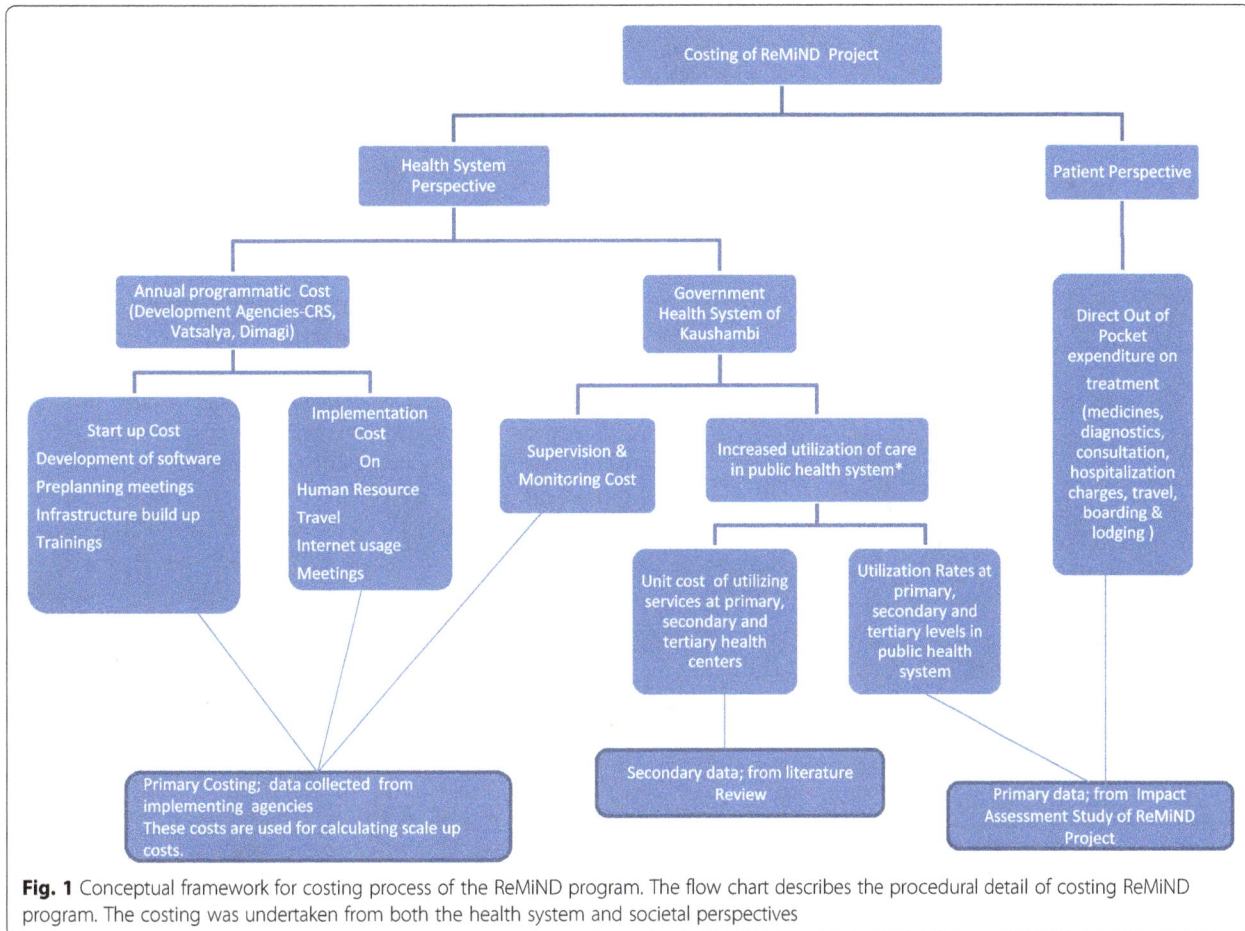

Fig. 1 Conceptual framework for costing process of the ReMiND program. The flow chart describes the procedural detail of costing ReMiND program. The costing was undertaken from both the health system and societal perspectives

Sensitivity analysis

The sensitivity analysis was carried out to understand the effect of variation in input costs on both the base case estimates i.e. annual cost of ReMiND program in two blocks of district Kaushambi and the scale up cost in entire state of Uttar Pradesh. Various case scenarios were considered. The choice of upper and lower bounds for the life of the mHealth application (5 to 15 years) was based on an extensive consultation with the state program managers and development partners. The choice of percentage variation in input prices was based on review of the costing studies done in India [35–37]. It was assumed that the mobile phone and internet data charges may fluctuate to 20%. The cost of training costs of ASHAs and supervisors were fluctuated 10% and 20% respectively; trainings for latter were done in private costlier locations, while a reduction in cost can be achieved if the same were done in Government set-up and monitoring activity was increased to 50% of total time.

A review of economic evaluation studies from India, reported the use of 3%, 3.5%, 8% and 10% as the rates to discount future costs [21]. Further, the WHO-CHOICE

and reference case developed by IDSi-BMGF for low and middle income countries recommends use of 3% discount rate [38, 39]. In view of this we used 3% discount rate in the base scenario. Further, since the inflation rate in India is relatively higher than most of the other developing countries [40], a discount rate below 3% was not justifiable. The other most commonly used discount rate for economic costing among developing countries are 5% and 8%. So, we varied the discount rate to 5% and 8%. The company has recently revised its hosting user charges from US$ 1 per beneficiary (pregnant women) per year to US$ 2 per ASHA worker (using mHealth application in phone) per month. In view of this, we undertook a scenario analysis during our scale up cost estimation for UP state to assess the overall and unit cost of ReMiND program in UP with changes in the hosting charges. The results of sensitivity analysis were presented in the form of tornado diagram. Sensit 1.51 software was used for the analysis.

Ethics and consent statement

The Institute Ethics Committee of the Post Graduate Institute of Medical Sciences (PGIMER), Chandigarh provided the ethical clearance for the study vide letter no. 'Program No IEC-01/2015-108'. Administrative approval was obtained from government health authorities of Uttar Pradesh state and Kaushambi district for obtaining health facility level data. In addition, written consent was obtained from all the participants who were interviewed in the study for obtaining the out of pocket expenditures and health system costs.

Results

Annual health system costs

The annual cost for rolling out ReMiND program in two blocks of district Kaushambi was INR 12.1 million (US $191,894). Out of this, start-up cost and implementation cost contributed 9% and 91% of the total annual cost respectively. Government health system contributed 4.8% of the total implementation cost. The unit costs of implementing ReMiND program were INR 31.4 (US $ 0.49) per capita and INR 1294 (US $ 20.5) per registered pregnant women. Figure 2 shows the proportional distribution of total expenditure on ReMiND program in district Kaushambi. An additional file provides detailed description of start-up and implementation costs contributing to annual intervention cost for ReMiND (see Additional file 1).

Start-up capital cost

The start-up cost for the ReMiND program was INR 1.1 million ($17,526). A major portion of this cost was for training of ASHAs and their supervisors (33%) followed by development of software & modules and its piloting (30.3%), mobile phones (29.2%), equipment (5.4%) and programmatic expenses (2.2%). Figure 3 shows the

proportional distribution of start-up costs of ReMiND program in district Kaushambi.

Recurrent implementation cost

The annual implementation cost of mHealth intervention in two blocks of Uttar Pradesh was INR 11 million (US $174,368). The costs were predominantly constituted by human resources (62.5%), followed by travel (15.4%), program support cost at national and state office of CRS (8.2%), utilities (5.2%), internet use (3.6%) and health system programme support cost (4.8%) (Fig. 4).

Government health system program cost

The cost of monitoring the intervention from the government health system as during the review meetings was estimated to be INR 94,750 (US $ 1496.8), INR 3133 (US $ 49.5) and INR 2230 (US $ 35.2) per year at block, district and state levels respectively. The costs included apportioned time value of government officials for supervisory activities, with small contribution from travel and overheads.

We estimated that health system in intervention area had to spend INR 430,582 (US $6802) in order to cater the increased coverage of MNCH services attributable to the intervention. The incremental cost borne by the health system during implementation of ReMiND program was INR 39.9 ($ 0.63) per pregnant woman. This cost included the additional cost borne by government on monitoring and supervision of the program; increased utilization of MNCH services by pregnant and lactating mothers and increased performance based incentives to ASHAs as a result of ReMiND program. However, there was no increase in ASHA payments,

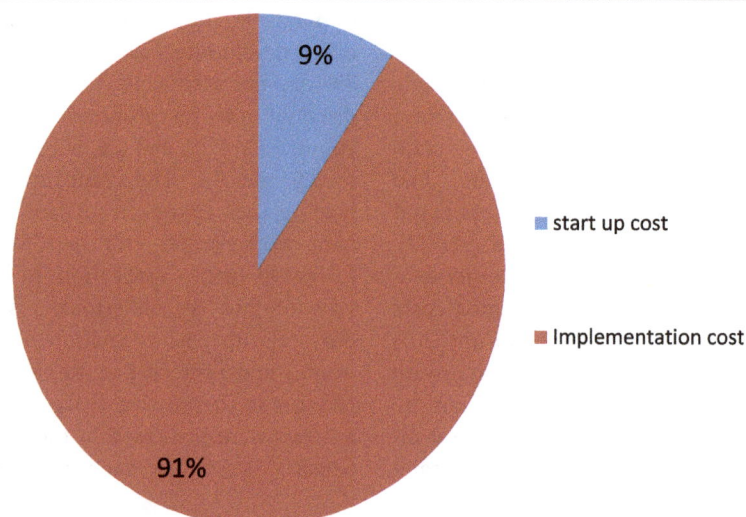

Fig. 2 Proportional distribution of total expenditure on ReMiND program from 2011 to 2015. The figure shows the proportional distribution of start up cost and implementation cost in the total expenditure of ReMiND program

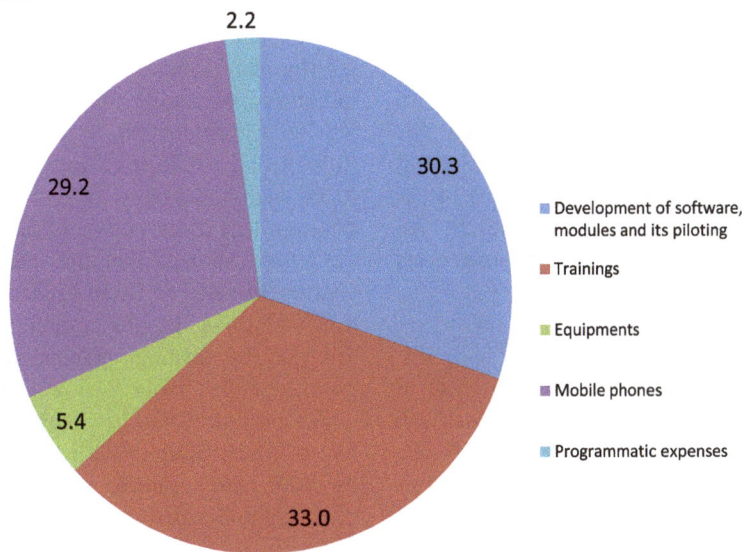

Fig. 3 Proportional distribution of start up costs of ReMiND program in intervention area of district Kaushambi. The figure shows the proportional contribution of different start up costs in the total start up cost of ReMiND program

hence the incremental health system cost represents the former two, i.e., cost of monitoring & supervision and cost of increase in service utilization. The detailed description of the start-up and implementation costs is given in the Additional file 1.

Out of pocket expenditure (Patient's perspective)
As discussed in methodology, to calculate cost of Re-MiND program from patient perspective, the proportion of people bearing OOP expenditure for seeking various MNCH services and the mean OOP expenditure at various levels of health centres in both public and private sector were taken from the Impact Assessment study

[14]. It was estimated that the incremental out of pocket expenditure for seeking various health care services in the intervention block was INR 15 million (US $ 240,333). The detailed out of pocket expenditures are shown in Additional file 2.

Scale up costs
In first case scenario where intervention has to be scaled up from two blocks in Kaushambi to 821 blocks in state using the existing human resources for monitoring and supervision, we estimated the scale-up would cost around INR 876 million (US$ 13.8 million). The unit cost of scale up in Uttar Pradesh state would be INR

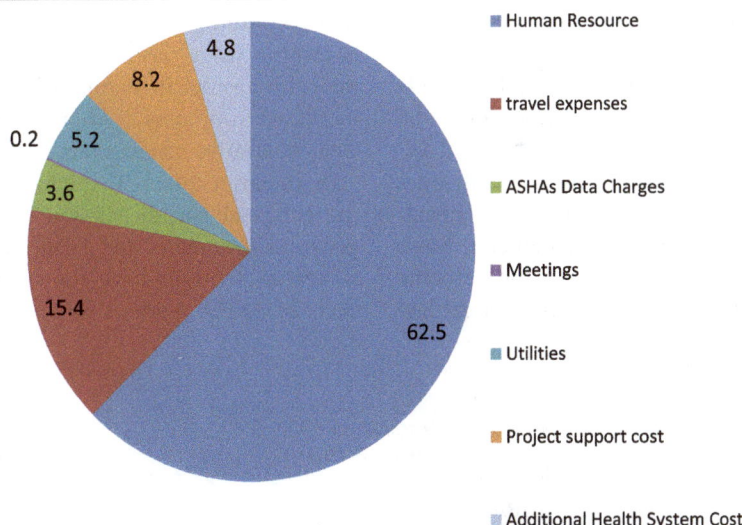

Fig. 4 Proportional distribution of annual cost of implementation of ReMiND program in district Kaushambi. The figure shows the proportional contribution of different recurrent costs in the annual implementation cost of ReMiND program

4.39 (US $0.07) per capita and INR 175.3 (US $2.77) per pregnant women. In second case scenario, additional human resource was assumed to be recruited for monitoring of ASHAs in every block of state. In this case, government has to spend around INR 993 million (US $15.7 million) with INR 4.97 (US $ 0.08) as per capita unit cost and INR 198.8 (US $ 3.14) as unit cost per pregnant woman (Refer Table 2). 'An additional file describes the details of scale up costs (see Additional file 3)'.

Sensitivity analysis

Sensitivity analysis was conducted to estimate costs in various alternate scenarios. Firstly, the total annual cost was estimated assuming that the development of software was done for two blocks of Kaushambi only. In this case, the start-up cost would be INR 4.6 million (USD 73,367) which is 30% of the total annual intervention cost of INR 15 million (USD 247,734). The incremental costs of intervention would be INR 1670 (USD 26.4) per pregnant woman and INR 40.52 (USD 0.64) per capita.

Secondly, the discount rates were varied to 5% and 8%, and the average life of program was taken as 5 and 15 years. On applying the discount rate of 5%, the incremental costs would be INR 1302 (USD 20.6) per pregnant woman and INR 31.60 (USD 0.49) per capita. At 8% discount rate, the incremental cost would be INR 1316 (USD 20.8) per pregnant woman and 31.93 (USD 0.50) per capita.

On assuming the life of programs to be 5 and 15 years, the incremental costs per pregnant woman would change to INR 1338 (USD 21.14) and 1287 (USD 20.34) respectively while per capita costs would be 32.5 (USD 0.51) and 31.23 (USD 0.49) respectively.

The tornado diagrams in Figs. 5 and 6 are the graphical representation of effect of multiple univariate input variables (represented as horizontal bars on y-axis) on the outcome variable (x-axis) i.e. annual cost of ReMiND program in two blocks of Kaushambi district and total cost of scale up of ReMiND project at the level of UP state respectively. The values shown along the both sides of black bars are range (lower and upper side) considered for varying a particular cost input parameter. More is the width of black bar, more sensitive is the outcome variable to change in input parameter. The vertical line

between the black horizontal bars shows the base case results. The tornado diagram in Fig. 5 shows that salaries (human resource cost) presents the highest uncertainty and maximum impact on the total annual cost of ReMiND program (90.7% swing) followed by travel cost (5.5% swing) while start up costs like training of ASHAs (0.3% swing), purchase of equipments (0.3% swing) and development of the software (0.0%) had little influence.

Figure 6 showed that the scale up of ReMiND intervention in state of Uttar Pradesh was most sensitive to the variations in the mobile internet data charges followed by hosting charges and purchase of mobile phones. Refer Table S4A and B in 'Additional file 4' which presented the base cost parameter values for different input variables with their upper and lower limits for both case scenarios i.e. program cost in two blocks of Kaushambi district and scale up cost in Uttar Pradesh state.

With the revised hosting charges at the rate of US$ 2 per ASHA worker per month, UP state will have to spend INR 559 million (US $ 8.8 million) per year. The per capita costs of ReMiND program in such a scenario will be INR 2.80 (US $ 0.04) per capita and INR 111.9 (US $ 1.76) per pregnant woman.

Discussion

Use of technology in health and other sectors has been promoted by GOI from the highest level [41]. Several other policy discourses have encouraged the application of mHealth. The High-Level Expert Group on Universal Health Coverage called for harnessing technology for promoting utilization of services [42]. Small to medium scale pilot interventions have been initiated in a variety of geographic settings in India involving a diverse range of health services such as maternal and child health to non-communicable diseases [43]. Various studies from elsewhere have also shown that the application of mHealth results in better delivery of health education, increased awareness & improved uptake of preventive as well as curative services [16, 44–46].

In Indian context, the introduction of ASHA under the National Health Mission holds strong potential for generating demand for health services [34]. However, several evaluations have shown that the knowledge and skills of ASHA workers to counsel pregnant women for

Table 2 Summary of scale up costs of mHealth intervention in Uttar Pradesh in two case scenarios

Cost Description	Scenario1 When currently employed staff is used for supervisory activities INR (US$)	Scenario 2 When additional human resource is employed at the level of blocks INR (US$)
Annual cost of scale up	87,63,69,067 (13,844,693)	99,38,73,262 (15,700,999)
Annual cost per beneficiary	175 (2.77)	198.8 (3.14)
Annual cost per capita	4.39 (0.07)	4.97 (0.08)

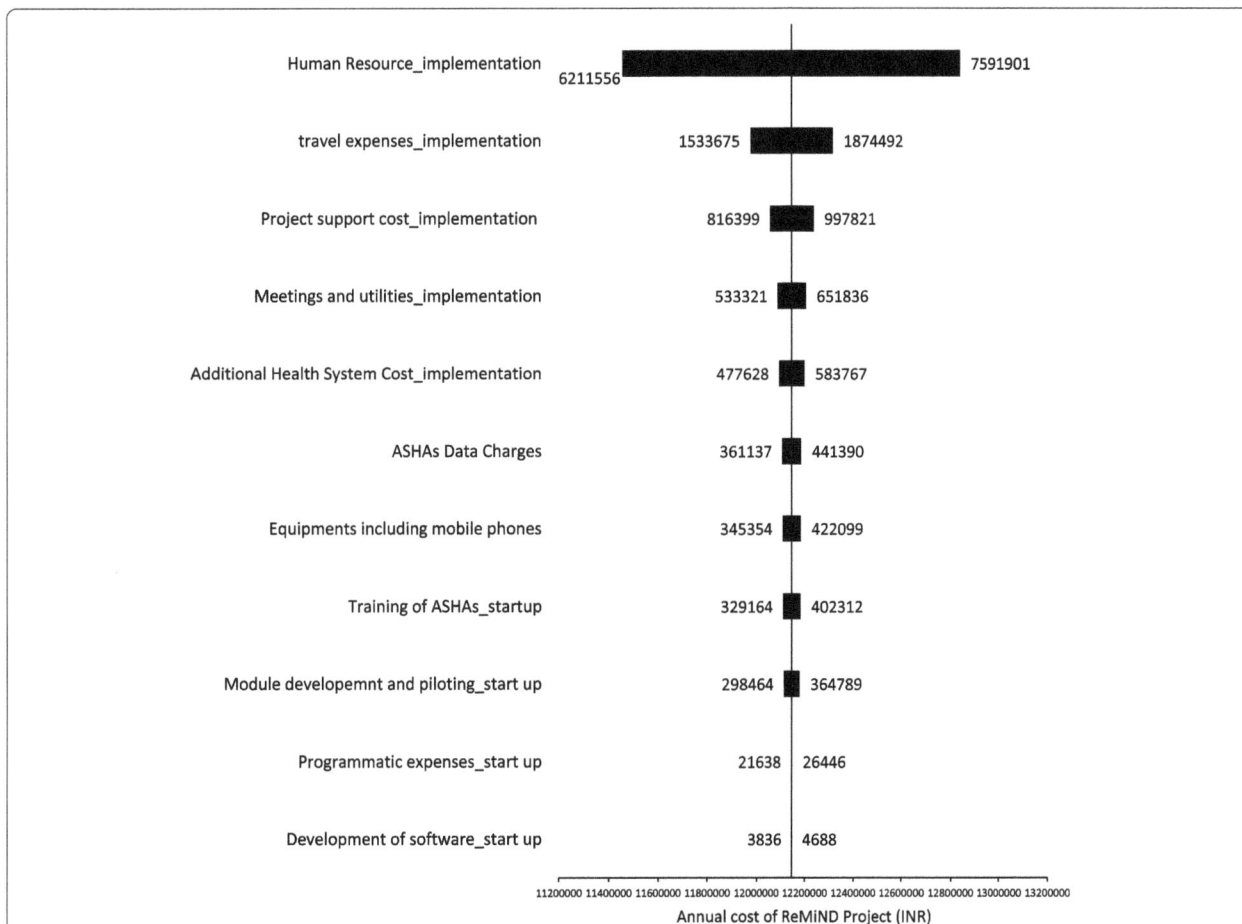

Fig. 5 Tornado diagram illustrates the sensitivity analysis for various input factors on the annual cost (INR) of ReMiND program. The figure shows the sensitivity analysis with the help of tornado diagram to show the effect of variation in different input factors on total annual cost of ReMiND program in two blocks of Kaushambi district

their health care needs during pregnancy and nursing babies requires strengthening [12]. In light of this, use of mobile technology for improving the quality of counselling can serve as a major strategy. This can further improve knowledge and awareness among communities which may directly augment demand for services. However, it is important to understand the feasibility and financial implications of implementing this intervention as part of routine care. Hence our economic analysis holds a significant value for the policy makers in order to estimate the economic implications for implementing and scaling up of such mHealth interventions. The researchers can also use costing studies for carrying out cost effectiveness analysis of such mHealth interventions.

Our study showed that the introduction of mHealth intervention costs INR 31.4 (US $ 0.49) per capita and INR 1294 (US $ 20.5) per pregnant woman registered. The unit costs for scale up within Uttar Pradesh state were INR 4.39 ($0.07) per capita and 175.3($ 2.77) per pregnant women. The overall annual scale up cost for Uttar Pradesh to implement the same intervention in the entire state would be at least INR 876 million (US $ 13.8 million) if no additional human resource were employed for the program monitoring and support. As per our knowledge, this is the first cost outcome analysis targeting MNCH services in India [44].

Fiscal sustainability

From the point of state budget, the total annual money allotted for reproductive & child health (RCH), maternal health (MH) and ASHA incentives for year 2015–16 in Uttar Pradesh were INR 14.6 billion, 6.99 billion and 1.22 billion respectively [47]. The introduction of mHealth intervention and its scale up in the entire state of Uttar Pradesh will represent 6.0%, 12.5% and 71.7% share in the total budget for RCH, MH and ASHA incentive program respectively. It is important to note, this scale up amount does not include introduction of any new cadre of supervisors, and rather considers training the already available cadre for supervision. As per the guidelines of Financial Management Group of National Health Mission-India's flagship health program, it is

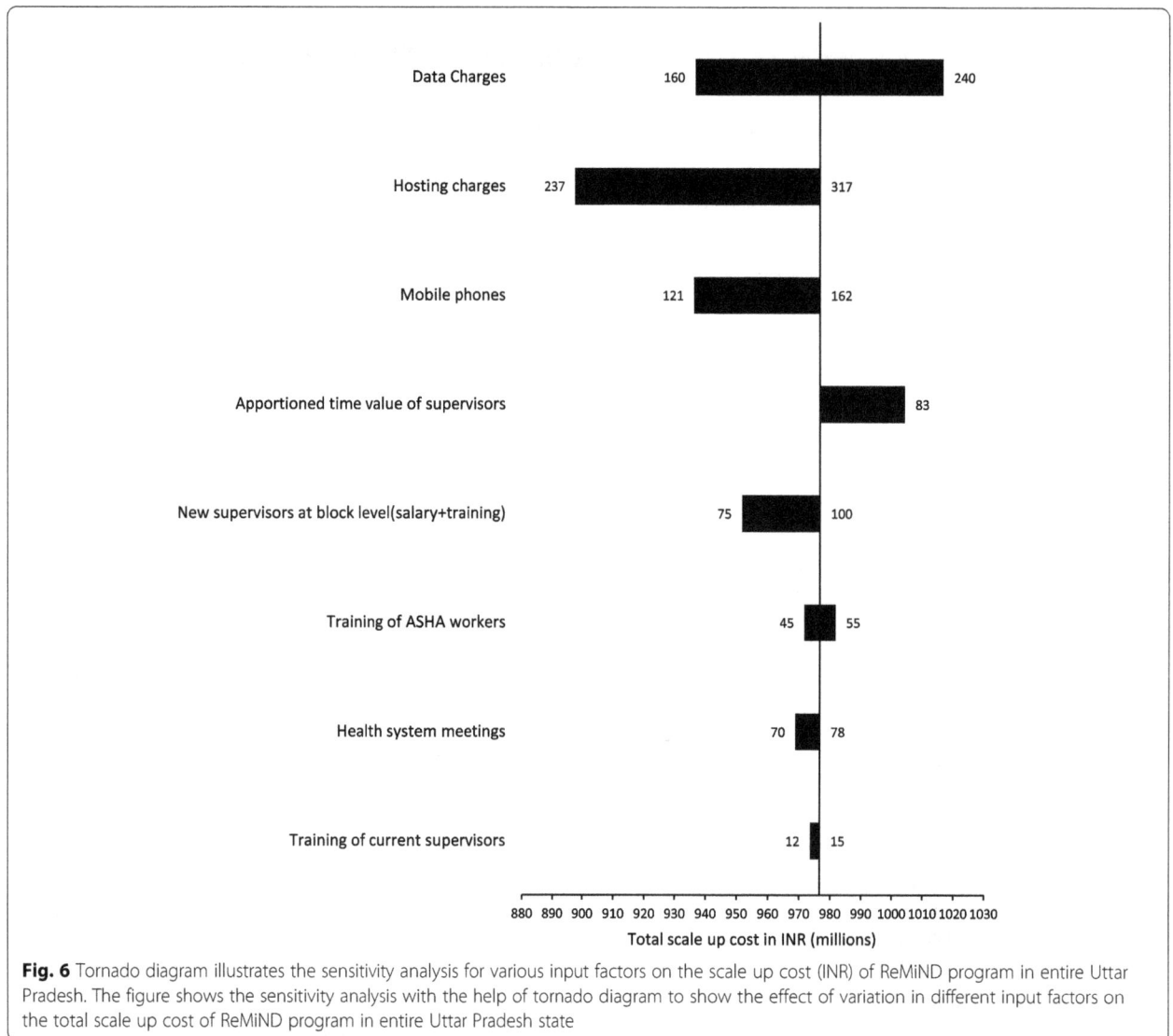

Fig. 6 Tornado diagram illustrates the sensitivity analysis for various input factors on the scale up cost (INR) of ReMiND program in entire Uttar Pradesh. The figure shows the sensitivity analysis with the help of tornado diagram to show the effect of variation in different input factors on the total scale up cost of ReMiND program in entire Uttar Pradesh state

recommended to increase the budget of high priority districts by 10–15% every year [48]. Considering the cost for scale up of ReMiND intervention to be 6% of the total budget allotted to 'Maternal and child health' line item under the NRHM budget of UP state, the intervention appears financially sustainable.

The World Health Report 2005 published a working paper series on scaling up of maternal and newborn interventions to reach universal health coverage by 2015. It estimated that for delivering the whole package of MNCH care (with 95% coverage) for countries in Health System Constraint Category 2 –where India fits – has an incremental cost of USD 1.53 per capita. On inflating this value to the current value of dollar by applying CPI rates in India, the current incremental cost would be USD 2.35 (INR 149.3). The WHO benefit package comprises of universal provision of comprehensive maternal, newborn and child health care services [49]. Our study

shows that scale-up of mHealth in UP state will incur an incremental cost of INR 4.77 (USD0.07) per capita, which is 3% of the total incremental value proposed by WHO for achieving universal coverage of MNCH services. This again shows that the scale-up of mHealth is sustainable from fiscal viewpoint.

Policy implications

The need to introduce a service or intervention in the benefit package of care is usually justified based on the burden of health problem which it addresses. However, the amenable burden or the reduction in the health problem which the intervention can potentially bring about is usually not considered. In light of this it is also important to understand that such mHealth application for RMNCH would thus be more useful in weaker states where the reasons for poor coverage are linked more with the demand for service. For example, the Coverage

Evaluation Survey reported that poorer states such as Bihar and Uttar Pradesh have low rates of RMNCH service utilization, a large portion of which is explained by lack of awareness and knowledge about the importance of services [36]. The findings from our impact assessment study suggested an increase in knowledge and thereby utilization of MNCH services after introduction of ReMiND program [14]. Hence, such an intervention which aims at improving counselling of ASHAs, which translates into improved knowledge of community and its demand for health services, is likely to be more beneficial in these states.

Also, ReMiND intervention and its scale up appear feasible from the financial and programmatic perspectives. Currently, a quarter of Indian population who could not access healthcare cited large distances from health facilities as the reason for not being able to access health care. In such situations, mHealth can offer a useful solution. Moreover, the increased penetration of mobile use in the rural areas as well as by community health workers makes it a feasible strategy. Second, mHealth can be used as platform for strengthening programs other than RMNCHA, which are implemented through community health workers. The Government of India's recently announced ambitious scheme of Ayushman Bharat which envisions the transformation of the existing sub-centres as Health and Wellness centres. The proposed health and wellness centres clearly outline a significant role of information technology and digital records for improving service delivery. Further, increased and timely utilization of services at these centres for primary care may decrease out of pocket expenditures on tertiary care. Global evidence suggest that mHealth solutions could lower the total annual per capita healthcare expenditure as it reduced in Brazil and Mexico by 20% and 25% respectively [50].

Also, the scale up cost of ReMiND program in UP would cost INR 993 million (US $15.7 million) if additional supervisors were to be recruited in each block for monitoring as was structured in ReMiND program while the cost would reduce to INR 876 million (US$ 13.8 million) if already employed staff was used for supervision. Dimagi Inc. charged US$ 1 per beneficiary per year as web hosting charges which has now changed to US$ 2 per ASHA worker (using mHealth application in phone) per month. This change in hosting charges would decrease the total scale up cost from INR 876.3 million to 559.8 million. Thus, it is likely that technological advances may further reduce the cost of ReMiND program. Therefore, m health solutions are emerging as useful and sustainable option from a fiscal point of view.

The mHealth program would also impact OOPE which can be understood by the theory of change explained elsewhere in a published study protocol [23].

The introduction of mHealth intervention as a job aid for community health volunteers improved their counselling skills and hence, increased knowledge among pregnant women towards early identification of the complications. This increased the demand for use of preventive and curative healthcare services. The impact assessment analysis showed that mHealth resulted in statistically significant increase in coverage iron and folic acid (IFA) supplementation (12.70%), identification and self-reporting of illnesses/complication during pregnancy (13.20%) and after delivery (19.5%) in the intervention area as compared to the control area. The coverage of > = 3 ANC visits, > = 2 tetanus toxoid, Full ANC, and ambulance usage also increased in the intervention area by 9.7%, 4.5%, 1% and 2.5% respectively, however, the change was statistically insignificant [14]. As far as utilization of public health facilities was concerned, while 50% of women with pregnancy related complications in intervention area sought care in public hospitals, nearly 72% women sought care in private health facilities in the control area [51]. Therefore, the increased uptake of primary and secondary health care services at initial stages of illness may result in reduction in subsequent tertiary care services thus, reducing OOPE on health care. The detailed description of the theory of change and results of impact assessment survey are provided as published literature [14, 23]. The out of pocket expenditures (OOPE) for seeking maternal, newborn and child care services in private and public health facilities in the intervention and control households in reported in the table in Additional file 2. It highlighted that the out of pocket expenditures on utilization of inpatient services for newborn and childhood illnesses were lesser in intervention areas than the control areas, there is limited data available in literature from India to assess the impact of mHealth interventions on out of pocket expenditures. However, assessment reports from other LMICs like Brazil and Mexico highlighted that mHealth could reduce OOPE by US$ 102 per mHealth user thus making healthcare more affordable [50].

Limitations

Our study had few limitations. Firstly, we could not obtain detailed year wise breakup of the expenses during the implementation phase, i.e., August 2012 to August 2015. We assumed that the same amount of expenses happened every year and averaged the cost, which might not be the case in the real situation. Second, in order to know the present worth of the capital involved in the study, we inflated the costs from year 2012 to 2015 considering the CPI Index for calculation of inflation and 3% discount rates. There is a possibility that advancement in technology over time may have actually reduced the price of capital items such as mobile phones, software etc. While this was not considered in the base case, we did undertake a sensitivity analysis to understand the impact of this assumption.

Third, since the retrospective data was collected and many of the officials from implementing agencies had left, there was a possibility of recall bias. However, as most of the data was retrieved from records, possibility of recall bas influencing the validity of our results was relatively less.

Fourth, the scale up cost implicitly included the costs of ASHAs' performance based incentives. However, based on our impact assessment analysis, we found that the ReMiND program increased the coverage of IFA supplementation, identification and self-reporting of illnesses/ complication during pregnancy & after delivery in the intervention area as compared to control area and none of these coverage indicators were linked to any performance based incentives paid to ASHAs [14]. Also, the data obtained from the district health office did not show any substantial difference in incentives received by ASHAs in the intervention and control areas. Therefore, the effect of ASHAs incentives on scale up cost was likely to be minimal on scale up costs.

The scale up cost analysis for Uttar Pradesh state was done from the health system perspective alone. It did not include cost for increased utilization of services because of following reasons. First, the choice of selection of two blocks was not random and specifically blocks were chosen from the worst performing high priority districts. The utilization rates of services in the other districts are likely to be better than the piloted blocks. Therefore, the effectiveness values obtained in these two blocks may not be generalized in the entire Uttar Pradesh state. Moreover, the contribution from the additional cost of increased utilization of services to overall cost is less than 3.5% in the 2 blocks where ReMiND was piloted. Thus, the effect on additional cost of utilization in entire state is expected to be even less than 3.5%. Hence, it is unlikely to make any significant difference in the scale up analysis. Also, scale-up costs were estimated in the ideal conditions without considering any bottlenecks in the implementation of programme which may deviate to some extent in the real life situations. The sudden changes like political & economic instability and introduction of newer programs may affect the program in one way or other. These uncertainties could not be accounted for in our analysis. Also, we acknowledge lack of data on time spent on supervisory and monitoring activities for which the data was taken from another study [29].

Finally, as there is a keen interest globally on the use of mobile health interventions, it is furthermore important to assess the cost- effectiveness of such interventions. Our analysis is a cost-outcome description and an attempt to study the scale-up costs to understand the fiscal challenges of scale-up. However, a full economic evaluation of ReMiND program from a societal perspective was also undertaken, the results of which has been published elsewhere [23, 52]. This economic analysis estimated the incremental cost of implementing ReMiND program per disability adjusted life year averted as a result of program's effectiveness on improving the maternal and child health outcomes. Overall, from a health system perspective, ReMiND incurred an incremental cost of INR 12,993 (USD 205) per DALY averted. From a societal perspective, ReMiND program was a cost saving intervention [52].

Conclusion

This study is the first cost analysis of a mHealth intervention for maternal & child health services in India. Our estimates on cost are useful for policy-makers and program managers in order to plan health programs. Overall the study findings on cost of mHealth are favourable from fiscal sustainability point of view.

Abbreviations
AF: Asha Facilitator; AMR: Annual Maintenance Rates; ASHA: Accredited Social Health Activist; BCM: Block Community Manager; CEAHH: Cost Effectiveness Analysis Household Survey; CHW: Community Health Workers; CPI: Consumer Price Index; CRS: Catholic Relief Services; DCPM: District Community Process Manager; HEO: Health Education Officer; IMR: Infant Mortality Rate; INR: Indian National Rupee; M & E: Monitoring and Evaluation; MH: Maternal health; mHealth: Mobile Health; MMR: Maternal Mortality Ratio; MNCH: Maternal, Newborn and Child Health; MoHFW: Ministry of Health and Family Welfare; NGO: Non- Government Organizations; NRHM: National Rural Health Mission; OOP: Out of Pocket; RCH: Reproductive & Child health; ReMiND: Reducing Maternal and Newborn Deaths; UP: Uttar Pradesh; USD: United States Dollar; WHO: World Health Organization

Acknowledgements
We gratefully acknowledge the implementing agencies of ReMiND program, namely; Catholic Relief Services, Vatsalya and Dimagi Inc., for providing data for undertaking costing of ReMiND program. We also recognize critical inputs from the Study Advisory Committee comprising Rajesh Kumar, Indrani Gupta, Stephen Jan, Krishna Rao, Pavitra Mohan, Meenu Singh, Jitendra Kumar, Rajani Ved, Ashok Jha, Neeta Rao, Suresh Dalpath, Prabhu Dayal, Rajesh Jha and Rajkumar Mishra.

Funding
The present study was funded by the United States' International Aid Agency (USAID), New Delhi, India. The funding agency has no role in the study design, collection of data, analysis or report writing.

Authors' contributions

Conception of study: SP. Study design and preparation of tool: AG, SP, PB. Data collection: AG, RN. Data Analysis: AG, SP. Written first Draft: AG. All authors reviewed the manuscript, provided critical inputs for revision, and approved the final version.

Competing interests

The authors' declare that they have no competing interests.

References

1. Ram U, Jha P, Ram F, Kumar K, Awasthi S, Shet A, Pader J, Nansukusa S, Kumar R. Neonatal, 1–59 month, and under-5 mortality in 597 Indian districts, 2001 to 2012: estimates from national demographic and mortality surveys. Lancet Glob Health. 2013;1(4):e219–26.
2. Press Information Bureau.Government of India. Ministry of Health and Family Welfare. List of High Priority Districts (HPDs) in the country http://pib. nic.in/newsite/PrintRelease.aspx?relid=118620. Accessed 24 May 2018.
3. Ministry of Home Affairs, Annual Health Survey Fact Sheet: Uttar Pradesh 2012–13 http://www.censusindia.gov.in/vital_statistics/AHSBulletins/AHS_Factsheets_2012-13/FACTSHEET-UTTAR_PRADESH.pdf. Accessed 4 Sept 2016.
4. UNICEF: The Situaton of Children in India: A profile. In.; May 2011.
5. Jaggi OP, Chattopadhyaya DP. Medicine in India: modern period. Oxford: Oxford University press; 2000.
6. NHM/MOHFW: InductionTraining Module for ASHAs in Urban Areas. In.
7. MoHFW, ASHA Training Modules, National health mission, Government of India http://nhm.gov.in/communitisation/asha/resources/asha-training-modules.html. Accessed 24 Aug 2016.
8. MoHFW, Training Modules for ASHA on NCD http://www.nhm.gov.in/communitisation/asha/resources/asha-training-modules.html. Accessed 24 Aug 2016.
9. Sundararaman T, Ved R, Gupta G, Samatha M. Determinants of functionality and effectiveness of community health workers: results from evaluation of ASHA program in eight Indian states. In: BMC proceedings: 2012: BioMed Central. 2012:O30.
10. Fathima FN, Raju M, Varadharajan KS, Krishnamurthy A, Ananthkumar S, Mony PK. Assessment of 'accredited social health activists'—a national community health volunteer scheme in Karnataka state, India. J Health Popul Nutr. 2015;33(1):137.
11. Saprii L, Richards E, Kokho P, Theobald S. Community health workers in rural India: analysing the opportunities and challenges accredited social health activists (ASHAs) face in realising their multiple roles. Hum Resour Health. 2015;13(1):95.
12. Bajpai N, Dholakia RH. Improving the performance of accredited social health activists in India. Mumbai: Columbia Global Centres South Asia. 2011.
13. Neogi S, Sharma J, Chauhan M, Khanna R, Chokshi M, Srivastava R, Prabhakar P, Khera A, Kumar R, Zodpey S. Care of newborn in the community and at home. J Perinatol. 2016;36(s3):S13.
14. Prinja S, Nimesh R, Gupta A, Pankaj B, Gupta M, Thakur JS. Impact of m-health application used by community health volunteers for improving utilization of maternal, newborn and child health care (MNCH) services in a rural area of Uttar Pradesh, India. Tropical Med Int Health. 2017. https://doi.org/10.1111/tmi.12895.
15. Little A, Medhanyie A, Yebyo H, Spigt M, Dinant GJ, Blanco R. Meeting community health worker needs for maternal health care service delivery using appropriate mobile technologies in Ethiopia. PLoS One. 2013;8(10):e77563.
16. Meankaew P, Kaewkungwal J, Khamsiriwatchara A, Khunthong P, Singhasivanon P, Satimai W. Application of mobile-technology for disease and treatment monitoring of malaria in the "better border healthcare Programme". Malar J. 2010;9:237.
17. Blanas DA, Ndiaye Y, MacFarlane M, Manga I, Siddiqui A, Velez O, Kanter AS, Nichols K, Hennig N. Health worker perceptions of integrating mobile phones into community case management of malaria in Saraya, Senegal. Int Health. 2015;7(3):176–82.
18. Ajay VS, Prabhakaran D. The scope of cell phones in diabetes management in developing country health care settings. J Diabetes Sci Technol. 2011;5(3):778–83.
19. Surka S, Edirippulige S, Steyn K, Gaziano T, Puoane T, Levitt N. Evaluating the use of mobile phone technology to enhance cardiovascular disease screening by community health workers. Int J Med Inform. 2014;83(9):648–54.
20. Kay M, Santos J, Takane M. mHealth: new horizons for health through mobile technologies. World Health Organ. 2011:66–71.
21. Prinja S, Chauhan AS, Angell B, Gupta I, Jan S. A systematic review of the state of economic evaluation for health care in India. Appl Health Econ Health Policy. 2015;13(6):595–613.
22. Kaushambi District : Census 2011 data http://www.census2011.co.in/census/district/545-kaushambi.html. Accessed 28 Aug 2016.
23. Prinja S, Nimesh R, Gupta A, Bahuguna P, Thakur JS, Gupta M, Singh T. Impact assessment and cost-effectiveness of m-health application used by community health workers for maternal, newborn and child health care services in rural Uttar Pradesh, India: a study protocol. Glob Health Action. 2016;9.
24. CRS. Baseline Study Summary: ReMiND - Reducing Maternal and Newborn Deaths. 2011–12. http://www.crs.org/sites/default/files/tools-research/baseline-study-summary-remind-reducing-maternal-newborn-deaths.pdf. Accessed 30 Aug 2016.
25. Annexure 6b: Module 6. Analysing Health Sector Financing and Expenditure http://www.who.int/hac/techguidance/tools/disrupted_sectors/module_06/en/index10.html. Accessed 10 Feb 2016.
26. Internal Revenue Service US: Yearly Average Currency Exchange Rates Translating foreign currency into U.S. dollars. In., Nov 2, 2015 edn.
27. Muennig P, Bounthavong M: Cost-effectiveness analysis in health: a practical approach: John Wiley & Sons; 2016.
28. Baltussen RM, Adam T, Tan-Torres Edejer T, Hutubessy RC, Acharya A, Evans DB, Murray CJ, World Health Organization. Making choices in health: WHO guide to cost-effectiveness analysis.
29. Larsen-Cooper E, Bancroft E, Rajagopal S, O'Toole M, Levin A. Scale matters: a cost-outcome analysis of an m-health intervention in Malawi. Telemedicine and e-Health. 2016;22(4):317–24.
30. Prinja S, Jeet G, Verma R, Kumar D, Bahuguna P, Kaur M, Kumar R. Economic analysis of delivering primary health care services through community health workers in 3 north Indian states. PLoS One. 2014;9(3):e91781.
31. Prinja S, Gupta A, Verma R, Bahuguna P, Kumar D, Kaur M, Kumar R. Cost of delivering health care services in public sector primary and community health centres in North India. PLoS One. 2016;11(8):e0160986.
32. Prinja S, Balasubramanian D, Jeet G, Verma R, Kumar D, Bahuguna P, Kaur M, Kumar R. Cost of delivering secondary-level health care services through public sector district hospitals in India. Indian J Med Res. 2017;146(3):354.
33. National Planning for Community Health Worker Programs http://www.mchip.net/sites/default/files/mchipfiles/03_CHW_Planning_0.pdf. Accessed 27 May 2018.
34. Policy and Guidelines. Guidelines for Community Processes 2014 http://nhsrcindia.org/index.php?option=com_content&view=article&id=152&Itemid=475. Accessed 2 June 2018.
35. Prinja S, Kaur G, Malhotra P, Jyani G, Ramachandran R, Bahuguna P, Varma S. Cost-effectiveness of autologous stem cell treatment as compared to conventional chemotherapy for treatment of multiple myeloma in India. Indian J Hematol Blood Transfus. 2017;33(1):31–40.
36. Kaur G, Prinja S, Malhotra P, Lad DP, Prakash G, Khadwal A, Ramachandran R, Varma S. Cost of treatment of multiple myeloma in a public sector tertiary Care Hospital of North India. Indian J Hematol Blood Transfus. 2018;34:1–7.

37. Kaur G, Prinja S, Ramachandran R, Malhotra P, Gupta KL, Jha V. Cost of hemodialysis in a public sector tertiary hospital of India, Clinical Kidney Journal, sfx152. https://doi.org/10.1093/ckj/sfx152.

38. Making choices in health: WHO guide to cost-effectiveness analysis http://apps.who.int/iris/bitstream/handle/10665/42699/9241546018.pdf;jsessionid=6AF3430426FB4D38FFD4FCB7393DBDB5?sequence=1. Accessed 2 June 2018.

39. Wilkinson T, Sculpher MJ, Claxton K, Revill P, Briggs A, Cairns JA, Teerawattananon Y, Asfaw E, Lopert R, Culyer AJ. The international decision support initiative reference case for economic evaluation: an aid to thought. Value Health. 2016;19(8):921–8.

40. The World Bank. Inflation, consumer prices (annual %) https://data.worldbank.org/indicator/FP.CPI.TOTL.ZG. Accessed 8 June 2018.

41. Narendra Modi speaks at AAPI Global Healthcare Summit. In.; 2014.

42. High Level Expert Group Report on Universal Health Coverage for India, Planning Commission of India http://planningcommission.nic.in/reports/genrep/rep_uhc0812.pdf. Accessed 24 Aug 2016.

43. Praveen D, Patel A, Raghu A, Clifford GD, Maulik PK, Abdul AM, Mogulluru K, Tarassenko L, MacMahon S, Peiris D. SMART Health India: development and field evaluation of a mobile clinical decision support system for cardiovascular diseases in rural India. JMIR mHealth and uHealth. 2014;2(4):e54.

44. Larsen-Cooper E, Bancroft E, Rajagopal S, O'Toole M, Levin A. Scale matters: a cost-outcome analysis of an m-health intervention in Malawi. Telemedicine and e-Health. 2015.

45. MacLeod BB, Phillips J, Stone A, Walji A, Awoonor-Williams JK. The architecture of a software system for supporting community-based primary health care with mobile technology: the mobile technology for community health (MoTeCH) initiative in Ghana. Online J Public Health Informat. 2012;4(1).

46. Lund S, Hemed M, Nielsen BB, Said A, Said K, Makungu M, Rasch V. Mobile phones as a health communication tool to improve skilled attendance at delivery in Zanzibar: a cluster-randomised controlled trial. BJOG Int J Obstet Gynaecol. 2012;119(10):1256–64.

47. Balasubramanian D, Prinja S, Aggarwal AK. Effect of user charges on secondary level surgical care utilization and out-of-pocket expenditures in Haryana state, India. PLoS One. 2015;10(5).

48. National Rural Health Mission 2005–12. Approval of state program implementation programme: Uttar Pradesh, 2013–14. In.

49. WHO, Estimating the cost of scaling-up maternal and newborn health interventions to reach universal coverage: methodology and assumptions. In.: Technical Working Paper. Prepared by the Department of Making Pregnancy Safer and Health Systems Financing for the World Health Report 2005: World Health Organization; 2005.

50. Socio-economic impact of mHealth. An assessment report for Brazil and Mexico https://www.pwc.in/assets/pdfs/consulting/strategy/socio-economic-impact-of-mhealth-brazil-and-mexico.pdf. Accessed 8 June 2018.

51. Delivery of maternal, neonatal and child health services in district Kaushambi, Uttar Pradesh (2011–2015): A descriptive report.

52. Prinja S, Bahuguna P, Gupta A, Nimesh R, Gupta M, Thakur JS. Cost effectiveness of mHealth intervention by community health workers for reducing maternal and newborn mortality in rural Uttar Pradesh, India. Cost Effectiveness and Resource Allocation : C/E, 16, 25. 2018. http://doi.org/10.1186/s12962-018-0110-2.

7

Maternal group B Streptococcus recto vaginal colonization increases the odds of stillbirth: evidence from Eastern Ethiopia

Tesfaye Assebe Yadeta[1,3,4*], Alemayehu Worku[2], Gudina Egata[3], Berhanu Seyoum[4], Dadi Marami[4] and Yemane Berhane[5]

Abstract

Background: Group B *Streptococcus* (GBS) causes a significant number of stillbirths. Despite this, there is little documented information on the association between stillbirth and pregnant women's GBS recto vaginal colonization in Sub Saharan Africa. As such, this study was aimed at identifying the association between stillbirth and pregnant women's GBS recto vaginal colonization in Eastern Ethiopia.

Methods: A health facility-based cross-sectional study was conducted among 1688 pregnant women who came for delivery service in Harar town, Eastern Ethiopia between June to October in 2016. Data were collected using a pre-tested structured questionnaire and checklist (which utilize clinical record). Group B *streptococcus* positivity of the pregnant women was confirmed by culture of recto vaginal swab using selective media. The association between GBS colonization and stillbirth was examined using multivariable logistic regression analysis. A statistical significance was declared at *p*-value ≤0.05.

Results: Of the 1688 pregnant women who participated in the study, 144 had stillbirths, representing a prevalence of 8.53% [(95% CI: (7.19, 9.86)]. Group B *Streptococcus* colonization at birth was detected in 231 women (13.68%; 95% CI 12.04, 15.32). Of these 144 stillbirths 59 (40.97%) were from colonized mothers and 72(59.03%) were from non-colonized mothers. Of these 59 stillbirth from colonized mothers, 32(54.23%) were intrapartum stillbirth, 27(45.77%) were antepartum stillbirth occur before exposed to intrapartum antibiotic prophylaxis (IAP). After controlling for potential confounders, the odds of having a stillbirth were 8.93 times higher among recto vaginal GBS colonized pregnant women [AOR = 8.93; 95% CI; (5.47, 14.56)].

Conclusions: This study demonstrated a significant association between maternal recto vaginal GBS colonization and stillbirth. Efforts to reduce stillbirth need to consider prevention of GBS colonization among pregnant women. Maternal vaccination may provide a feasible strategy to reduce stillbirth due to GBS.

Keywords: Stillbirth, GBS, Maternal recto vaginal colonization, Harar, Ethiopia

Background

The prevention of stillbirth remains a major global challenge. Of the estimated 2·6 million stillbirths that occur globally every year, 98% occur in low-income and middle-income countries [1]. Efforts to reduce stillbirths in low-income countries have not shown much progress.

Sub-Saharan Africa harbors the highest stillbirth rates with Ethiopia ranking fifth among the ten countries with the highest stillbirth rates in the world [1, 2].

Stillbirth is a major cause of psychosocial distress, grief and guilt to families [3]. In Sub Saharan Africa, mothers who have stillbirth are often subjected to severe psychosocial pressure; especially women who experience repeated stillbirth, can be out casted, dishonored and subjected to divorce [4, 5].

The causes of stillbirth vary greatly from country to country. In low income countries about one-third of all

* Correspondence: tesfaye.assebe@yahoo.com
[1]School of Nursing and Midwifery, College of Health and Medical Sciences, Haramaya University, Harar, Ethiopia
[3]School of Public Health, College of Health and Medical Sciences, Haramaya University, Harar, Ethiopia
Full list of author information is available at the end of the article

stillbirths are attributed to maternal infection during pregnancy [6]. Group B *Streptococcus* colonization and vertical transmission can cause fetal infection and still-birth as a direct result of toxin-induced cytolysis [7, 8]. Group B *Streptococcus* is estimated to account for 15% of all infection related stillbirths globally [9] and Africa harbor 73.68% of the estimated GBS caused stillbirth [10]. Other factors associated with stillbirth include: higher maternal age, residence, lower economic status, lower education level, poor antenatal care (ANC) uptake, antepartum hemorrhage, essential hypertension, pre-eclampsia, obstetric complication during labour, preterm delivery, low birth weight, and fetal mal-presentation [11, 12].

Stillbirths due to GBS are preventable [9, 13]. However, most of Sub-Saharan African countries do not have guidelines for the prevention of GBS infection, which could increase associated health risks to the mother and fetus [14]. The inaction could be related to a lack of evidence from the region. As such, this study assessed the association between GBS colonization and stillbirth in Eastern Ethiopia.

Methods
Study setting
This study was performed in three health facilities (Hiwot Fana Specialized University Hospital, Jugal Hospital and Arategna Health Center) in Harar town, Eastern Ethiopia. Harar is located 510 km east of the capital city of Ethiopia, Addis Ababa. Ethiopia is a low-income country with a total fertility rate of 4.6 per woman [15], stillbirth rates of 25.5 per 1000 birth [11], a neonatal mortality rate of 29 per 1000 live births [15] and 34.3% of neonatal deaths are due to infection [16].

Study design and sampling
A cross-sectional study was done between June and October 2016. The study participants were pregnant women came for delivery services at labour and delivery rooms of the selected health facilities. This study is part of a larger study conducted to assess GBS colonization among a total of 1688 singltone pregnant women. Women who recieved antibiotics in the last 2 weeks during their pregnancy prior to specimen collection and women who came due to vaginal bleeding prior to labour began, were excluded from this study [17, 18]. Study participants were taken proportional to the client load of the selected health facilities.

Data collection
Data were collected using a pretested and structured questionnaire. In addition, a checklist was used to extract data from the medical record, and a laboratory test was performed to detect GBS colonization from a recto-vaginal swab. The data collection tools were developed by reviewing previous related data collection instruments [15, 19]. The original questionnaire was prepared in English language and later translated into the local languages (Amharic and Afan Oromo) for data collection. Forward and backward translations were performed by language experts.

A six-day training was given to attending midwives and the supervisors who worked as data collectors. The training for data collectors and supervisors addressed issues related to data collection procedures and tools, interviewing techniques, medical record review and specimen collection procedures. Two medical microbiologists were read, confirm and interpret laboratory test results. Three medical laboratory technologists involved in media preparation and sterilization processes. A research manual was prepared to guide training, data collection and management.

Measurement
Stillbirth was the dependent variable in this study and this information was obtained from medical records. It was labelled as "yes" and "no" with a code of 1 and 0, respectively. ANC follow-up, hypertensive disease, women's GBS test result, prolonged labour, birth weight and gestational age were independent variables.

Age of the mother was documented based on maternal reply and later grouped as 15–19, 20–24, 25–29 and 30–34 and 35+ with code 1, 2, 3, 4 and 5, respectively for analysis. Maternal education was grouped as "literate" for those who could read and write and all others as "illiterate" and was coded 0 and 1, respectively. Number of births (parity) were grouped as one primiparity (one delivery), multiparous (2–4 delivery) and grand multiparous (≥ 5 deliveries) and code with 1, 2 and 3, respectively [20]. To determine the economic status of the families, wealth index was used. The wealth distribution was generated by applying principal components analysis to 33 household variables. The wealth status was determined by using three groups, poor as 1, middle as 2, and better as 3 [21].

Hypertesive disease and prolonged labour were obtained from the medical record and labeled as "yes" and "no" and coded with 1 and 0, respectively. Birth weight was categorized as < 2500 g and ≥ 2500 g and labeled as "yes" and "no" and code with 1 and 0, respectively. Similarly, gestational age was categorized as < 37 weeks and ≥ 37 weeks and labeled as "yes" and "no" and code with 1 and 0, respectively.

The specimens were collected by the attending midwives from the lower third of the vagina and rectum of women using a sterile cotton applicator. The specimens collection were performed at admission to the labour and delivery room of the selected health facilities. The laboratory procedure was done following the Center for Disease Control and Prevention (CDC) recommendation and Standard Operating Procedures described elsewhere [22, 23]. Details of specimen transportation and processing have been published previously [24]. A positive GBS reading was labeled as "yes" and a negative reading was labeled as "no".

Statistical analysis

Initially crude odds ratio (COR) along with 95% confidence interval was estimated to assess the association between each independent variable and the outcome variable. Variables with p-value ≤0.20 in the bivariable analyses were considered in the multivariable logistic regression model. Important variables deemed to be considered were also included, though they did not reach a p-value less than 0.20. Multicollinearity was tested using the Variance Inflation Factor (VIF) test, the tolerance test and values of the standard error. No multicollinearity problem was found. Correlation matrix and covariate matrix were tested for the final model. The final model selections were performed by: log likelihood ratio test, Akaike's information criterion, and Bayesian information criterion. The Hosmer-Lemeshow goodness-of-fit tests were used to test for model fitness [25]. The logistic regression model was used to assess the association between women's GBS recto vaginal colonization and the outcome variable (stillbirth) by controlling for other potential confounding variables. Adjusted Odds Ratio (AOR) along with 95% confidence interval was estimated to assess the strength of the association. Statistical significance was declared at a p-value ≤0.05.

Ethical approval and consent to participate

The study material was reviewed and approved by the Institutional Health Research Ethics Review Committee of the College of Health and Medical Sciences at Haramaya University. permission was obtained from each of the health facilities involved in the study. Women detected to have GBS colonization were provided antibiotic prophylaxis and women who had a stillbirth received counseling. Neonates with health problems were treated and immediate referral was also facilitated.

Results

The study enrolled a total of 1688 pregnant women. The age of participants ranged from 15 to 46 years with the mean (standard deviation) of 26.59 (± 5.63) years. Almost all (95.73%) of the participants were married, 47.04% had no formal education, and 44.14% were rural residents (Table 1). A large proportion (33.23%) of the pregnant women had never attended ANC at a health facility. The mean number of deliveries was 2.6 (with a range from 1 to 14). About 11 % of pregnant women had experienced hypertension, 23.22% had experienced prolonged labour, and 15.26% had low birth weight. Group

Table 1 Socio-demographic characteristics of the study participants Harar town, Eastern Ethiopia, 2016

Characteristics	Frequency (n)	Percent (%)
Residence of mothers		
Urban	943	55.86
Rural	745	44.14
Age of mothers in year		
≤ 19	301	17.83
20–24	510	30.21
25–29	461	27.31
30–34	275	16.29
≥ 35	141	8.35
Ethnicity		
Oromo	1214	71.92
Amhara	267	15.82
Harari	95	5.63
Somali	15	0.89
Other[a]	97	5.75
Religion		
Muslim	1286	76.18
Orthodox christian	308	18.25
Protestant	89	5.27
Catholic	5	0.3
Marital status		
Married	1616	95.73
Others[b]	72	4.27
Educational status		
Literate	894	52.96
Illiterate	794	47.04

Others[a] Gurage, Tigre, Silte,...; others[b] single, separated, divorced, widowed

B *Streptococcus* colonization at birth was detected in 231 (13.68%; 95% CI 12.04, 15.32) (Table 2).

The overall, 144 had stillbirths, representing a proportion of 8.53% [(95% CI: (7.19, 9.86)]. Of these 144 stillbirths 59 (40.97%) were from colonized mothers, 72(59.03%) were from non-colonized mothers. Of these 59 stillbirth from colonized mothers, 32(54.23%) were intrapartum stillbirth, 27(45.77%) were antepartum stillbirth occur before exposed to IAP (Table 3).

The multivariable logistic regression analysis revealed the odds of stillbirth was 8.93 times higher among recto vaginal GBS colonized pregnant women compared to those who had no colonization [AOR = 8.93; 95% CI; (5.47, 14.56)]. In addition, the odds for pregnant women who attended ANC follow-up was lower by 47% [AOR =0.53; 95% CI;(0.34, 0.82)]. The odds for pregnant women with hypertensive disorders was AOR = 4.66; 95% CI; (2.77, 7.8), for those with prolonged labor was AOR = 3.65; 95% CI: (2.38, 5.60), for

Table 2 Pregnancy, labour, and delivery related characteristics of the study participants Harar town, Eastern Ethiopia, 2016

Characteristics	Frequency (n)	Percent (%)
Para		
1	722	42.77
2–4	755	44.73
≥ 5	211	12.50
ANC follow up		
No	561	33.23
Yes	1127	66.77
Anemia		
No	1535	90.94
Yes	153	9.06
Hypertensive disease		
No	1502	88.98
Yes	186	11.02
Prolonged labour		
No	1296	76.78
Yes	392	23.22
Birth weight		
≥ 2500 g	1422	84.24
< 2500 g	266	15.76
Gestational age		
≥ 37 weeks	1540	91.23
< 37 weeks	148	8.77
GBS test result		
Negative	231	13.68
Positive	1457	86.32
IAP received		
No	964	57.11
Yes	724	42.89

IAP intrapartum antibiotic prophylaxis

those with low birth weight was AOR = 1.81; 95% CI: (1.09, 3.03), and preterm delivery AOR = 4.24; 95% CI: (2.41, 7.45) (Table 3).

Discussion

This study showed a strong association between still-births and maternal GBS colonization, even after controlling for other potential confounders. Other studies have also reported similar findings [26, 27]. It is evident that GBS cytolysis breaches maternal-fetal barriers ultimately causing intrauterine fetal death [7]. The stillbirths due to recto vaginal colonization of pregnant women are due to ascending infection. The genome sequencing studies have demonstrated the GBS isolated at birth from the skin of newborns were genetically identical to maternal GBS colonizing isolates [26].

Intrapartum antibiotic prophylaxis is highly effective in preventing newborn's GBS colonization [28]. However, there are limitations in the clinical benefit of IAP in reducing stillbirth. Antibiotics, for prophylaxis must be administered before the potential exposure, but stillbirth may occur before labour started [29]. In this study, 45.77% of stillbirths occurred before labour began.

Furthermore, identifying pregnant women who need IAP has been challenging for lower- and middle-income countries since most pregnant women did not attend ANC and most deliveries occur at home [30]. However, recent achievements in increasing coverage for the ANC and institutional/ facility delivery could improve the possibility of introducing screening, prevention and treatment interventions in routine ANC and delivery services.

Maternal vaccination could also be cost-effective to prevention programs since it can induce population-level herd immunity, address limitations in the clinical benefit of IAP in reducing stillbirth and late onset of neonatal GBS disease [31, 32]. Maternal immunization could protect the infant and fetus from invasive GBS disease. A clinical trials study, in South Africa, evaluated GBS polysaccharide-protein conjugate vaccine among pregnant women. The vaccine was well tolerated, had similar safety profiles with placebo, and induced capsular-specific antibody responses, in a women. Infant born from vaccinated pregnant women, resulted in higher GBS serotype-specific antibody concentrations [31, 33].

The burden of stillbirth on families, especially women, is severe and long lasting, yet stigma and taboo hinder this burden even in high-income countries. Mothers may be unlikely to seek medical care and such stillbirths could go unreported, thereby skewing or minimizing the actual reported cases of stillbirth [34]. Since women coming to health facilities for delivery could be those with better access to health services and perhaps more aware of the benefits of seeking health services for improved newborn health, the occurrence of stillbirth is likely to be an underestimation. One could also argue those women who opted for institutional delivery could be those with health problems the reported stillbirth represents an overestimation.

Antenatal care follow up was one of the predictors' of stillbirth. Similar findings were reported in other studies conducted in different part of the world [11, 35]. Despite this, ANC follow up was a protective for GBS related stillbirth. Only 32% of pregnant women had four recommended ANC visits in Ethiopia [15]. To achieve the sustainable development goal to end all preventable stillbirth and neonatal mortality, health promotion programs must better target those communities where maternal health care utilization is low. Urgent effective interventions are therefore needed to improve the ANC coverage as part of a stillbirth and neonatal reduction strategy.

Table 3 Factors associated with stillbirth among pregnant women, Harar, Eastern Ethiopia, 2016

Characteristics	Stillbirth	Live birth	Crude OR			Adjusted OR		
	n = 144(%)	n = 1544(%)	OR	95% CI		OR	95% CI	
GBS colonization								
No	5.83	94.17	1			1		
Yes	25.54	74.46	5.53	3.83	7.99	8.93***	5.47	14.56
ANC follow up								
No	15.15	84.85	1			1		
Yes	5.24	94.76	0.3	0.21	0.43	0.53**	0.34	0.82
Anemia								
No	7.88	92.12	1			1		
Yes	15.03	84.97	2.06	1.27	3.34	0.79	0.42	1.45
Hypertensive disorder								
No	6.32	93.68	1			1		
Yes	26.34	73.66	5.29	3.59	7.79	4.66***	2.77	7.84
Prolonged labour								
No	6.10	93.90	1			1		
Yes	16.58	83.42	3.06	2.15	4.34	3.65***	2.38	5.60
Para								
1	8.17	91.83	1			1		
2–4	8.21	91.79	1.00	0.69	1.45	1.46	0.88	2.42
≥ 5	10.90	89.10	1.31	0.82	2.28	1.29	0.58	2.92
Age of women								
≤ 19	10.63	89.37	1			1		
20–24	6.86	93.14	0.6	0.37	1.02	1.11	0.60	2.05
25–29	9.33	90.67	0.86	0.53	1.4	1.10	0.58	2.11
30–34	5.82	94.18	0.51	0.27	0.96	0.42	0.19	0.95
≥ 35	12.77	87.23	1.23	0.66	2.27	0.76	0.30	1.92
Resident								
Urban	5.20	94.80	1			1		
Rural	12.75	87.25	2.66	1.86	3.81	1.27	0.69	2.33
Educational status								
literate	6.26	93.74	1			1		
illiterate	11.08	88.92	1.86	1.31	2.64	1.13	0.69	1.83
Wealth status								
Poor	14.03	85.97	1			1		
Middle	7.00	93.00	0.46	.30	0.68	1.06	0.58	1.91
Better	4.45	95.55	0.28	0.17	0.45	0.65	0.29	1.44
Birth weight								
≥ 2500 g	5.98	94.02	1			1		
< 2500 g	22.18	77.82	4.48	3.11	6.44	1.81*	1.09	3.03
Gestational age								
≥ 37 weeks	5.97	94.03	1			1		
< 37 weeks	35.14	64.86	8.52	5.72	12.69	4.24***	2.41	7.45
IAP received								
No	7.37	92.63	1			1		
Yes	8.53	91.47	1.41	1.00	1.98	1.01	0.67	1.51

IAP intrapartum antibiotic prophylaxis, *OR* odds ratio, *CI* confidence intervals; * = *p*, 0.05; ** = *p*, 0.01; *** = *p*, 0.001

In this study preterm is significantly associated with still-birth, and this was consistent with previous study [35]. Furthermore, GBS ascending infection, resulting in infection of fetal membranes, decidua and fetus, causing premature rupture of the membrane. Prolonged exposure of the fetus to maternal bacterial flora without any protective membrane barrier enhances the transmission. Host inflammatory response stimulation of prostaglandin and protease synthesis are increases uterine contractility and results in preterm delivery [36]. Vascular insufficiency in pre-eclampsia reduces blood flow to the placenta, leading to hypoxia of the fetus which may also be associated with stillbirth [37, 38]. In prolonged labour, there is also an increased chance that a fetus will suffer from asphyxia due to umbilical cord compression, placental abruption, maternal low blood pressure and birth trauma. Problems with the placenta pose risks to the fetus, including lack of oxygen and nutrients, which can impair fetal growth and could also lead to low birth weight and preterm delivery [12, 39].

The strengths of this study were that a relatively high number of participants included and the study obtained swab samples from both the rectum and vagina, which help to improve the yield [40]. All swabs were transported in Amie's transport media to the Medical Microbiology Laboratory within 4 h of collection [41]. Selective and differential media were used to isolate and GBS [23].

Measurement and diagnostic biases were minimized by assigning two medical microbiology experts to measure and read the results. Thus, the procedures used was believed to help to reasonably estimate the association. As limitations, the data obtained from the medical records may be potential sources of biases. This has been minimized through verifying the data by the study team before discharging the mother and newborn. Moreover, collecting of microbiological evidence of invasive GBS infection from a normally sterile site, such as fetal blood from the umbilical cord or from the heart, lung aspirate, cerebrospinal fluid or fetal tissues as recommended [42] were not done due to resource constraints. Moreover, immunologic and placenta investigations were also not possible in this setting. Finally, unaccounted and residual confounding could have had an effect on the association found [43, 44].

Conclusions

This study identified a strong association between maternal recto vaginal colonization of GBS and stillbirth. Efforts to reduce stillbirth need to consider prevention of colonization by GBS among pregnant women. Further stillbirth reduction efforts need to consider introducing effective prevention strategies and improving the quality of the ANC and intrapartum care. Maternal vaccination may provide feasible strategy to reduce stillbirth due to GBS.

Abbreviations

ANC: Antenatal care; CDC: Center of disease control and prevention; GBS: Group B streptococcus; IAP: Intrapartum antibiotic prophylaxis; LMICS: Low-and-middle income countries; SDG: Sustainable development goal; SOPS: Standard Operating Procedures

Acknowledgements

The authors would like to thank Haramaya University for financial support, Addis Continental Institute of Public Health for technical support, the study participants, data collectors, and staff of the Department of Medical Laboratory Sciences, College of Health and Medical Sciences for their kind cooperation.

Funding

This study was financially supported by Haramaya University.

Authors' contributions

TA, AW, GE, BS and YB conceived and designed the paper, involved in data collection, performed the statistical analysis, interpret the results, wrote and reviewed the manuscript. DM interprets the result, wrote and reviewed the manuscript. All authors read and approved the final version of manuscript before submission.

Competing interests

The authors declare that they have no competing interests.

Author details

[1]School of Nursing and Midwifery, College of Health and Medical Sciences, Haramaya University, Harar, Ethiopia. [2]Department of Epidemiology and Biostatistics, School of Public Health, Addis Ababa University, Addis Ababa, Ethiopia. [3]School of Public Health, College of Health and Medical Sciences, Haramaya University, Harar, Ethiopia. [4]Department of Medical Laboratory Sciences, College of Health and Medical Sciences, Haramaya University, Harar, Ethiopia. [5]Department of Epidemiology, Addis Continental Institute of Public Health, Addis Ababa, Ethiopia.

References

1. Lawn JE, Blencowe H, Waiswa P, Amouzou A, Mathers C, Hogan D, Flenady V, Frøen JF, Qureshi ZU, Calderwood C. Stillbirths: rates, risk factors, and acceleration towards 2030. Lancet. 2016;387(10018):587–603.
2. Wang H, Bhutta ZA, Coates MM, Coggeshall M, Dandona L, Diallo K, Franca EB, Fraser M, Fullman N, Gething PW. Global, regional, national, and selected subnational levels of stillbirths, neonatal, infant, and under-5 mortality, 1980-2015: a systematic analysis for the Global Burden of Disease Study 2015. Lancet. 2016;388(10053):1725.

3. Gopichandran V, Subramaniam S, Kalsingh MJ. Psycho-social impact of stillbirths on women and their families in Tamil Nadu, India–a qualitative study. BMC pregnancy and childbirth. 2018;18(1):109.

4. Kiguli J, Namusoko S, Kerber K, Peterson S, Waiswa P. Weeping in silence: community experiences of stillbirths in rural eastern Uganda. Glob Health Action. 2015;8(1):24011.

5. Sisay MM, Yirgu R, Gobezayehu AG, Sibley LM. A qualitative study of attitudes and values surrounding stillbirth and neonatal mortality among grandmothers, mothers, and unmarried girls in rural Amhara and Oromiya regions, Ethiopia: unheard souls in the backyard. Journal of Midwifery & Women's Health. 2014;59(s1).

6. Engmann C, Garces A, Jehan I, Ditekemena J, Phiri M, Mazariegos M, Chomba E, Pasha O, Tshefu A, McClure E. Causes of community stillbirths and early neonatal deaths in low-income countries using verbal autopsy: an international, multicenter study. J Perinatol. 2012;32(8):585.

7. Randis TM, Gelber SE, Hooven TA, Abellar RG, Akabas LH, Lewis EL, Walker LB, Byland LM, Nizet V, Ratner AJ, Group B. Streptococcus β-hemolysin/cytolysin breaches maternal-fetal barriers to cause preterm birth and intrauterine fetal demise in vivo. J Infect Dis. 2014;210(2):265–73.

8. Waldorf KMA, Gravett MG, McAdams RM, Paolella LJ, Gough GM, Carl DJ, Bansal A, Liggitt HD, Kapur RP, Reitz FB. Choriodecidual group B streptococcal inoculation induces fetal lung injury without intra-amniotic infection and preterm labor in Macaca nemestrina. PLoS One. 2011;6(12):e28972.

9. Madhi SA, Dangor Z. Prospects for preventing infant invasive GBS disease through maternal vaccination. Vaccine. 2017.

10. Lawn JE, Bianchi-Jassir F, Russell NJ, Kohli-Lynch M, Tann CJ, Hall J, Madrid L, Baker CJ, Bartlett L, Cutland C. Group B streptococcal disease worldwide for pregnant women, stillbirths, and children: why, what, and how to undertake estimates? Clin Infect Dis. 2017;65(suppl_2):S89–99.

11. Berhie KA, Gebresilassie HG. Logistic regression analysis on the determinants of stillbirth in Ethiopia. Maternal health, neonatology and perinatology. 2016;2(1):10.

12. Chuwa FS, Mwanamsangu AH, Brown BG, Msuya SE, Senkoro EE, Mnali OP, Mazuguni F, Mahande MJ. Maternal and fetal risk factors for stillbirth in northern Tanzania: a registry-based retrospective cohort study. PLoS One. 2017;12(8):e0182250.

13. Bhutta ZA, Das JK, Bahl R, Lawn JE, Salam RA, Paul VK, Sankar MJ, Blencowe H, Rizvi A, Chou VB. Can available interventions end preventable deaths in mothers, newborn babies, and stillbirths, and at what cost? Lancet. 2014; 384(9940):347–70.

14. Seale AC, Bianchi-Jassir F, Russell NJ, Kohli-Lynch M, Tann CJ, Hall J, Madrid L, Blencowe H, Cousens S, Baker CJ. Estimates of the burden of group B streptococcal disease worldwide for pregnant women, stillbirths, and children. Clin Infect Dis. 2017;65(suppl_2):S200–19.

15. Central Statistical Agency (CSA) [Ethiopia] and ICF: Ethiopia Demographic and Health Survey 2016. In. Addis Ababa, Ethiopia, and Rockville, Maryland, USA: CSA and ICF; 2016.

16. Debelew GT, Afework MF, Yalew AW. Determinants and causes of neonatal mortality in Jimma zone, Southwest Ethiopia: a multilevel analysis of prospective follow up study. PLoS One. 2014;9(9):e107184.

17. McNanley AR, Glantz JC, Hardy DJ, Vicino D. The effect of intrapartum penicillin on vaginal group B streptococcus colony counts. Am J Obstet Gynecol. 2007;197(6):583. e581–4.

18. Bailey P, Lobis S, Maine D, Fortney JA. Monitoring emergency obstetric care: a handbook: World Health Organization; 2009.

19. Getachew A, Ricca J, Cantor D, Rawlins B, Rosen H, Tekleberhan A, Bartlett L, Gibson H. Quality of care for prevention and management of common maternal and newborn complications: a study of Ethiopia's hospitals. Baltimore: Jhpiego; 2011.

20. Mgaya AH, Massawe SN, Kidanto HL, Mgaya HN. Grand multiparity: is it still a risk in pregnancy? BMC pregnancy and childbirth. 2013;13(1):241.

21. Vyas S, Kumaranayake L. Constructing socio-economic status indices: how to use principal components analysis. Health Policy Plan. 2006;21(6):459–68.

22. Cheesbrough M: District laboratory practice in tropical countries: Cambridge university press; 2006.

23. Verani JR, McGee L, Schrag SJ: Prevention of perinatal group B streptococcal disease: revised guidelines from CDC, 2010. 2010.

24. Yadeta TA, Worku A, Egata G, Seyoum B, Marami D, Berhane Y. Vertical transmission of group B Streptococcus and associated factors among pregnant women: a cross-sectional study, eastern Ethiopia. Infection and drug resistance. 2018;11:397.

25. Blizzard L, Hosmer W. Parameter estimation and Goodnessâ€ of â €fit in log binomial regression. Biom J. 2006;48(1):5–22.

26. Seale AC, Koech AC, Sheppard AE, Barsosio HC, Langat J, Anyango E, Mwakio S, Mwarumba S, Morpeth SC, Anampiu K. Maternal colonization with Streptococcus agalactiae and associated stillbirth and neonatal disease in coastal Kenya. Nature microbiology. 2016;1:16067.

27. Nan C, Dangor Z, Cutland C, Edwards M, Madhi S, Cunnington M. Maternal group B Streptococcus-related stillbirth: a systematic review. BJOG Int J Obstet Gynaecol. 2015;122(11):1437–45.

28. Lin F-YC, Weisman LE, Azimi P, Young AE, Chang K, Cielo M, Moyer P, Troendle JF, Schneerson R, Robbins JB. Assessment of intrapartum antibiotic prophylaxis for the prevention of early-onset group B streptococcal disease. Pediatr Infect Dis J. 2011;30(9):759.

29. Arnold KC, Flint CJ. Use of prophylactic antibiotics in labor and delivery. In: Obstetrics Essentials. edn: Springer; 2017. p. 129–33.

30. Nishihara Y, Dangor Z, French N, Madhi S, Heyderman R: Challenges in reducing group B Streptococcus disease in African settings. Arch Dis Child 2016:archdischild-2016-311419.

31. Madhi SA, Koen A, Cutland CL, Jose L, Govender N, Wittke F, Olugbosi M, Sobanjo-ter Meulen A, Baker S, Dull PM. Antibody kinetics and response to routine vaccinations in infants born to women who received an investigational trivalent group B Streptococcus polysaccharide CRM197-conjugate vaccine during pregnancy. Clin Infect Dis. 2017;65(11):1897–904.

32. Kwatra G, Adrian PV, Shiri T, Izu A, Cutland CL, Buchmann EJ, Madhi SA. Serotype-specific cell-mediated immunity associated with clearance of homotypic group B Streptococcus rectovaginal colonization in pregnant women. J Infect Dis. 2016;213(12):1923–6.

33. Madhi SA, Cutland CL, Jose L, Koen A, Govender N, Wittke F, Olugbosi M, Sobanjo-ter Meulen A, Baker S, Dull PM. Safety and immunogenicity of an investigational maternal trivalent group B streptococcus vaccine in healthy women and their infants: a randomised phase 1b/2 trial. Lancet Infect Dis. 2016;16(8):923–34.

34. Kobayashi M, Vekemans J, Baker CJ, Ratner AJ, Le Doare K, Schrag SJ, Group B. Streptococcus vaccine development: present status and future considerations, with emphasis on perspectives for low and middle income countries. F1000Research. 2016;5.

35. Ashish K, Wrammert J, Ewald U, Clark RB, Gautam J, Baral G, Baral KP, Målqvist M. Incidence of intrapartum stillbirth and associated risk factors in tertiary care setting of Nepal: a case-control study. Reprod Health. 2016;13(1):103.

36. Vornhagen J, Armistead B, Santana-Ufret V, Gendrin C, Merillat S, Coleman M, Quach P, Boldenow E, Alishetti V, Leonhard-Melief C. Group B streptococcus exploits vaginal epithelial exfoliation for ascending infection. J Clin Invest. 2018;128(5).

37. Myatt L, Muralimanoharan S, Maloyan A. Effect of preeclampsia on placental function: influence of sexual dimorphism, microRNA's and mitochondria. In: Advances in Fetal and Neonatal Physiology edn: Springer; 2014. p. 133–46.

38. Stark MJ, Dierkx L, Clifton V, Wright IM. Alterations in the maternal peripheral microvascular response in pregnancies complicated by preeclampsia and the impact of fetal sex. J Soc Gynecol Investig. 2006;13(8):573–8.

39. Gordon A, Raynes-Greenow C, McGeechan K, Morris J, Jeffery H. Risk factors for antepartum stillbirth and the influence of maternal age in New South Wales Australia: a population based study. BMC pregnancy and childbirth. 2013;13(1):12.

40. Moussa TA, Elsherif RH, Mohamed YA, Dawoud ME, AboElAref AM. Group B streptococcus colonization of pregnant women: comparative molecular and microbiological diagnosis. Comp Clin Pathol. 2013;22(6):1229–34.

41. El Aila NA, Tency I, Claeys G, Saerens B, De Backer E, Temmerman M, Verhelst R, Vaneechoutte M. Genotyping of Streptococcus agalactiae (group B streptococci) isolated from vaginal and rectal swabs of women at 35-37 weeks of pregnancy. BMC Infect Dis. 2009;9(1):153.

42. Seale AC, Blencowe H, Bianchi-Jassir F, Embleton N, Bassat Q, Ordi J, Menéndez C, Cutland C, Briner C, Berkley JA. Stillbirth with group B Streptococcus disease worldwide: systematic review and meta-analyses. Clin Infect Dis. 2017;65(suppl_2):S125–32.

43. Glass TA, Goodman SN, Hernán MA, Samet JM. Causal inference in public health. Annu Rev Public Health. 2013;34:61–75.

44. Khong TY, Mooney EE, Ariel I, Balmus NC, Boyd TK, Brundler M-A, Derricott H, Evans MJ, Faye-Petersen OM, Gillan JE. Sampling and definitions of placental lesions: Amsterdam placental workshop group consensus statement. Archives of pathology & laboratory medicine. 2016;140(7):698–713.

8

Breech birth at home: outcomes of 60 breech and 109 cephalic planned home and birth center births

Stuart James Fischbein[1] and Rixa Freeze[2]*

Abstract

Background: Research on outcomes of out-of-hospital breech birth is scarce. This study evaluates the outcomes of singleton term breech and cephalic births in a home or birth center setting.

Methods: This is a retrospective observational cohort study of 60 breech and 109 cephalic planned out-of-hospital term singleton births during a 6 year period with a single obstetrician. Outcomes measured included mode of delivery; birth weights; 1 & 5-min Apgar scores; ante-, intra-, and post-partum transports; perineal integrity; and other maternal and neonatal morbidity.

Results: 50 breech and 102 cephalic presentations were still in the obstetrician's care at the onset of labor; of those, 10 breech and 11 cephalic mothers required transport during labor. 76% of breech and 92.2% of cephalic births were planned to occur at home, with the remainder at a freestanding birth center. When compared to the cephalic group, the breech group had a higher rate of antepartum and in-labor transfer of care and cesarean section. Among completed out-of-hospital births, the breech group had a significantly higher rate of 1-min Apgar scores < 7 but no significant difference at 5 min. Rates of vaginal birth for both groups were high, with 84% of breech and 97.1% of cephalic mothers giving birth vaginally in this series. Compared to primiparas, multiparas in both groups had less perineal trauma and higher rates of out-of-hospital birth, vaginal birth, and spontaneous vaginal birth. No breech infant or mother required postpartum hospital transport, while one cephalic infant and one cephalic mother required postpartum transport. Of the babies born out-of-hospital, there was one short-term and one longer-term birth injury among the breech group and one short-term brachial plexus injury in the cephalic group.

Conclusions: A home or birth center setting leads to high rates of vaginal birth and good maternal outcomes for both breech and cephalic term singleton presentations. Out-of-hospital vaginal breech birth under specific protocol guidelines and with a skilled provider may be a reasonable choice for women wishing to avoid a cesarean section—especially when there is no option of a hospital breech birth. However, this study is underpowered to calculate uncommon adverse neonatal outcomes.

Keywords: Breech, Vaginal breech delivery, Delivery mode, Home birth, Birth center, Out-of-hospital birth, Upright birth, Physiological birth, Autonomy, Informed consent

* Correspondence: rixa.freeze@gmail.com
[2]Wabash College, 211 Center Hall, Crawfordsville, IN 47933, USA
Full list of author information is available at the end of the article

Background

The options for term vaginal breech birth (VBB) have rapidly declined in the western world. This decline began in the 1980s and has led to the removal of training of breech skills from most residency programs. This trend was codified, in large part, by the 2000 Term Breech Trial (TBT), which found poorer outcomes for planned vaginal breech births compared to planned cesareans for term singleton babies [1]. Counseling for term breech pregnancies often steers women towards cesarean section and only addresses short-term risks to the baby [2]. The TBT has drawn criticism for flaws in its study design, case selection, and intrapartum care practices across the 174 participating centers [3–6]. In addition, the 2-year follow-up study found no long-term difference in death or neurodevelopmental delay among a subset of the overall TBT cohort [7].

Since that time there have been well over 100 single-center, multi-center, and birth certificate/national registry studies published on term breech outcomes, some of which recommend routine cesarean and others which support the option of a planned vaginal birth. The RCOG's 2017 breech guideline is the most up-to-date compilation of the body of post-TBT literature [8]. The most influential study since the TBT has been the 2006 PREMODA study, a multicenter prospective observational study of 2526 planned vaginal and 5579 planned cesareans births [9]. With a cohort nearly four times the size of the TBT and with strict selection criteria and protocols, the PREMODA study did not find any significant differences in outcomes between planned vaginal breech birth (pVBB) and planned cesarean section (pCS).

Cochrane reviews have also moved from certainty regarding recommended mode of delivery for term breech immediately following the TBT [10] to complex uncertainty, acknowledging in 2015 that performing a cesarean should "be weighed against factors such as the mother's preferences for vaginal birth and risks such as future pregnancy complications in the woman's specific healthcare setting" [11]. The 2015 review also noted that the TBT data are not generalizable to dissimilar settings or in places where delivery techniques and protocols "differ materially." Due to these developments since the TBT, the national obstetric societies of the USA (ACOG), Canada (SOGC), UK (RCOG), and Australia & New Zealand (RANZCOG) have all reversed their early-2000 guidelines recommending routine cesarean beginning in 2006 and now currently support properly selected VBB for term singleton fetuses [8, 12–14].

The 2015 Cochrane review also recommended research on how to "improve the safety of breech delivery." The most notable research and innovations have come from midwives and obstetricians around the world exploring breech birth with mothers in upright positions

[15–24]. In particular, Louwen's 2017 study of 740 term breech births in Frankfurt (433 pVBB and 314 pCS) found that upright vaginal breech birth leads to a shorter 2nd stage, fewer cesareans, less intervention, fewer maneuvers, and fewer injuries to mother and baby, compared to on-the-back positions [15]. In addition to research indicating that cesarean section might not be the universal solution for term breech presentation, there is growing awareness of the importance of vaginal birth and of the risks of cesarean section on the long-term health of the baby and mother [25–30].

Medical ethics recognizes that patient autonomy in decision making should be honored [31]. In 2016 ACOG produced a committee opinion strongly supporting maternal autonomy, including the right of pregnant women to refuse a recommended treatment [32]. Despite good evidence, ethical arguments, and organizational support for the option of vaginal breech birth, there has been a concerted effort to eliminate VBB in most American hospitals, including outright bans. As hospitals continue to restrict or ban vaginal breech birth, some women will give birth at home or in birth centers to avoid a mandatory cesarean section. Some women also choose to give birth unassisted (with no care provider). Some state legislatures, including in CA where SJF practices, have recently restricted midwives from attending OOH breech births, further narrowing women's options.

Research on outcomes of planned breech home or birth center birth is sparse; the two main datasets that include a subset of home breech births are the MANA Statistics Project and the National Vital Statistics System Natality Data Files [33–36]. Both show an increased risk of adverse outcomes for breech birth at home compared to cephalic babies. Citing the outcomes reported in Cheyney 2014 [36], ACOG considers fetal malpresentation an absolute contraindication to planned home birth [37]. These datasets did not have information about practitioner education or skill level in breech, selection criteria, labor management protocols, or maternal motivations for seeking an out-of-hospital breech birth. Without this information, it is difficult to determine what causes the higher rates of adverse outcomes. Our study examines outcomes for vaginal breech birth outside of a hospital for well-selected women attended by an experienced practitioner.

Methods

This paper is a retrospective analysis of a series of planned out-of-hospital births: 60 term breech and 109 term cephalic presentations. All were under the care of a single obstetrician and occurred between August 2010 and April 2017. We excluded VBACs from this analysis to eliminate the confounding factor of a scarred uterus; we hope to analyze both cephalic & breech VBACs in a separate paper. The birth team consisted of an obstetrician (SJF), a licensed midwife, and a midwifery student. SJF has been in private practice in greater Los Angeles since 1986 and has attended close to 200 vaginal breech births. In 2010, SJF's admitting hospital instituted a breech and VBAC ban, prompting SJF to continue offering these birth options in an out-of-hospital setting.

Equipment brought to each birth included IV fluids and tubing, sterile gloves, gauze, pads, betadine, suture material, and instruments. The birth team also supplied an inflatable birth pool. Medications included antibiotics, lidocaine, oxytocin, misoprostol, oral methylergonovine, vitamin K, and oxygen. In this series SJF also carried a portable GE Voluson ultrasound, a Masimo pulse oximeter, a Mityvac vacuum, Piper forceps, Simpson forceps, and Tucker-McLean forceps. All licensed practitioners were certified in neonatal resuscitation and cardio-pulmonary resuscitation.

The women in this series were all in good health and received prenatal care with an obstetrician, a midwife, or a collaboration of both. Most of the cephalic clients self-selected the option of home birth at an early gestational age and experienced continuity of care throughout their pregnancies. In contrast, most of the breech mothers entered into SJF's care late in pregnancy after discovering the breech presentation and after unsuccessful attempts to turn the baby.

Most women with breech babies tried chiropractic Webster technique, acupuncture with moxabustion, inversions, and Spinning Babies exercises [38]. Most were offered external cephalic version (ECV). Clients who were not good candidates, who declined ECV, or for whom ECV was unsuccessful were counseled regarding all available options for giving birth to their breech baby. In the Los Angeles metropolitan area, this included scheduled cesarean section (easily available), cesarean section at the onset of labor (not easily available), vaginal breech birth in a hospital where breech-skilled physicians were on call intermittently (rarely available), or an OOH breech birth with SJF (available 24/7 except when he was out of town).

Women in both cohorts were not excluded for conditions that were unlikely to affect labor such as diet-controlled gestational diabetes, mild chronic hypertension, or age over 35. Cephalic babies did not have an upper estimated fetal weight (EFW) limit, while breech babies did. Planned OOH births could occur from 36 weeks + 0 days onward. The data were not analyzed prior to completion of the 50th breech birth.

Term breech clients were selected and labor was managed according to these 8 basic criteria (asterisks indicate criteria shared among cephalic clients):

1) Frank or complete breech presentation
2) Flexed or neutral head (confirmed by ultrasound)
3) EFW between 5 and 9.5lbs (~ 2250–4300 g)
4) Clinically adequate maternal pelvis by history and/ or exam
5) No gross anomalies*
6) Spontaneous labor; no induction or augmentation*
7) Fetal and maternal tolerance of labor*
8) Well-informed and motivated parents*

The midwifery model of care encourages settings where women feel "free, safe, and private" [39]. Breech and cephalic labors were managed identically with two minor exceptions: for breech, water birth was discouraged and an initial vaginal exam was offered upon SJF's arrival. In all 152 labors women were encouraged to eat and drink, ambulate, change positions, and choose their birth location and position. Both breech and cephalic women had the option of a shower and tub for labor analgesia; water birth for breech births was not preferred due the higher likelihood of assistance.

Fetal monitoring was performed intermittently with a Nicolet Elite 200 Handheld Doppler. Auscultation was individualized but the usual protocol was every 30–60 min in active labor, every 15–30 min in transition and every 5–10 min in second stage. With the breech labors SJF offered an initial vaginal exam in labor to confirm fetal position. Otherwise, vaginal exams were kept to a minimum, often withheld until maternal guttural vocalizations signaled an urge to push.

Pushing only began when maternal urge became irresistible; pushing was spontaneous rather than coached. Breech mothers were encouraged to labor down before active pushing began. Passage of pasty meconium was considered a positive sign of descent. Breech mothers were counseled about the benefits of upright and hands-off techniques. On-the-back positioning for breech was used on an as-needed basis and with maternal consent. Delayed cord clamping (usually until the placenta was birthed or later) and immediate and uninterrupted skin-to-skin were routine for both groups. Footage of a primip frank breech birth with SJF is available to view at https://vimeo.com/45678615 [40]. The baby was 39 ½ weeks gestation, weighed 2890 g, and had 1 & 5 min Apgars of 8 and 9.

This project received approval from the Wabash College IRB (IRB# 1610303). Written or verbal consent from participants was not required since the project used de-identified data extracted from medical records.

Data were analyzed using Stata version 14.1. We employed Fisher's exact test for categorical data and t-test for continuous data. A p-value of < 0.05 was considered statistically significant.

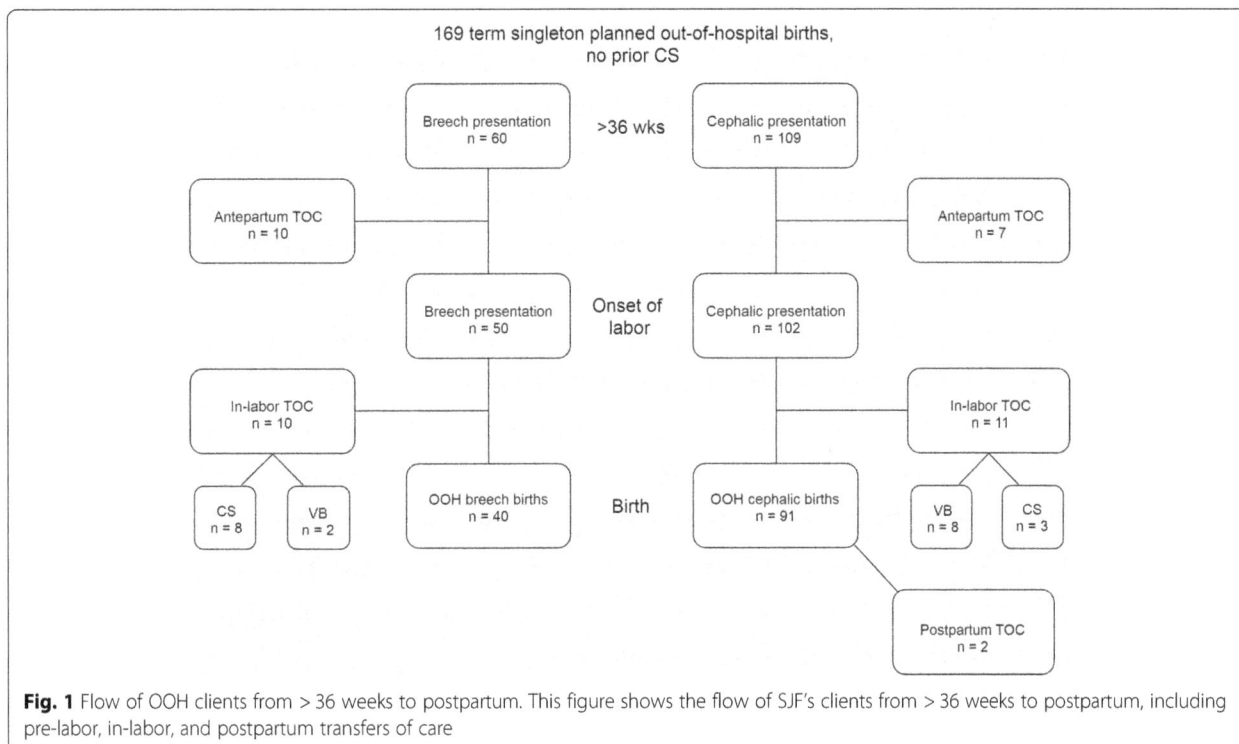

Fig. 1 Flow of OOH clients from > 36 weeks to postpartum. This figure shows the flow of SJF's clients from > 36 weeks to postpartum, including pre-labor, in-labor, and postpartum transfers of care

Results

A total of 169 pregnant women entered into care at term (see Fig. 1). Antepartum transfer of care (TOC) occurred for 10 breech mothers (16.7%) and 7 cephalic mothers (6.4%; see Table 1). The cephalic mother complaining of decreased fetal movement at 37 weeks had a poor biophysical profile and underwent an urgent cesarean section. The IUFD at 39 weeks was due to an avulsion of a velamentous umbilical cord insertion.

Table 1 Reasons for antenatal transfer of care to a hospital-based provider

Indication for transfer	Breech n = 60	Cephalic n = 109
> 41 wks, suspected macrosomia	1	
Cholestasis	1	
SJF out of town	3	
Oligohydramnios	2	
SPROM > 5 days, NIL (not in labor)	1	
> 42 wks, NIL	2	1
37 wks, preeclampsia		1
39 wks, IUFD		1
43 wks, polyhydramnios		1
39 wks, increasing hypertension		1
37 wks, decreased fetal activity, NIL		1
DVT (blood clot)		1
Total antenatal transfers	10 (16.7%)	7 (6.4%)

After these 17 transfers of care, there were 50 breech and 102 cephalic full-term women still under SJF's care when they went into spontaneous labor. Table 2 presents maternal, fetal, and obstetric characteristics of these two groups at the onset of labor.

A significantly higher proportion of the breech group were first-time mothers compared to the cephalic group. The mean gestational age was not statistically significant. Breech babies had a significantly lower mean birthweight than cephalic babies (3274 g vs 3606 g), possibly due to the upper EFW limit for breech but not for cephalic presentations. This trend is visible in the number of babies below the 10th or above the 90th birth weight percentiles.

57% of the breech babies were female, similar to a reported rate of 56.7% among Dutch babies born during the 40th gestational week [41]. We are missing complete data on maternal age, pre-pregnancy weight, pregnancy weight gain, and length of 1st stage and therefore did not include those factors in this analysis.

Table 3 examines the location of birth and the mode of birth for both groups, sorted by parity. The overall cesarean rate was 16% in the breech group and 2.9% in the cephalic group; all cesareans were among primiparous clients. All multips in both groups had 100% rates of spontaneous vaginal birth. Of the 41 breech primips, 31 (75.6%) gave birth vaginally OOH, compared to 50 of the 60 cephalic primips (83.3%). Four breech primips were assisted with Piper forceps, all in the early years of the series before SJF adopted upright breech techniques.

Table 2 Maternal, fetal, and obstetric characteristics of the study population at onset of labor

Characteristic	Breech n = 50	Cephalic n = 102	P value
Parity			0.006
Primipara	41 (82.0%)	59 (57.8%)	
Multipara	9 (18.0%)	43 (42.2%)	
Type of breech			
Frank	45 (90.0%)	NA	
Complete	5 (10.0%)	NA	
Planned location of birth			
Home	38 (76.0%)	94 (92.2%)	
Birth center	12 (24.0%)	8 (7.9%)	
Mean birthweight (range)[a]	3274 g (2410–4224)	3606 g (2325–5046)	0.0002
Birthweight percentiles[b]			
< 10th	10 (20.8%)	11 (11.0%)	
> 90th	1 (2.1%)	16 (16.0%)	
Mean wks gestation (range)[c]	39.9 (37–42)	40.1 (35–44)	0.154

[a] Birthweights were not recorded for 2 cephalic and 2 breech infants; one infant from each group was a hospital transport
[b] Compared against percentile tables in Talge 2014 [69]
[c] Weeks gestation were recorded as a rounded average, i.e. 37 weeks = 36 4/7 to 37 3/7

Upright positioning for breech birth (hands & knees, kneeling, or standing) occurred in 11 (27.5%) of the forty successful OOH breech births, while the other 29 (72.5%) used a modified lithotomy position.

Only 5 (10%) of the 50 breech women had babies in a complete breech position; 4 of these had an OOH vaginal breech birth and the 5th transferred to a hospital for arrest at 7 cm. Of the 45 frank presentations, 36 gave birth vaginally OOH and the other 9 women (all primips) transferred in labor, leading to 2 operative vaginal breech births and 7 cesareans.

In-labor transports
We do not have access to complete medical records for the in-labor transports, which limits our ability to analyze some outcomes on an intention-to-treat basis. All 10 in-labor breech transports were primiparas and were transported for arrested labor/descent at or beyond 6 cm (n = 7) or during second stage (n = 3) (Table 4). None were emergent when the decision to transport was made. Six had a non-emergent cesarean section upon admission; these babies did well and none required NICU admission. The seventh mother transferred for a stalled labor at 7 cm and prolonged rupture of membranes. She was afebrile with normal maternal vital signs and reassuring structured intermittent fetal auscultation at the time of recommended transfer. She transferred to a local hospital that did not offer the option of a vaginal breech birth and was thus admitted for a planned cesarean section with the fetal heartrate in the 150–160 s range without decelerations. The fetal monitoring was not felt to require urgent cesarean delivery; however, more than two hours after admission there was a prolonged bradycardia in the operating room and a cesarean was

Table 3 Location of birth and mode of birth for breech & cephalic mothers, categorized by parity

	Breech primip n = 41	Breech multip n = 9	Total breech n = 50	Cephalic primip n = 60	Cephalic multip n = 42	Total cephalic n = 102
Birth location						
OOH	31 (75.6%)	9 (100%)	40 (80.0%)	50 (83.3%)	41 (97.6%)	91 (89.2%)
Hospital (TOC)	10 (24.4%)	0	10 (20.0%)	10 (16.7%)	1 (2.4%)	11 (10.8%)
Mode of birth						
Cesarean	8 (19.5%)	0	8 (16.0%)	3 (5.0%)	0	3 (2.9%)
Vaginal	33 (80.5%)	9 (100%)	42 (84.0%)	57 (95.0%)	42 (100%)	99 (97.1%)
SVD	*27 (65.9%)*	*9 (100%)*	*36 (72.0%)*	*37 (61.7%)*	*42 (100%)*	*79 (77.5%)*
Forceps/vacuum	*6 (14.6%)*	*0*	*6 (12.0%)*	*20 (33.3%)*	*0*	*20 (19.6%)*

Table 4 Indications for in-labor hospital transfer

Indication for transfer	Breech $n = 50$	Cephalic $n = 102$
Arrest of active labor (6–9 cm)	7	6
Arrest of labor in 2nd stage	3	
Maternal exhaustion and pain relief		3
Decelerations in early labor		2
Total in-labor transfers	10 (20.0%)	11 (10.8%)

performed under spinal anesthesia. Neonatal resuscitation was unsuccessful.

The last three breech mothers were transported, all in stable condition, to a physician who offered the option of augmentation in one of the local hospitals. Two gave birth vaginally after epidural and oxytocin augmentation. Both of these births were prolonged, described as difficult, and entailed the use of Piper forceps and/or vacuum extraction and episiotomies with extensions. The third had an emergent cesarean section for fetal bradycardia immediately after placement of an intrauterine pressure catheter (IUPC). All 3 of these babies required NICU admission with 2 transported to another facility equipped with neonatal therapeutic hypothermia capability. Both babies born vaginally have recovered fully; the baby delivered by emergent CS has mild developmental delay.

There were 11 laboring cephalic women who were transported in labor, only one emergently. Six women transported for arrest of active labor. After epidural and oxytocin, two had spontaneous vaginal births, two had a vacuum extraction, and two had cesareans. One of the cesareans was due to a twin fetus papyraceous presenting in front of the live fetus and obstructing descent. (The mother had a selective fetal reduction early in pregnancy; her pregnancy was then treated as a singleton gestation.) The other cesarean occurred after a long delay at 10 cm with no descent. Three additional women transported for maternal exhaustion, one with back pain and asynclitism. All three had spontaneous vaginal births after epidural and oxytocin. The two final women were transported for audible decelerations in early labor. One was a multiparous woman with prolonged ROM and GBS+ status; she was transferred emergently and gave birth rapidly in the hospital. The other had a non-reassuring fetal heart rate tracing at 3 cm and was taken for cesarean section.

Length of 2nd stage
We have partial data (27/50) on length of 2nd stage for the breech births that actually occurred OOH. In SJF's practice, second stage is defined as beginning at complete dilation. Many breech and cephalic labors included a passive or "laboring down" phase before active maternal pushing began. Breech mothers were

encouraged to labor down for as long as possible. SJF's records do not distinguish between passive and active second stages. Of the 19 primiparous mothers, 2nd stage ranged from 19 to 228 min (mean: 94, SD: 58). Two of these 19 mothers had second stages exceeding 2 ½ hours (170 and 228 min). Of the 8 multiparous mothers, 2nd stage lasted between 5 and 34 min (mean: 17, SD 9.7). Second stage data are not available for the remaining breech mothers or for the cephalic births.

Perineal integrity
We do not have full data on perineal outcomes for in-labor transports, so we can only report on completed OOH births (Tables 5 and 6). In the breech group there were 5 episiotomies performed plus two 3rd degree and one 4th degree laceration, all in primiparous mothers and repaired on site. None of the multiparous breech mothers required episiotomies or experienced any perineal trauma.

Of the cephalic mothers giving birth OOH, a vacuum extractor was used 16 times and outlet forceps twice. Episiotomy was performed on 8 of these 18 operative vaginal deliveries. (This rate of operative delivery is skewed upward by calls to the author from local midwives requesting assistance for their own clients already in the second stage of labor.) There were two 3rd degree lacerations, both in the primiparous group and repaired on site, and no 4th degree lacerations.

Estimated blood loss
We are missing data on estimated blood loss (EBL) for the majority of the breech and cephalic transports, thus we have calculated mean EBL for completed OOH births only. Mean EBL among the breech group was 314 ccs, compared to 386 ccs in the cephalic group; this difference was not statistically significant ($p = 0.15$). There were 4 breech mothers (10.0%) and 16 cephalic mothers (16.2%) with an EBL between 500 and 1000 ccs. No breech mother had an EBL > 1000 ccs and none required postpartum transport. Six cephalic women had an EBL > 1000 ccs; five of those stabilized at home and required no further acute treatment. The sixth mother was transported after birth by ambulance for an EBL of > 1500 ccs; once at the hospital, she stabilized with no

Table 5 Perineal outcomes of completed OOH births

Perineal integrity	Breech ($n = 40$)	Cephalic ($n = 91$)
Intact	25 (62.5%)	51 (56.0%)
1st degree tear	4 (10.0%)	23 (25.3%)
2nd degree tear	3 (7.5%)	5 (5.5%)
Episiotomy	5 (12.5%)	10 (11.0%)
3rd degree tear	2 (5.0%)	2 (2.2%)
4th degree tear	1 (2.5%)	0

Table 6 OOH breech perineal outcomes, categorized by parity and by maternal position

Perineal integrity	Parity		Maternal position	
	Primip (n = 31)	Multip (n = 9)	Upright (n = 11)	Lithotomy (n = 29)
Intact	16 (51.6%)	9 (100%)	10 (90.9%)	15 (51.7%)
1st degree tear	4 (12.9%)	0	1 (9.1%)	3 (10.3%)
2nd degree tear	3 (9.7%)	0	0	3 (10.3%)
Episiotomy	5 (16.1%)	0	0	5 (17.2%)
3rd degree tear	2 (6.5%)	0	0	2 (6.9%)
4th degree tear	1 (3.2%)	0	0	1 (3.4%)

need for blood transfusion and recovered without other morbidity.

Apgar scores and neonatal morbidity

As with EBL, we only have information on Apgar scores for completed OOH births (Table 7). The rate of 1-min Apgars < 7 and mean 1- and 5-min Apgars were significantly different between the breech and cephalic groups. Although low 5-min Apgars were twice as common in the breech group, this difference was not significantly significant.

All four Piper forceps assisted OOH breech births had 1-min scores < 7 but 5-min scores of 7 or better. Three other breech babies had 5-min scores < 7 with scores of 6, 6, and 2. This last baby had a terminal bradycardia for suspected umbilical cord compression just before birth and required respiratory assistance and cardiac resuscitation. Paramedics were called. By ten minutes the Apgar score was 8, the baby was doing well, and transport was deemed unnecessary.

Besides the three low 5-min Apgars, there were two neonatal morbidities in the breech group. One baby suffered a fractured humerus during an assisted all-fours breech birth. Pediatrics was consulted and no immediate attention was required. The infant recovered without incident. A second baby suffered a brachial plexus injury at an assisted breech delivery in lithotomy position for another terminal bradycardia just as the rump was protruding. She had momentary assisted ventilation. At the time of publication she is doing well but still has a significant residual Erb's palsy 6 months after birth.

Seven cephalic babies had 1-min Apgar scores < 7 (7.8%) and 5 of these were vacuum assisted. There were only 3 cephalic babies with 5-min Apgar scores < 7, all

Table 7 1- and 5- min Apgar scores for completed OOH births

OOH Apgar scores	Breech (n = 40)	Cephalic (n = 90[a])	P value
1-min < 7	16 (40.0%)	7 (7.8%)	< 0.0001
5-min < 7	3 (7.5%)	3 (3.3%)	0.371
1-min average	6.3 (range 1–9)	8.0 (range 2–9)	< 0.0001
5-min average	8.4 (range 2–10)	8.9 (range 4–10)	0.0167

[a] Apgar scores are missing for one baby in the cephalic group

vacuum assisted. The first woman had a prolonged second stage over 4 h, at which point the midwife requested SJF's assistance. The second was a primiparous woman at 41.5 weeks with persistent occiput transverse position; assistance was requested by a local midwife and a vacuum vaginal birth was achieved over a midline episiotomy. The third baby was also a vacuum for a prolonged second stage and maternal exhaustion with a shoulder dystocia of < 1 min; the baby had a mild brachial plexus injury that has since resolved. All babies did well and none required transport.

Postpartum transport

No breech mothers or babies required postpartum transport. In the cephalic group there was one newborn postpartum transport for persistent tachypnea; the infant had a spontaneous pneumothorax that resolved within 24 h. The other postpartum transport was the previously mentioned woman with an EBL of 1500 ccs that resolved without transfusion.

Discussion

High rates of vaginal birth are possible for both breech and cephalic presentations in a home or birth center setting, similar to or greater than levels reported in two recent large studies of out-of-hospital births (Table 8; see also [42, 43]). The cesarean rate among our cephalic group was lower than reported in other home and birth data, but the rate of operative vaginal birth was much higher, likely due to SJF being called by local midwives to assist with obstructed 2nd stage labors, situations that otherwise would have required hospital transport.

As expected, the cesarean rate was higher for the breech group than for the cephalic group. However, our breech group had lower cesarean rates compared to other home and hospital studies. The 222 planned home breech births reported in Cheyney 2014 had a vaginal birth rate of 57.2%, compared to 84% in this series. However, is unknown how many of the breech presentations in the Cheyney cohort were diagnosed before labor and thus how many were actually planned home breech births.

Table 8 Outcomes compared to recent home and birth center studies (all numbers in %)

Source (n = pVBB at onset of labor)	Breech group (n = 50)	Cephalic group (n = 102)	Cheyney 2014 Home birth (n = 16,984)	Stapleton 2013 Birth center (n = 14,881)
In-labor TOC	20	10.8	10.9	12
PP TOC (mother or baby)	0	2	2.4	5
Cesarean section	16	2.9	5.2	6
Assisted vaginal birth	12	19.6	1.2	1
Spontaneous vaginal birth	72	77.5	93.6	93
5-min Apgar < 7	*7.5*	*3.3*	1.5	NR
EBL > 500 ccs	*10*	*16.2*	15.5	NR
EBL > 1000 ccs	*0*	*6.6*	4.8	NR
Intact perineum	*62.5*	*56*	49.2	NR
1st or 2nd degree	*17.5*	*30.8*	40.9	NR
Episiotomy	*12.5*	*11*	1.4	NR
3rd or 4th degree	*7.5*	*2.2*	1.2	NR

Italicized numbers indicate completed OOH births only (data not available for hospital transfers)

EBL was lower for the breech group and slightly higher for the cephalic group compared to the home births in Cheyney 2014. Women planning OOH generally have good perineal outcomes; 80% of the breech group, 86.8% of the cephalic group, and 90.1% of the Cheyney cohort experienced either moderate (intact perineum or 1st/2nd degree lacerations) or no perineal trauma. However, as stated previously, our data on perineal integrity include only the completed OOH births.

If we look at planned hospital VBB (Table 9), successful vaginal birth rates range from 56.7 to 71% in a sampling of single-center, multi-center, and national registry studies [1, 9, 15, 44–46]. We attribute the high vaginal success rates in our series to the collaboration between the obstetrician and midwife and to a setting that allowed the mother to have an undisturbed, physiological labor.

With the exception of the PREMODA study, all studies listed in Table 9 had higher rates of low 5-min Apgars for pVBB compared to pCS. Our breech cohort followed a similar (albeit nonsignificant) pattern, although outcomes were compared to planned cephalic births rather than planned cesarean breech births.

Although our numbers are too small to calculate statistical significance, upright positioning for breech birth may be more protective to the perineum than on-the-back positioning. This mirrors the findings reported in Louwen 2017 [15] and warrants further examination.

There is disagreement in breech literature and guidelines on optimal length of second stage. The TBT allowed up to 3.5 h for 2nd stage [1]. In the PREMODA cohort, over 18% of women had a passive second stage longer than 1 h, while 94% of the active 2nd stages were under 30 min. However, oxytocin was used in the large majority of all births (8.9% of all labors were induced, and oxytocin was used in 74.1% of all non-induced labors); this high rate of oxytocin could have affected the duration of 2nd stage [9]. The SOGC guidelines, which draw heavily from the PREMODA study, recommend a total of 2 ½ hours with no more than 60 min of active 2nd stage [13]. In the Louwen study on upright vs supine breech, supine breeches averaged 1.77 h and

Table 9 Rate of successful vaginal birth and low Apgar scores compared to hospital studies of pVBB

Source	Country, dates	Type of study	# of pVBB	Vaginal birth rate	5-min Apgar < 7
Breech group	USA, 2010–2017	single center retro.	50	84.0%	7.5%[a]
TBT 2000	International, 1997–2000	multi center RCT	1042	56.7%	3.0%
PREMODA 2006	France & Belgium, 2001–2002	multi center pros.	2526	71.0%	1.48%
Vlemmix 2014	Netherlands, 1999–2007	registry retro.	27,817	58.7%	2.2%
Vistad 2015	Norway, 1991–2011	registry retro.	17,500	64.0%	2.4%
Burgos 2015	Spain, 2003–2012	single center retro.	891	57.5%	2.2%
Louwen 2017	Germany, 2004–2011	single center retro.	433	62.1%	2.5%

[a] Completed OOH births only—data not available for hospital transfers

retro. = retrospective

pros. = prospective

upright breeches averaged 1.02 h for 2nd stage. 17.1% of the supine breeches and 7.4% of the upright breeches had a 2nd stage exceeding 3 h [15]. SJF follows a midwifery model of care for managing first and second stage, eschewing rigid time limits in favor of individualized care and ongoing assessment of maternal and fetal status. This approach explains some of the longer second stages with a small number of the breech primips. Decisions to transport (for breech) or to offer operative delivery (for cephalic) are based on the mother's request—usually for exhaustion—or on SJF's recommendations due to lack of fetal progress/descent.

Breech mothers seeking care with SJF were significantly more likely to be primips compared to cephalic mothers. Uotila et al. observed a similar difference in parity between their breech and cephalic cohorts and proposed it might be due to ECV having higher success rates in multips, thus leaving more primips with persistent breech presentations [47].

We found a significant difference in birth weights between the two groups. We hypothesize the difference is likely due to having an upper weight limit for breech babies but not for cephalic babies. However, Molkenboer found that term breech presentations had a significantly lower mean birth weight compared to matched cephalic presentations, suggesting a possible causal relationship between birth weight and type of presentation [48].

One difference in breech labor protocols between a hospital and OOH setting is in fetal monitoring techniques; at home, intermittent monitoring with a handheld Doppler is the standard of care. We encourage further research comparing intermittent with continuous fetal monitoring for breech labors.

The advisability of augmentation for breech labors is still debated. Although the TBT and the PREMODA study both allowed augmentation, neither the RCOG nor the SOGC guidelines recommend augmentation for uterine dystocia in a spontaneous labor without epidural analgesia [1, 8, 9, 13]. Our experience confirms that, at least for out-of-hospital breech labors, a cesarean section is more prudent than augmentation; all three transports admitted for augmentation in a hospital setting had complicated neonatal courses. Whatever the indication for hospital transfer, women deserve systemic collaboration, good communication, and a smooth, nonjudgmental transition from home or birth center to hospital. (See the transfer guidelines created by the Home Birth Summit Collaboration Task Force [49]).

Strengths & Limitations
Although fetal and maternal outcomes for care transfers were usually reported back informally by the parents, medical records for these women were not available for review, making further analysis of these hospital transfers

impossible. Thus we have incomplete data on the transfers and were unable to do an intention-to-treat analysis on some outcomes.

We recognize that our cephalic and breech groups are not directly comparable, not only due to presentation but also due to differences in parity and EFW restrictions. However, because of the inherent preferences of their client base, out-of-hospital practitioners do not generally have access to a large cohort of women with breech presentations who choose a planned cesarean. With these limitations in mind, we chose to set out-of-hospital breech outcomes in the context of cephalic births occurring during the same time period with the same obstetrician. Using a cephalic cohort as a comparison group also has precedent in the medical literature [47, 48, 50–57].

The relatively small sample size of both groups limits the ability to extrapolate our findings, and our numbers are underpowered for calculating the relatively rare events of severe morbidity or mortality. However, this is the largest study of planned OOH vaginal breech birth with a single care provider. It provides a rich glimpse into what is possible for a breech birth with a trained practitioner who follows clear protocol guidelines and who respects the physiological process of birth. On the other hand, SJF offers a unique service and most women seeking OOH birth will not have access to a highly skilled obstetrician.

The high rates of vaginal birth in both breech and cephalic groups in our series may not be achievable in most hospital settings. The midwifery model of care used in this series does not lend itself well to the high-volume, shift-oriented practices in many hospitals. Instead, the midwifery model stresses preventative care, well-developed relationships, longer prenatal visits, personalized attention, and uninterrupted one-on-one care during labor, birth, and postpartum.

The breech mothers in our study faced the added stress and disruption of their birth plans, being forced to change providers and/or planned location of birth last minute. The impact of this dramatic upheaval for the breech mothers was not independently assessed, but it should not be ignored as a factor potentially affecting outcomes.

We acknowledge that many consider breech birth to be high-risk and home or birth center birth to be an absolute contraindication for breech presentation. However, hospitals in many countries have consistently failed or refused to offer VBB since the TBT, despite evidence that it remains a reasonable option for well-selected women. Women continue to value vaginal birth highly. When hospitals or providers refuse to offer vaginal breech birth, some women will seek care outside the hospital.

We warn of the dangers of restricting or outlawing vaginal breech birth at home or birth centers; this will result in some women giving birth unassisted, which is arguably less safe than breech birth with a trained practitioner. Instead, we encourage a model where women are fully informed of the risks (both absolute and relative) and benefits of their options and are allowed to make the final decision of where and how to give birth. Two such models are Amish birth centers allowing breeches, twins, and vaginal birth after cesarean (VBAC) [58] and state midwifery regulations that do not force the midwife to abandon care for breech, twin, or VBAC clients.[1]

Informed consent is now a fundamental principle of modern medicine, law, and ethics. This includes access to the full range of information about a treatment's risks, benefits, and alternatives and the patient's ability to freely consent to or refuse a proposed treatment [59–65]. For women with breech presentations, this means the right to refuse surgery in favor of a vaginal breech birth. ACOG's May 2016 practice bulletin strongly upholds pregnant women's right to refuse medical treatment. It reads:

[A] decisionally capable pregnant woman's decision to refuse recommended medical or surgical interventions should be respected. The use of coercion is not only ethically impermissible but also medically inadvisable because of the realities of prognostic uncertainty and the limitations of medical knowledge. As such, it is never acceptable for obstetrician–gynecologists to attempt to influence patients toward a clinical decision using coercion [32].

Forcing women to have cesareans for breech presentations also violates U.S. legal rulings that uphold the right of competent adults to refuse surgery.[2]

Breech birth requires training and skill; it deserves respect and caution but not fear. We strongly recommend that hospitals stop banning vaginal breech birth and that residency training programs reinstitute training in vaginal breech birth as a core obstetric skill. Even today, around 1/4 to 1/3 of all breech presentations are undiagnosed before labor [66], highlighting the need for skilled attendants when it might not be advisable or possible to do a cesarean.

Conclusions

Planned vaginal breech birth should remain an accessible option for all women, especially taking into account the short-and long-term risks of cesarean section to the baby, the mother, and the mother's future babies. While universal cesarean for breech might prevent a very small number of fetal deaths, it comes at the price of overriding maternal autonomy and subjecting both mother and baby to another set of risks—risks that she might not be comfortable with [67]. We cannot overemphasize the importance many women place on giving birth vaginally. Bassaw et al. eloquently conclude in their 2004 study of breech outcomes at a tertiary hospital in Trinidad:

A policy of planned vaginal birth for selected breech fetuses with a low threshold to proceed to caesarean section may still be in the best interest of both mother and child. The individual woman's wishes must be taken into consideration as for some, labour is an integral and treasured experience and a vaginal delivery is a life event of enormous magnitude [68].

As our study demonstrates, out-of-hospital vaginal breech birth with carefully selected patients, specific protocol guidelines, and a skilled provider results in high rates of vaginal birth and good maternal outcomes. However, the absolute risks of neonatal morbidity and mortality are difficult to quantify due to the small samples sizes in this study and to our inability to include some outcomes from hospital deliveries occurring after intrapartum transfer. Whether a planned OOH breech birth is considered reasonable or safe is an individualized judgment call based on the history and values of the expectant family and on the birth options available within their communities. Reviving vaginal breech skills in all settings and respecting maternal autonomy would benefit both practitioners and the women they care for.

Endnotes

[1]See, for example, Wis. Admin. Code SPS § 182.03(4).

[2]See, for example: Union Pacific Railway Co. v. Botsford, 141 U.S. 250, 251 (1891); Schloendorff v. Society of New York Hospital, 105 NE. 92, 93 (N.Y. 1914); Cruzan V. Director, Missouri Dept. of Health, 497 U.S. 261, 270 (1990); In re Brown, 478 So.2d 1033 (Miss. 1985); Cruzan V. Harmon, 160 S.W.2d 408, 417 (Mo. 1988); Matter of Guardianship of L.W., 482 N.W.2d 60, 65 (Wis. 1992); In re Fiori, 673 A.2d 905, 910 (Pa. 996); Stouffer v. Reid, 993 A.2d 104, 109 (Maryl. 2010).

Abbreviations

CS: Cesarean section; EBL: Estimated blood loss; ECV: External cephalic version; EFW: Estimated fetal weight; IUFD: Intrauterine fetal demise; IUPC: Intrauterine pressure catheter; OOH: Out-of-hospital (i.e., home or birth center); pCS: Planned cesarean section; pVBB: Planned vaginal breech birth; TBT: Term Breech Trial; TOC: Transfer of care; VBAC: Vaginal birth after cesarean; VBB: Vaginal breech birth

Authors' contributions

SJF extracted the data from medical records and did a preliminary analysis of the data. RF performed the statistical analysis and obtained ethics approval.

Both authors helped write and edit the manuscript. Both authors read and approved the final manuscript.

Competing interests

The authors declare that they have no competing interests.

Author details

[1]Birthing Instincts, Inc., Los Angeles, CA, USA. [2]Wabash College, 211 Center Hall, Crawfordsville, IN 47933, USA.

References

1. Hannah ME, Hannah WJ, Hewson SA, Hodnett ED, Saigal S, Willan AR. Planned caesarean section versus planned vaginal birth for breech presentation at term: a randomised multicentre trial Term Breech Trial Collaborative Group. Lancet. 2000;356(9239):1375–83.
2. Delotte J, Schumacker-Blay C, Bafghi A, Lehmann P, Bongain A. Medical information and patients' choices. Influences on term singleton breech deliveries. Gynecol Obstet Fertil. 2007;35(9):747–50.
3. Glezerman M. Five years to the term breech trial: the rise and fall of a randomized controlled trial. Am J Obstet Gynecol. 2006;194(1):20–5.
4. Lawson GW. The term breech trial ten years on: primum non nocere? Birth. 2012;39(1):3–9.
5. Su M, McLeod L, Ross S, Willan A, Hannah WJ, Hutton E, et al. Factors associated with adverse perinatal outcome in the term breech trial. Am J Obstet Gynecol. 2003;189(3):740–5.
6. Goffinet F, Azria E, Kayem G, Schmitz T, Deneux-Tharaux C. Re: the risks of planned vaginal breech delivery versus planned caesarean section for term breech birth: a meta-analysis including observational studies: Let's avoid simplistic radicalism when reality is complex. BJOG. 2016;123(1):145–7.
7. Whyte H, Hannah ME, Saigal S, Hannah WJ, Hewson A, Amankwah K, et al. Outcomes of children at 2 years after planned cesarean birth versus planned vaginal birth for breech presentation at term: the international randomized term breech trial. Am J Obstet Gynecol. 2004;191(3):864–71.
8. Royal College of Obstetricians and Gynaecologists. Management of Breech Presentation: green-top guideline no. 20b. BJOG. 2017;124(7):e151–77.
9. Goffinet F, Carayol M, Foidart JM, Alexander S, Uzan S, Subtil D, et al. Is planned vaginal delivery for breech presentation at term still an option? Results of an observational prospective survey in France and Belgium. Am J Obstet Gynecol. 2006;194(4):1002–11.
10. Hofmeyr GJ, Hannah ME. Planned Caesarean section for term breech delivery. Cochrane Database Syst Rev. 2001;1(1):CD000166.
11. Hofmeyr GJ, Hannah M, Lawrie TA. Planned caesarean section for term breech delivery. Cochrane Database Syst Rev. 2015;(7):CD000166. https://doi.org/10.1002/14651858.CD000166.pub2.
12. ACOG Committee on Obstetric Practice. ACOG Committee opinion no. 340. Mode of term singleton breech delivery. Obstet Gynecol. 2006;108(1):235–7 Interim update August 2018: Committee Opinion No. 745.
13. Kotaska A, Menticoglou S, Gagnon R, Farine D, Basso M, Bos H, et al. SOGC clinical practice guideline: vaginal delivery of breech presentation: no. 226, June 2009. Int J Gynaecol Obstet. 2009;107(2):169–76.
14. Royal Australian and New Zealand College of Obstetricians and Gynaecologists (RANZCOG). The management of breech presentation at term. C-Obs 11. 2016.
15. Louwen F, Daviss BA, Johnson KC, Reitter A. Does breech delivery in an upright position instead of on the back improve outcomes and avoid cesareans? Int J Gynaecol Obstet. 2017 Feb;136(2):151–61.
16. Evans J. Understanding physiological breech birth. Essentially MIDIRS. 2012; 3(2):17–21.
17. Burger M, Safar P. Delivery from breech presentation with the delivery chair. Initial experiences with a new obstetric method. Gynakol Geburtshilfliche Rundsch. 1996;36(2):69–74.
18. Bogner G, Strobl M, Schausberger C, Fischer T, Reisenberger K, Jacobs VR. Breech delivery in the all fours position: a prospective observational comparative study with classic assistance. J Perinat Med. 2015 Nov;43(6): 707–13.
19. Banks M. Breech birth woman-wise. Hamilton: Birthspirit Books; 1998.
20. Tully G. Breech birth, quick guide. Minneapolis: Maternity House Publishing, Inc; 2016.
21. Walker S, Scamell M, Parker P. Standards for maternity care professionals attending planned upright breech births: a Delphi study. Midwifery. 2016;34: 7–14.
22. Borbolla Foster A, Bagust A, Bisits A, Holland M, Welsh A. Lessons to be learnt in managing the breech presentation at term: an 11-year single-Centre retrospective study. Aust N Z J Obstet Gynaecol. 2014;54(4):333–9.
23. Walker S, Scamell M, Parker P. Principles of physiological breech birth practice: a Delphi study. Midwifery. 2016;43:1–6.
24. Walker S, Breslin E, Scamell M, Parker P. Effectiveness of vaginal breech birth training strategies: an integrative review of the literature. Birth. 2017;44(2): 101–9.
25. van Dillen J, Zwart JJ, Schutte J, Bloemenkamp KW, van Roosmalen J. Severe acute maternal morbidity and mode of delivery in the Netherlands. Acta Obstet Gynecol Scand. 2010;89(11):1460–5.
26. Schutte JM, Steegers EA, Santema JG, Schuitemaker NW, van Roosmalen J. Maternal mortality committee of the Netherlands society of obstetrics. Maternal deaths after elective cesarean section for breech presentation in the Netherlands. Acta Obstet Gynecol Scand. 2007;86(2):240–3.
27. Neu J, Rushing J. Cesarean versus vaginal delivery: long-term infant outcomes and the hygiene hypothesis. Clin Perinatol. 2011;38(2):321–31.
28. Thavagnanam S, Fleming J, Bromley A, Shields MD, Cardwell CR. A meta-analysis of the association between caesarean section and childhood asthma. Clin Exp Allergy. 2008;38(4):629–33.
29. Cardwell CR, Stene LC, Joner G, Cinek O, Svensson J, Goldacre MJ, et al. Caesarean section is associated with an increased risk of childhood-onset type 1 diabetes mellitus: a meta-analysis of observational studies. Diabetologia. 2008;51(5):726–35.
30. Almgren M, Schlinzig T, Gomez-Cabrero D, Gunnar A, Sundin M, Johansson S, et al. Cesarean delivery and hematopoietic stem cell epigenetics in the newborn infant: implications for future health? Am J Obstet Gynecol. 2014; 211(5):502.e1,502.e8.
31. ACOG Committee on Ethics. ACOG Committee opinion no. 439: informed consent. Obstet Gynecol. 2009;114(2 1):401–8.
32. American College of Obstetricians and Gynecologists' Committee on Ethics. Committee opinion no. 664: refusal of medically recommended treatment during pregnancy. Obstet Gynecol. 2016;127(6):e175–82.
33. Bovbjerg ML, Cheyney M, Brown J, Cox KJ, Leeman L. Perspectives on risk: assessment of risk profiles and outcomes among women planning community birth in the United States. Birth. 2017;22:209–21.
34. Johnson KC. Daviss B. outcomes of planned home births with certified professional midwives: large prospective study in North America. BMJ. 2005; 330:1416.
35. Grunebaum A, McCullough LB, Brent RL, Arabin B, Levene MI, Chervenak FA. Perinatal risks of planned home births in the United States. Am J Obstet Gynecol. 2015;212(3):350.e1,350.e6.
36. Cheyney M, Bovbjerg M, Everson C, Gordon W, Hannibal D, Vedam S. Outcomes of care for 16,924 planned home births in the United States: the midwives Alliance of North America statistics project, 2004 to 2009. J Midwifery Womens Health. 2014;59(1):17–27.
37. Committee on Obstetric Practice. Committee opinion no. 697: planned home birth. Obstet Gynecol. 2017;129(4):e117–22.
38. Spinning Babies [Internet]; 2017 [cited September 1, 2017]. Available from: https://spinningbabies.com.
39. Midwives Model of Care Brochure [Internet]: Citizens for Midwifery; 2008 [cited September 1, 2017]. Available from: http://cfmidwifery.org/PDF/mmoc_brochure.pdf.
40. Aurora's frank breech home birth [Internet]: Jodie Myers; 2012 [cited Sep 1, 2017]. Available from: https://vimeo.com/45678615.

41. Rietberg CCT, Elferink-Stinkens PM, Visser GHA. Ch. 6: There are more girls than boys in breech position. In: Term breech delivery in the Netherlands [thesis]. Utrecht: Utrecht University; 2006. p. 71–79.

42. Fischbein SJ. "home birth" with an obstetrician: a series of 135 out of hospital births. Obstet Gynecol Int. 2015;2(4):00046.

43. Janssen PA, Lee SK, Ryan EM, Etches DJ, Farquharson DF, Peacock D, et al. Outcomes of planned home births versus planned hospital births after regulation of midwifery in British Columbia. CMAJ. 2002;166(3):315–23.

44. Vlemmix F, Bergenhenegouwen L, Schaaf JM, Ensing S, Rosman AN, Ravelli AC, et al. Term breech deliveries in the Netherlands: did the increased cesarean rate affect neonatal outcome? A population-based cohort study. Acta Obstet Gynecol Scand. 2014;93(9):888–96.

45. Vistad I, Klungsoyr K, Albrechtsen S, Skjeldestad FE. Neonatal outcome of singleton term breech deliveries in Norway from 1991 to 2011. Acta Obstet Gynecol Scand. 2015;94(9):997–1004.

46. Burgos J, Rodriguez L, Cobos P, Osuna C, Del Mar Centeno M, Larrieta R, et al. Management of breech presentation at term: a retrospective cohort study of 10 years of experience. J Perinatol. 2015;35(10):803–8.

47. Uotila J, Tuimala R, Kirkinen P. Good perinatal outcome in selective vaginal breech delivery at term. Acta Obstet Gynecol Scand. 2005;84(6):578–83.

48. Molkenboer JF, Vencken PM, Sonnemans LG, Roumen FJ, Smits F, Buitendijk SE, et al. Conservative management in breech deliveries leads to similar results compared with cephalic deliveries. J Matern Fetal Neonatal Med. 2007;20(8):599–603.

49. Vedam S, Leeman L, Cheyney M, Fisher TJ, Myers S, Low LK, Ruhl C. Transfer from planned home birth to hospital: improving interprofessional collaboration. J Midwifery Womens Health. 2014;59(6):624–34.

50. Ouattara A, Some AD, Ouattara H, Lankoande J. Prognosis for term breech presentations in Africa (Bobo Dioulasso, Burkina Faso). Med Sante Trop. 2016;26(2):155–8.

51. Belfrage P, Gjessing L. The term breech presentation. A retrospective study with regard to the planned mode of delivery. Acta Obstet Gynecol Scand. 2002;81(6):544–50.

52. Amoa AB, Sapuri M, Klufio CA. Perinatal outcome and associated factors of persistent breech presentation at the Port Moresby general hospital, Papua New Guinea. P N G Med J. 2001;44(1–2):48–56.

53. Meye JF, Mayi S, Zue AS, Engongah-Beka T, Kendjo E, Ole BS. Neonatal prognosis for breech infants delivered vaginally at the Josephine bongo maternity Hospital in Libreville. Gabon Sante. 2003;13(2):81–4.

54. Mukuku O, Kimbala J, Kizonde J. Breech vaginal delivery: a study of maternal and neonatal morbidity and mortality. Pan Afr Med J. 2014;17:27.

55. Nordin NM. An audit of singleton breech deliveries in a hospital with a high rate of vaginal delivery. Malays J Med Sci. 2007;14(1):28–37.

56. Sibony O, Luton D, Oury JF, Blot P. Six hundred and ten breech versus 12,405 cephalic deliveries at term: is there any difference in the neonatal outcome? Eur J Obstet Gynecol Reprod Biol. 2003;107(2):140–4.

57. Toivonen E, Palomaki O, Huhtala H, Uotila J. Selective vaginal breech delivery at term - still an option. Acta Obstet Gynecol Scand. 2012;91(10):1177–83.

58. Deline J, Varnes-Epstein L, Dresang LT, Gideonsen M, Lynch L. Frey JJ,3rd. Low primary cesarean rate and high VBAC rate with good outcomes in an Amish birthing center. Ann Fam Med. 2012;10(6):530–7.

59. Whitney SN, McCullough LB. Physicians' silent decisions: because patient autonomy does not always come first. Am J Bioeth. 2007;7(7):33–8.

60. Chavkin W, Diaz-Tello F. When Courts Fail: Physicians' Legal and Ethical Duty to Uphold Informed Consent. Columbia Med Rev. 2017;1(2):6–9.

61. Goldberg H. Informed decision making in maternity care. J Perinat Educ. 2009;18(1):32–40.

62. Hammami MM, Al-Gaai EA, Al-Jawarneh Y, Amer H, Hammami MB, Eissa A, et al. Patients' perceived purpose of clinical informed consent: Mill's individual autonomy model is preferred. BMC Med Ethics. 2014;15:2 6939-15-2.

63. Kotaska A. Informed consent and refusal in obstetrics: a practical ethical guide. Birth. 2017;44(3).

64. Moulton B, King JS. Aligning ethics with medical decision-making: the quest for informed patient choice. J Law Med Ethics. 2010 Spring;38(1):85–97.

65. Sprung CL, Winick BJ. Informed consent in theory and practice: legal and medical perspectives on the informed consent doctrine and a proposed reconceptualization. Crit Care Med. 1989;17(12):1346–54.

66. Walker S, Cochrane V. Unexpected breech: what can midwives do? Pract Midwife. 2015;18(10):26–9.

67. Homer CS, Watts NP, Petrovska K, Sjostedt CM, Bisits A. Women's experiences of planning a vaginal breech birth in Australia. BMC Pregnancy Childbirth. 2015;15:89 015-0521-4.

68. Bassaw B, Rampersad N, Roopnarinesingh S, Sirjusingh A. Correlation of fetal outcome with mode of delivery for breech presentation. J Obstet Gynaecol. 2004;24(3):254–8.

69. Talge NM, Mudd LM, Sikorskii A, Basso O. United States birth weight reference corrected for implausible gestational age estimates. Pediatrics. 2014;133(5):844–53.

9

Vitamin D plasma concentrations in pregnant women and their preterm newborns

Milene Saori Kassai[1], Fernanda Ramirez Cafeo[2], Fernando Alves Affonso-Kaufman[2], Fabíola Isabel Suano-Souza[1,2]* ⓘ and Roseli Oselka Saccardo Sarni[1]

Abstract

Background: Vitamin D deficiency is a global public health issue. More than half of pregnant women are affected by vitamin D insufficiency/deficiency. Studies suggest an association between low vitamin D concentrations during pregnancy with intrauterine growth restriction and prematurity. This study aimed to describe the concentrations of 25(OH)D (25-hydroxyvitamin D) of mothers who delivered preterm newborns compared to women with full-term pregnancy deliveries, as well as to relate 25(OH)D blood concentrations of mothers with those of their newborns.

Method: This cross-sectional study was conducted with 66 mothers who had given birth to preterm babies and their preterm newborns (PTNB, < 32 weeks), and 92 women who had given birth at the full-term of their pregnancy and their newborns (FTNB). Data were collected on the characteristics of mothers (gestational age, diseases, and habits) and newborns (anthropometry and adequacy for gestational age). Ten milliliters of blood were drawn from the mothers and the umbilical cord of newborns at birth to identify the 25(OH)D, parathyroid hormone, calcium, phosphorus, and alkaline phosphatase concentrations.

Results: Mothers in the PTNB group had significantly lower mean 25(OH)D blood levels (21.7 ± 10.8 ng/mL vs. 26.2 ± 9.8 ng/mL; $p = 0.011$) and were three times more likely to have insufficiency when compared to mothers in the FTNB group (OR = 2.993; 95%CI 1.02–8.74). Newborns in the PTNB group also had lower 25(OH)D concentrations compared to FTNB group (25.9 ± 13.9 ng/dL vs. 31.9 ± 12.3 ng/dL; $p = 0.009$). There was a directly proportional correlation between mother and newborn umbilical cord 25(OH)D concentrations in PTNB ($r = 0.596$; $p < 0.001$) and FTNB ($r = 0.765$; $p < 0.001$).

Conclusion: Mothers who delivered preterm babies and their preterm newborns had lower 25(OH)D concentrations compared to women who had given birth at the full-term of their pregnancy. In both groups, 25(OH)D concentrations of the mothers correlated directly with those of the newborns, and this correlation was higher in the full-term birth group. Nevertheless, the recommended universal vitamin D supplementation in pregnant women to curb the risk of preterm birth is still incipient. More studies are required to clarify the particularities of vitamin D metabolism further and define the adequate 25(OH)D concentrations throughout pregnancy.

Keywords: Vitamin D, Newborns, Pregnancy, Umbilical cord

* Correspondence: fsuano@gmail.com
[1]Department of Pediatrics, Faculdade de Medicina do ABC, Avenida Lauro Gomes, 2000. Vila Sacadura Cabral, Santo André, São Paulo 09060-870, Brazil
[2]Department of Pediatrics, Universidade Federal de São Paulo - Escola Paulista de Medicina, Rua Botucatu, 898, Vila Clementino, São Paulo 04023-062, Brazil

Background

Vitamin D is a prohormone associated with improved bone metabolism and strengthens the immune, respiratory, endocrine and cardiovascular systems [1]. The maintenance of blood concentrations depends predominantly on exposure to sunlight (conversion of cutaneous 7-dehydrocholesterol caused by exposure to ultraviolet B rays) and, to a lesser extent, the intake of vitamin D of either animal-derived (cholecalciferol) or plant-derived (ergocalciferol) food sources. Ethnicity, latitude, season, sunscreen and body mass index also influence vitamin D concentrations [2].

The 25-hydroxyvitamin-D [25(OH)D] and 1,25-dihydroxyvitamin-D [1.25(OH)$_2$D] can be measured. However, serum concentrations of 25(OH)D are used both as D2 and D3 to evaluate the nutritional state of patients regarding vitamin D levels. Calcitriol [1.25(OH)$_2$D] is the active form, but its half-life is very short and limits patient blood concentration measurement. Vitamin D deficiency can modify bone metabolism markers such as parathyroid hormone, calcium, phosphor and alkaline phosphatase [1, 2].

The 25(OH)D cutoff points currently in use for the general population are > 30 ng/mL, 20 to 30 ng/mL and < 20 ng/dL for sufficiency, insufficiency, and deficiency, respectively, and are based on bone outcomes [3]. Recommended levels are higher than 30 ng/mL for specific groups, such as pregnant women.

Insufficient 25(OH)D levels are a global public health issue, and pregnant women are a significant at-risk group. More than half of pregnant women evidence 25(OH)D concentrations comparable to vitamin D insufficiency [4]. A fetus relies exclusively on the mother's 25(OH)D concentrations, which affect the placental transfer of calcium and phosphorus, as well as hormonal and immunological balance, all of which are fundamental processes for bone development and fetoplacental integrity [5].

Observational studies suggest correlation between low concentrations of 25(OH)D (25 hydroxyvitamin D) during pregnancy and a higher risk of complications for the mother, such as pre-eclampsia, gestational diabetes, and bacterial vaginosis, as well as complications for the newborn [6, 7], such as intrauterine growth restriction [8], a higher risk of developing allergies [7] and obesity over the long-term [9].

Some international scientific organizations recommend that pregnant women take supplemental doses of vitamin D, ranging from 600 to 1,000 UI daily doses [10–12]. However, the World Health Organization has not universally adopted this practice [13]. The Brazilian Department of Health also does not recommend routine tests for 25(OH)D serum concentrations during prenatal care, nor vitamin D supplements for pregnant women.

Some studies evaluated 25(OH)D concentrations in Brazilian pregnant women [10, 11, 14]. However, no studies have been published on women who have prematurely given birth with a gestational age of fewer than 32 weeks.

This study aims to describe 25(OH)D, parathyroid hormone, calcium, phosphorus and alkaline phosphatase plasma concentrations of women who have delivered preterm (< 32 weeks) compared to women with full-term pregnancy deliveries, as well as to compare the 25(OH)D concentrations in mother with those of their newborn infants in both groups.

Methods

Study design

This cross-sectional study was conducted between March 2016 and May 2017 at the Municipal Hospital of São Bernardo do Campo University, São Paulo, Brazil (latitude: 23° 41′ 38″ S) with a convenience sample of 66 mothers who had delivered preterm and their newborns (PTNB, < 32 weeks), and 92 mothers full-term pregnancy deliveries and their newborns (FTNB group, 37 to 41 6/7 weeks), who were adequate for gestational age and with a birth weight > 2500 g. The full-term birth group was included during the spring and summer months of the Southern Hemisphere (September 2016 and March 2017).

Mothers with kidney disease, rheumatic disease, diabetes mellitus type 1, acquired immune deficiency syndrome (AIDS), and those using immunosuppressants (such as corticosteroids) were excluded. Newborns with significant malformations, genetic disorders, and neonatal hypoxia were also excluded.

The Research Ethics Committee of the ABC Faculty of Medicine approved the project under opinion N° 1.060.653, dated 13/05/2015. Mothers included in the study agreed to the procedures of the research and signed the informed consent form.

Data collected

Mother's health and prenatal care

Standardized questionnaires were applied to the mothers, which included questions about their socioeconomic conditions, education, habits (tobacco and alcohol use, medications), pre-existing conditions and obstetric disease (pre-existing pre-pregnancy conditions or those developed during pregnancy), use of vitamin or mineral supplements (iron, folic acid, vitamin D and multivitamins), skin color (white, mixed ethnicity or black), exposure to sunlight, and the regular use of sunscreen.

Their prenatal cards were reviewed for laboratory tests, ultrasounds, date of mothers' last menstrual period, and the anthropocentric measurements of the fetus during the obstetric monitoring of pregnancy. Pre-pregnancy body mass index (BMI) and weekly weight gain adequacy during pregnancy were based on weight and height measurements (kg/m^2) [15].

Newborn data

Information about the child's weight, length, and head circumference was retrieved within the first 24 h of life. The gestational age was preferably calculated according to the date of the mothers' last menstrual period, failing which it was based on the data from the ultrasound taken during the first trimester and, ultimately, according to clinical evaluation of the newborn [16]. The newborns were classified as small, adequate and large for their gestational age using INTERGROWTH-21st standards as a reference [17].

Laboratory tests

Blood samples were collected from the mothers on delivery at the obstetrics center. Ten (10) mL of the mothers' blood were drawn by arm venipuncture and, in the case of the newborns, from the umbilical cord vein. The material was immediately placed in tubes (one dry and one with EDTA) and submitted to the hospital's clinical analysis laboratory, where they were centrifuged and then transported under refrigeration to the ABC School of Medicine to measure the level of 25(OH)D (electrochemiluminescence, Roche, Mannheim, Germany), intact parathyroid hormone (PTH; electrochemiluminescence, Roche, Mannheim, Germany), calcium, phosphorus, and alkaline phosphatase (colorimetric method). In the case of mothers, 25(OH)D concentrations < 30 ng/mL were considered insufficient, and PTH > 65 pg/mL were deemed to be elevated [3].

All calculations followed the best clinical practice. The mean of 19.9 ng/mL (SD: 0.948 ng/mL and an intra-control CV of 4.8%) was the referred reproducible value to measure the 25(OH)D. For the same parameter, the intermediate precision was 19.9 ng/mL (SD: 1.23 ng/mL and an intra-control CV of 6.2%). For PTH, an average of 54.6 pg/mL was referred for repeatability with SD: 0.657 pg/mL and an intra-control CV of 1.2%. The mean intermediate precision was 54.6 pg/mL with a DP of 1.11 pg/mL and CV of 2.0%.

Data analysis

A spreadsheet was drafted on Microsoft Excel® with data on identification, general characteristics, data from the questionnaires regarding mothers and newborns, anthropometric data and the results of the laboratory tests. The spreadsheet was revised, consolidated and analyzed using the statistical package SPSS 25.0 (IBM®) to display the results.

The categorical variables were compared using the Chi-squared test in the bivariate analysis. Continuous analyses were tested for their normality through their distribution in histograms and a kurtosis evaluation. Since they were parametric, they were shown according to their means (standard deviation) and compared according to Student's t-test for independent variables. Pearson's coefficient was adopted to analyze correlations.

The comparison of the clinical and laboratory variables evidenced that the seasons during which the mothers were pregnant and exposure to sunlight differed between the groups. Thus, a stratified analysis of the frequency of 25(OH)D insufficiencies during spring and summer was conducted with multivariate analysis, using a logistic regression according to the Enter mode method to assess the adjusted effect of prematurity on the odds ratios of 25(OH)D insufficiency.

Pearson's correlation assessed the correlation between mothers' and newborns' 25(OH)D concentrations in both groups assessed by Pearson's correlation. The significance level adopted was 5%. The sample employed in the study proved sufficient to detect a difference of 5 ng/mL 25(OH)D between the groups [18] by adopting bidirectional $\alpha = 0.05$ and $\beta = 0.20$.

Results

Table 1 shows the general characteristics of the mothers and newborns in both the preterm and full-term birth groups. There was no difference between the groups regarding mother's age, ethnicity, number of pregnancies, sunscreen use, alcohol use, tobacco use, pre-pregnancy body mass index, or use of vitamin D or iron supplements. Mothers in the PTNB group had a lower frequency of folic acid supplementation [Yes: 46 (70.8%) vs 92 (87.6%); p = 0.038], prenatal care [< 6 visits: 54 (81.8%) vs 20 (21.7%); p < 0.001) and regular exposure to sunlight [Yes: 5 (7.6%) vs 54 (58.7%); p < 0.001].

The main complications associated with premature births were pregnancy-related hypertensive disorders (27) (40.9%; p < 0.001). Among women with pregnancy-related hypertensive disorders, 21 (77.8%) were taking methyldopa.

The mean of gestational age and birth weight in newborns of the PTNB group were 29.8 ± 2.4 weeks (p < 0.001) and 1250 ± 354.6 g (p < 0.001), respectively. In this group, 14 (21.2%) were small for their gestational age (Table 1). All these variables show a statistically significant difference concerning the FTNB group (Table 1).

The mothers in the PTNB group had lower mean values (21.7 ± 10.8 ng/mL vs. 26.2 ± 9.8 ng/mL, p = 0.011) and higher percentage of 25(OH)D insufficiency and deficiency when compared with the FTNB group (p = 0.018) (Table 2). Logistic regression showed that mothers who had delivered preterm babies were three times more likely to have insufficient 25(OH)D (OR = 2.993; 95%CI 1.02–8.74) (Table 3).

Table 1 Description of the general characteristics of the mothers, preterm newborns (PTNB) and full-term newborns (FTNB)

Variables		PTNB Group N = 66	FTNB Group N = 92	p-value
Characteristics of the mothers				
Age (n = 158)	Years	26.0 ± 7.3	26.03 ± 6.8	0.987[a]
Ethnicity (n = 158)	White	18 (27.3%)	35 (38.0%)	0.151[b]
	Black	6 (9.1%)	3 (3.3%)	
	Mixed ethnicity	42 (63.6%)	54 (58.7%)	
Schooling (n = 150)	< 4 years	5 (8.5%)	2 (2.2%)	0.194[b]
	4 to 8 years	50 (84.7%)	81 (89.0%)	
	> 8 years	4 (6.8%)	8 (8.8%)	
Number of pregnancies (n = 158)	Number	2.2 ± 1.5	2.3 ± 1.5	0.761[a]
Alcohol use (n = 158)	Yes	5 (7.6%)	4 (4.3%)	0.492[b]
Tobacco use (n = 158)	Yes	13 (19.7%)	10 (10.9%)	0.169[b]
Vitamin D Suplementation (n = 158)	Yes	6 (9.1%)	5 (5.4%)	0.528[b]
Folic Acid (n = 158)	Yes	46 (70.8%)	92 (87.6%)	0.038[b]
Iron (n = 158)	Yes	50 (75.8%)	76 (82.6%)	0.320[b]
Frequent use of sunscreen (n = 158)	Yes	9 (13.6%)	23 (25.0%)	0.108[b]
Regular exposure to sunlight (n = 158)	Yes	5 (7.6%)	54 (58.7%)	< 0.001[b]
Pregnancy-induced illness (n = 158)	Hypertension	27 (40.9%)	14 (15.2%)	< 0.001[b]
	Gestational diabetes	3 (4.5%)	2 (2.2%)	0.650[b]
	Urinary tract infection	14 (21.2%)	32 (34.8%)	0.077[b]
Prenatal care (n = 158)	Yes (> 6 check-ups)	12 (18.2%)	71 (78.3%)	< 0.001[b]
	Yes (< 6 check-ups)	42 (63.6%)	16 (17.4%)	
	No (no check-ups)	12 (18.2%)	4 (4.3%)	
Pre-pregnancy BMI (n = 116)	> 30 kg/m^2	6 (19.4%)	19 (22.4%)	0.905[b]
	25 to 29.9 kg/m^2	8 (25.8%)	22 (25.9%)	
	18.5 to 24.9 kg/m^2	16 (51.6%)	39 (45.9%)	
	< 18.5 kg/m^2	1 (3.2%)	5 (5.9%)	
Pregnancy weight gain	High	18 (58.1%)	55 (65.5%)	0.720[b]
	Adequate	7 (22.4%)	14 (16.7%)	
	Low	6 (19.4%)	15 (17.9%)	
Season (n = 158)	Spring	14 (21.2%)	48 (52.2%)	< 0.001[b]
	Summer	24 (36.4%)	44 (47.8%)	
	Fall	16 (24.2%)	0 (0.0%)	
	Winter	12 (18.2%)	0 (0.0%)	
Newborn Characteristics				
Gender (n = 158)	Male	35 (53.0%)	50 (54.3%)	0.727[b]
Type of birth (n = 158)	Vaginal	17 (25.8%)	48 (52.2%)	0.001[b]
Gestational Age (n = 158)	Weeks	29.8 ± 2.4	39.3 ± 1.2	< 0.001[a]
Birth weight (n = 158)	Grams	1250 ± 354.6	3317 ± 449.4	< 0.001[a]
Size for gestational age (n = 158)	Small for GA	14 (21.2%)	0.0 (0.0%)	< 0.001[b]
	Adequate for GA	47 (71.2%)	83 (90.2%)	
	Large for GA	5 (7.6%)	9 (9.8%)	

[a]Average and standard deviation. Level of significance of Student's t-test
[b]Number (percentage). Level of significance of the chi-squared test

Table 2 Description of general characteristics of preterm newborns (PTNB) and full-term newborns (FTNB) included in this study

Variables			PTNB Group (n = 66)	FTNB Group (n = 92)	p-value
Mother					
25(OH)D (n = 144)		ng/mL	21.7 ± 10.8	26.2 ± 9.8	0.011[a]
Deficiency		n (%)	27 (43.5%)	23 (28.0%)	0.018[b]
Insufficiency		n (%)	25 (40.3%)	29 (35.4%)	
Sufficiency		n (%)	10 (16.1%)	30 (36.6%)	
Parathyroid hormone (n = 121)		pg/mL	50.1 ± 40.7	51.1 ± 37.6	0.890[a]
Calcium (n = 145)		mg/dL	7.8 ± 1.2	8.7 ± 1.0	< 0.001[a]
Phosphorus (n = 144)		mg/dL	3.4 ± 1.5	3.3 ± 0.9	0.718[a]
Alkaline phosphatase (n = 145)		U/L	178.0 ± 81.6	269.1 ± 77.4	< 0.001[a]
Umbilical cord					
25(OH)D (n = 140)		ng/mL	25.9 ± 13.9	31.9 ± 12.3	0.009[a]
Deficiency		n (%)	25 (41.7%)	17 (21.3%)	0.033[b]
Insufficiency		n (%)	13 (21.7%)	24 (30.0%)	
Sufficiency		n (%)	22 (36.7%)	39 (48.4%)	
Calcium (n = 139)		mg/dL	9.3 ± 1.1	10.2 ± 1.0	< 0.001[a]
Phosphorus (n = 138)		mg/dL	5.9 ± 2.1	5.0 ± 1.2	0.002[a]
Alkaline phosphatase (n = 140)		U/L	363.3 ± 185.1	324.1 ± 344.4	0.431[a]

[a]Level of significance of the Student's t-test. [b]Level of significance of Chi-square test

No correlation was observed between 25(OH)D insufficiency and pregnancy complications (PIH, DM, and m UTI) nor habits during pregnancy (tobacco use, alcohol use, and iron, folic acid, and vitamin D supplementation) among women in the PTNB group (data not shown).

The 25(OH)D levels of newborns were also lower in the PTNB group compared to the FTNB group (25.9 ± 13.9 ng/dL vs. 31.9 ± 12.3 ng/dL; $p = 0.009$) (Table 2). Vitamin D insufficiency and deficiency was higher in the PTNB group compared to the FTNB group ($p = 0.033$) (Table 2).

There was a directly proportional correlation between 25(OH)D concentrations of mother and newborn umbilical cord in the PTNB group ($r = 0.596$; $p < 0.001$) and the FTNB group ($r = 0.765$; $p < 0.001$) (Fig. 1). An inverse correlation was found between PTH and 25(OH)D concentrations in all mothers ($r = -0.230$; $p = 0.012$). However, no statistically significant difference was observed between the groups concerning PTH (23.2% vs. 12.3%; $p = 0.090$).

Table 3 Odds ratio of 25(OH)D insufficiency in the mothers included in this study

Variable	Beta	Confidence Interval 95%	p-value
Season (Spring/Summer)	0.831	0.21 to 3.30	0.793
Exposure to sunlight (no)	1.158	0.48 to 2.74	0.739
Prematurity	2.993	1.02 to 8.74	0.045

With regard to the other bone metabolism-related markers, we found that the PTNB group had lower levels of calcium (7.8 ± 1.2 mg/dL vs. 8.7 ± 1.0 mg/dL; $p < 0.001$) and alkaline phosphatase (178.0 ± 81.6 U/L vs. 269.1 ± 77.4 U/L; $p < 0.001$) when compared to the FTNB group (Table 2).

Discussion

This study found that mothers who had given birth prematurely had a lower concentration of 25(OH)D compared to those who had given birth the end of their full term. The 25(OH)D levels of the newborns, in both groups, correlated with those of the mothers. However, this correlation was more significant in the FTNB group.

Vitamin D sufficiency (> 30 ng/mL) was found in 20.8% of mothers and 42.3% of newborns. Some studies in Brazil describe the 25(OH)D concentrations during pregnancy [10, 11, 14]. The prevalence of insufficiency/deficiency evidenced by them (range: 44.1% to 58.9%) was lower than this study, taking to account term birth (63.4%) and preterm birth (83.9%). Lower exposure to sunlight, no intake of supplements, low socioeconomic level, and African descent are considered at risk for insufficiency [4]. There are currently no data available for Brazil regarding preterm newborns and their mothers.

The cross-sectional study model does not allow the attribution of a cause and effect relationship. Therefore, we cannot infer whether a vitamin D deficiency was the cause of preterm birth. However, a meta-analysis that

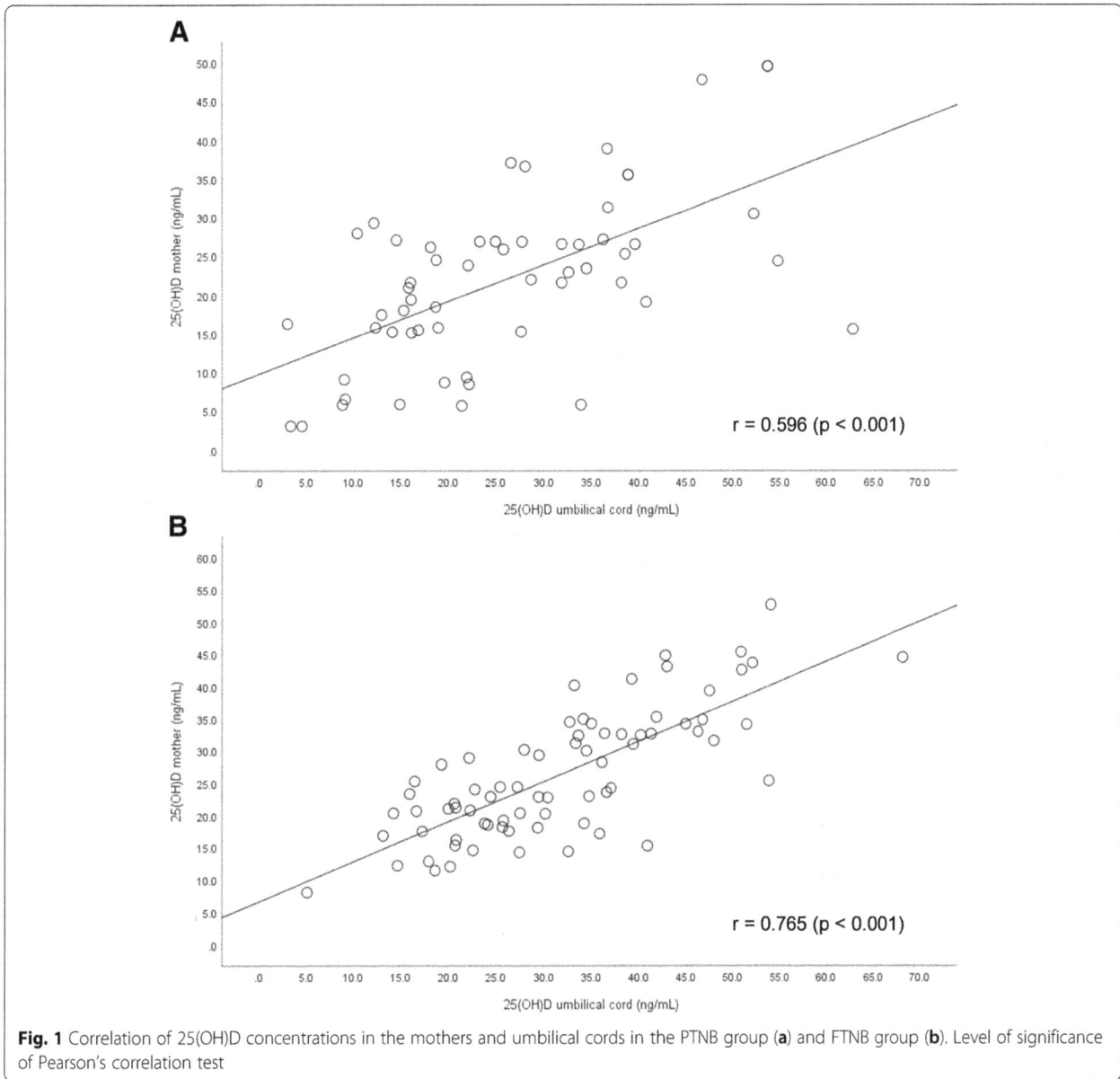

Fig. 1 Correlation of 25(OH)D concentrations in the mothers and umbilical cords in the PTNB group (**a**) and FTNB group (**b**). Level of significance of Pearson's correlation test

included only longitudinal studies confirmed that mothers with 25(OH)D concentrations below 30 ng/mL were 83% more likely to give birth prematurely [19].

The transport and metabolism of vitamin D of mothers and newborns have several particularities that should be considered when interpreting the results of this study. First, vitamin D is transported in the blood by the vitamin D-binding protein (DBP) (90%) and albumin (10%), and only 0.03% of it is unbound. The liver increases its DBP production, and lower levels of circulating albumin [20] are observed during pregnancy. The method adopted in this study to analyze 25(OH)D only allows for the evaluation of the DBP-bound percentage.

Secondly, the production of epimers related to the metabolism of vitamin D [ex: 3-epi25(OH)D3 and

3-epi-1.25α(OH)$_2$D3] rise during pregnancy, as well as in infants during the first 3 months of life [21]. This elevation is more significant in preterm newborns [21]. Until recently, it was not possible to measure the level of epimers in the blood or understand their function. However, recent studies have shown their affinity with 25(OH)D receptors, as well as 1,25(OH)D receptors, and also inhibit the production of PTH. Therefore, they play a role in the metabolism of vitamin D situations, such as prematurity [22].

Studies have shown the benefits of taking vitamin D supplements to reduce the probability of preterm birth [6]. In 2016, Wagner et al. observed a 60% decline in premature births in U.S. mothers with 25(OH)D concentrations above 40 ng/dL. The authors concluded that a prescribed supplementation of at least 4000 UI/day was required [23] to achieve these levels.

PTH concentrations are influenced by dietary factors (calcium intake), 1,25(OH)D levels and peptide levels related to PTH (PHTrP) produced in the parathyroid of the fetus and the placental tissue, and that step up vitamin D synthesis. While no difference in the mean PTH levels was observed between the groups, inverse correlation was found between PTH and 25(OH)D concentrations in all mothers. From a physiological perspective, the opposite was expected, as PTH levels tend to increase in the third trimester of pregnancy [24, 25]. A study that assessed the development of PTH concentrations in pregnant adolescents found an increase of 16.3 pg/mL between the 26th week of pregnancy and the moment of birth [26].

A difference between the levels of calcium, phosphorus and alkaline phosphatase in the blood was found between mothers who delivered preterm babies and those with full-term pregnancy deliveries. However, none of these markers correlated significantly with the 25(OH)D concentrations found in newborns and their mothers, suggesting that the factors involved in this alteration may be more related to maternal hemodilution than to vitamin D [27].

The 25(OH)D concentrations found in the mothers were lower than in their newborns and correlated with those of the newborns in both groups. In the meta-analysis published by Saraf et al., 2016 [4], forty studies confirmed a correlation between 25(OH)D concentrations in mothers and the umbilical cords of newborns, and the correlation coefficient ranged from 0.42 to 0.96. Only three studies found higher levels in the umbilical cords than in the mothers. According to the findings of this study, the closer a mother is to the end of her full-term pregnancy, the stronger the correlations of vitamin D levels between mother and newborn will be. All the three studies that found higher levels in newborns showed a higher prevalence of vitamin D insufficiency/deficiency. These findings suggest that gestational age and vitamin D sufficiency interact with the flow of vitamin D from mother to newborn.

Given the particularities of vitamin D metabolism during pregnancy, the lack of well-established cut-off points, and the limited number of studies evaluating the short and long-term safety of supplementation for mothers and their children, it is not currently advisable to universally recommend vitamin D supplementation to pregnant women. The identification of at-risk expecting mothers and the measurement of other vitamin D metabolism markers can provide clues regarding which pregnant women indeed evidence low levels and should take supplements.

Recently, a randomized, double-blind, placebo-controlled trial in Bangladesh assessed the effects of weekly prenatal vitamin D supplementation during pregnancy and postpartum. The authors did not find improvement in fetal or infant growth until 1 year of age [28].

To date, this is the first study conducted in Brazil that has evaluated 25(OH)D concentrations in a group of mothers who gave birth before the 32nd week of pregnancy and their newborns.

The lack of an evaluation of dietary factors, especially mothers' calcium intake, the difficulty of collecting part of the prenatal care data and accurately establishing the cause of preterm delivery can all be considered limitations of this study.

Conclusions

In conclusion, mothers who had delivered preterm babies (less than 32 weeks) and their premature newborns had lower 25(OH)D concentrations compared to women with full-term pregnancy deliveries. In both groups, 25(OH)D concentrations of the mothers correlated directly with those of the newborns, and this correlation was higher in the full-term birth group. Nevertheless, the recommended universal vitamin D supplementation in pregnant women to curb the risk of preterm birth is still incipient. More studies are required to clarify the particularities of vitamin D metabolism further and define the adequate 25(OH)D concentrations throughout pregnancy.

Abbreviations
25(OH)D: Vitamin D; FTNB: Full-term newborn; PTH: Intact parathyroid hormone; PTNB: Preterm newborn

Acknowledgments
We are grateful to the multidisciplinary team of Municipal University Hospital of São Bernardo do Campo for their support to the implementation of the Project, and the clinical analysis laboratory of the ABC School of Medicine for their analyses.

Funding
Financial Support: Foundation for Research Support of the State of São Paulo (FAPESP). Process number 2015/15399–1. (Certificate of presentation for Ethical Appreciation: 44213315.1.0000.0082).

Authors' contributions
MSK, FISS, and ROS: contributed with the outline, design, and data acquisition, analysis and interpretation. FRC and FAK contributed with data acquisition, analysis, and interpretation. All authors approved the final version of the manuscript.

Competing interests

The authors declare that they have co competing interests.

References

1. Afzal S, Brøndum-Jacobsen P, Bojesen SE, Nordestgaard BG. Vitamin D concentration, obesity, and risk of diabetes: a Mendelian randomization study. Lancet Diabetes Endocrinol. 2014;2:298–306.
2. van Schoor N, Lips P. Global overview of vitamin D status. Endocrinol Metab Clin N Am. 2017;46:845–70.
3. Gel-H F, Bouillon R, Clarke B, Chakhtoura M, Cooper C, McClung M, Singh RJ. Serum 25-Hydroxyvitamin D levels: variability, knowledge gaps, and the concept of a desirable range. J Bone Miner Res. 2015;30:1119–33.
4. Saraf R, Morton SM, Camargo CA Jr, Grant CC. Global summary of maternal and newborn vitamin D status - a systematic review. Matern Child Nutr. 2016;12:647–68.
5. Olmos-Ortiz A, Avila E, Durand-Carbajal M, Díaz L. Regulation of calcitriol biosynthesis and activity: focus on gestational vitamin D deficiency and adverse pregnancy outcomes. Nutrients. 2015;7:443–80.
6. Zhou SS, Tao YH, Huang K, Zhu BB, Tao FB. Vitamin D and risk of preterm birth: up-to-date meta-analysis of randomized controlled trials and observational studies. J Obstet Gynaecol Res. 2017;43:247–56.
7. Amegah AK, Klevor MK, Wagner CL. Maternal vitamin D insufficiency and risk of adverse pregnancy and birth outcomes: a systematic review and meta-analysis of longitudinal studies. PLoS One. 2017;12:e0173605.
8. Tian Y, Holzman C, Siega-Riz AM, Williams MA, Dole N, Enquobahrie DA, Ferre CD. Maternal serum 25-Hydroxyvitamin D concentrations during pregnancy and infant birthweight for gestational age: a three-cohort study. Paediatr Perinat Epidemiol. 2016;30:124–33.
9. Feng H, Xun P, Pike K, Wills AK, Chawes BL, Bisgaard H, Cai W, Wan Y, He K. In utero exposure to 25-hydroxyvitamin D and risk of childhood asthma, wheeze, and respiratory tract infections: a meta-analysis of birth cohort studies. J Allergy Clin Immunol. 2017;139:1508–17.
10. Pereira-Santos M, Queiroz-Carvalho G, David-Couto R, Barbosa Dos Santos D, Marlucia Oliveira A. Vitamin D deficiency and associated factors among pregnant women of a sunny city in Northeast of Brazil. Clin Nutr ESPEN. 2018;23:240–4.
11. Figueiredo ACC, Cocate PG, Adegboye ARA, Franco-Sena AB, Farias DR, de Castro MBT, et al. Changes in plasma concentrations of 25-hydroxyvitamin D and 1,25-dihydroxyvitamin D during pregnancy: a Brazilian cohort. Eur J Nutr. 2018;57:1059–72.
12. Boyle VT, Thorstensen EB, Thompson JMD, McCowan LME, Mitchell EA, Godfrey KM, Poston L, Wall CR, Murphy R, Cutfield W, Kenealy T, Kenny LC, Baker PN. The relationship between maternal 25-hydroxyvitamin D status in pregnancy and childhood adiposity and allergy: an observational study. Int J Obes. 2017;41:1755–60.
13. Guideline. Vitamin D supplementation in pregnant women. Geneva: World Health Organization; 2012.
14. Chrisostomo KR, Skare TL, Kulak J Jr, Urbanetz AA, Chrisostomo ER, Nisihara R. The prevalence and clinical associations of hypovitaminosis D in pregnant women from Brazil. Int J Gynaecol Obstet. 2018;143(1):66–70. https://doi.org/10.1002/ijgo.12575.
15. Institute of Medicine (US) and National Research Council (US) Committee to Reexamine IOM Pregnancy Weight Guidelines. In: Rasmussen KM, Yaktine AL, editors. Weight gain during pregnancy: Reexamining the Guidelines. Washington (DC): National Academies Press (US); 2009.
16. Ballard JL, Khoury JC, Wedig K, Wang L, Eilers-Walsman BL, Lipp R. New Ballard score, expanded to include extremely premature infants. J Pediatr. 1991;119:417–23.
17. Villar J, Cheikh Ismail L, Victora CG, Ohuma EO, Bertino E, Altman DG, et al. International fetal and newborn growth consortium for the 21st century (INTERGROWTH-21st). International standards for newborn weight, length,
18. and head circumference by gestational age and sex: the newborn cross-sectional study of the INTERGROWTH-21st project. Lancet. 2014;384:857–68.
18. Hurley SB. Outlining the clinical research: an epidemiological approach. 2nd ed. Porto Alegre: Artmed; 2003.
19. Amegah AK, Nsoh M, Ashley-Amegah G, Anaman-Togbor J. What factors influences dietary and non-dietary vitamin D intake among pregnant women in an African population? Nutrition. 2018;50:36–44. https://doi.org/10.1016/j.nut.2017.11.003.
20. Tsuprykov O, Chen X, Hocher CF, Skoblo R, Lianghong Yin, Hocher B. Why should we measure free 25(OH) vitamin D? J Steroid Biochem Mol Biol. 2018;180:87–104. https://doi.org/10.1016/j.jsbmb.2017.11.014.
21. Bailey D, Perumal N, Yazdanpanah M, Al Mahmud A, Baqui AH, Adeli K, Roth DE. Maternal-fetal-infant dynamics of the C3-epimer of 25-hydroxyvitamin D. Clin Biochem. 2014;47:816–22.
22. Ooms N, van Daal H, Beijers AM, Gerrits GP, Semmekrot BA, van den Ouweland JM. Time-course analysis of 3-epi-25-hydroxyvitamin D3 shows markedly elevated levels in early life, mainly from vitamin D supplementation in preterm infants. Pediatr Res. 2016;79:647–53.
23. Wagner CL, Baggerly C, McDonnell S, Baggerly KA, French CB, Baggerly L, Hamilton SA, Hollis BW. Post-hoc analysis of vitamin D status and reduced risk of preterm birth in two vitamin D pregnancy cohorts compared with South Carolina March of Dimes 2009-2011 rates. J Steroid Biochem Mol Biol. 2016;155:245–51.
24. McDonnell SL, Baggerly KA, Baggerly CA, Aliano JL, French CB, Baggerly LL, Ebeling MD, Rittenberg CS, Goodier CG, Mateus Niño JF, Wineland RJ, Newman RB, Hollis BW, Wagner CL. Maternal 25(OH)D concentrations ≥40 ng/mL associated with 60% lower preterm birth risk among general obstetrical patients at an urban medical center. PLoS One. 2017;12:e0180483.
25. Wagner CL, Taylor SN, Dawodu A, Johnson DD, Hollis BW. Vitamin D and its role during pregnancy in attaining optimal health of mother and fetus. Nutrients. 2012;4:208–30.
26. Young BE, McNanley TJ, Cooper EM, McIntyre AW, Witter F, Harris ZL, O'Brien KO. Vitamin D insufficiency is prevalent and vitamin D is inversely associated with parathyroid hormone and calcitriol in pregnant adolescents. Bone Miner Res. 2012;27:177–86.
27. Abrams SA. In utero physiology: role in nutrient delivery and fetal development for calcium, phosphorus, and vitamin D. Am J Clin Nutr. 2007;85:604S–7S.
28. Roth DE, Morris SK, Zlotkin S, Gernand AD, Ahmed T, Shanta SS, et al. Vitamin D supplementation in pregnancy and lactation and infant growth. N Engl J Med. 2018;379:535–46.

10

Sociocultural determinants of nomadic women's utilization of assisted childbirth in Gossi, Mali: a qualitative study

M.A. Ag Ahmed[1]* ⓘ, L. Hamelin-Brabant[2] and M.P. Gagnon[3]

Abstract

Background: In sub-Saharan Africa (SSA), nomads account for 30 to 60 million people. Their mobility, due to a constant search for pastures and water points, makes health services less accessible to them. Few nomadic women use assisted delivery, which increases the risk of maternal mortality. The reasons behind this limited use have been poorly documented. The objective of this study was to understand the sociocultural determinants of assisted childbirth by nomadic women.

Methods: We conducted a qualitative research in the health area of Gossi (Mali), mainly populated by nomads. Data were collected through a literature review, 26 semi-structured interviews, a non-participant observation, and a logbook. Nomadic women who gave birth in the past three months were included in the study, whether they used assisted delivery or not. A thematic content analysis was performed with QDA Miner software.

Results: The study identified a complex combination of determinants resulting in the use or non-use of assisted childbirth by the nomads of Gossi. Several participants recognized the value of assisted delivery but gave birth at home. They identified sociocultural determinants related to their representations and bodily experiences; the risks and emotions (fear, stress, anxiety) associated with pregnancy; the onset of labor and delivery; and their weak autonomy in terms of movement, decision-making, and economic agency. Nomadic women are not free in their movements, and in order to seek care, they require the permission and support of a man (husband, brother, or father). Furthermore, the participants are housewives, and men control family resources and make decisions regarding all financial matters. Assisted delivery is often only considered when there are complications.

Conclusion: This research has made it possible to understand the sociocultural determinants of the use of assisted childbirth among nomadic women, which should be taken into account when organizing health services for these populations.

Background

Despite significant progress in reducing its ravages, maternal mortality remains a major concern for public health [1, 2]. Worldwide, the maternal mortality ratio (MMR) fell from 385 to 216 deaths per 100,000 live births between 1990 and 2015, a drop of 44% [3]. However, almost all of these maternal deaths (99%) occur in developing countries (DCs) [4]. Unlike other regions of the world, Sub-Saharan Africa (SSA), with about 62% of global maternal deaths [5], did not experience significant

improvement [6]. Moreover, SSA still has the highest MMR in the world, with 546 deaths per 100,000 live births [7], and the World Health Organization (WHO) estimates the number of women living with untreated obstetric fistula to be over 2 million in Asia and SSA [6]. These high maternal mortality rates have severe health and social consequences for the survival of children and for the financial health of the family.

Despite the efforts made, the situation in Mali is not different from that of other SSAs. According to the latest Demographic Health Survey (DHS V), conducted in 2012, the MMR is 368 maternal deaths per 100,000 live births, while the WHO estimated it at 587 per 100,000 live births in 2015 [7]. These figures also mask

* Correspondence: intoucaina@yahoo.fr
[1]Université Laval, 1050 Avenue de la Médecine, room 3696, Québec G1V 0A6, Canada
Full list of author information is available at the end of the article

significant disparities between income levels and be-tween rural and urban populations [8, 9]. In particular, the risk for nomadic women of dying from maternal causes is very high [10].

There are multiple causes of this high maternal mortality [11]. In DCs, obstetric complications are the main cause of maternal death [12]. In fact, they will occur in about 40% of all pregnant women [13] and apparently cause about 80% of their deaths [14]. More than half of these deaths are related to direct causes, such as hemorrhage (27%), infections (10%), hypertension during pregnancy (14%), and abortions (7%) [15]. Next, indirect obstetric causes represent 27% of maternal deaths. It turns out that these obstetric complications cannot be predicted [16]. All women are therefore at risk of developing a life-threatening obstetric complication during pregnancy.

This high maternal mortality is not acceptable because most maternal deaths are due to preventable causes or modifiable behaviors [17, 18]. There is scientific evidence in particular regarding the potential for skilled care at birth as a means of preventing maternal deaths [14]. According to some estimates, it can reduce maternal mortality from 16 to 33% [19], which makes it the most effective intervention to save women's lives [20].

Furthermore, if it is agreed that assisted childbirth is a relevant strategy for avoiding maternal deaths [21, 22], it is also clear that women do not have the same opportunities to use it because of their sociocultural and economic differences or differences in the places where they live. Indeed, several factors can delay the use of maternal healthcare or make its use impossible [17, 18]. For this reason, despite scientific evidence attesting to the effectiveness of assisted childbirth and the efforts made by several countries to make quality health services available, women continue to give birth at home. In fact, coverage for assisted childbirth is 66% worldwide, but is only 49% for SSA and South Asia [23], compared to 97–99% in high-income countries [24].

For nomadic pastoralists in SSA, the use of healthcare services is very limited when compared to the general population [25]. This is due to several constraints, on the one hand, stemming from their environment and their way of life and, on the other, from important social and spatial disparities. Although underestimated in demographic statistics [26], these nomadic pastoralists are numerous, comprising an estimated 20 to 30 million people in the Sahel [25]. They are defined by Wiese [27] as anyone living in a tent, taking care of livestock, and practicing transhumance. In Mali, nomadic pastoralists are mainly Tuareg, Moor, and Fulani peoples. They live more frequently in low-rainfall desert areas where they migrate throughout the year along well-defined and almost identical routes depending on their rights of

access and use, as well as the availability of resources for themselves and their animals [25].

In Mali, the use of assisted childbirth was already limited among nomadic pastoralists, but further deteriorated with the conflicts in the north and center of the country where they live. In fact, in these regions, about 7% of health facilities in Timbuktu, 4% in Gao, and 69% in Kidal were still closed in 2016 due to the security situation [28]. Assisted childbirth proportions in Mali, while reaching 58.4% for the whole country, decrease to 2.6% in Timbuktu, 2.4% in Gao, and 3.3% in Kidal [29]. However, even before the outbreak of war in northern Mali in 2009, these proportions were 35% for Timbuktu, 29% for Gao, and 29% for Kidal, compared to 66% at the national level. In SSA, these trends are confirmed for nomads. In Tanzania, assisted childbirth rates among nomadic women of Dagota were lower than those of the sedentary Iraqw tribe [30]. Similarly, in Ethiopia, of 478 Afar nomadic mothers interviewed, 83.3% gave birth to their last child at home without skilled care [31].

The reasons why these nomadic women do not use assisted childbirth seem difficult to identify as they vary from one context to another. Several authors in SSA refer to determining factors, which could be geographical, economic, cultural, technical, social, or political [10, 27, 32–34], whereas only a few studies explore them for Mali in particular. However, some studies, whose results will be discussed later, have been carried out in Mali [35], Chad [36], Ethiopia [31, 37–40], Kenya [41], and Sudan [42]. These studies have identified some sociocultural, geographic, and financial determinants that could limit the use of maternal healthcare by nomadic women.

The objective of this study is therefore to contribute to this very limited knowledge in order to improve the use of assisted childbirth by nomads in Mali. More specifically, it aims to describe and reach an insight into the sociocultural determinants of the use of assisted childbirth by nomadic women in the commune of Gossi.

This study was guided by the conceptual model of determinants of delivery service use proposed by Gabrysch and Campbell [43], who were themselves inspired by that of Thaddeus and Maine [44], which seems to be the most operational and best-suited model to understand the determinants of the use of assisted childbirth. Furthermore, it is adapted to the context of DCs [45]. It has the advantage of taking into account not only the risks of complications, but also the normal situations of using maternal care (preventive for instance). For these authors, the factors involved in the decision to use preventive maternal care significantly differ from those determining research in emergency obstetric care in the case of complications. In the second case, the severity of the complication may prevail over cost or distance considerations. In the event of life-threatening danger, even those who consider that normal delivery does not justify expenses and travel to a health center may attempt to overcome these barriers, despite high costs [43]. However, for normal delivery or preventive care, the time might be longer and the decision-making mechanism different in such cases.

In addition, this framework seems to distinguish intention to use care from behavior, i.e. actual use of care. For Gabrysch and Campbell [43], four groups of factors influence intention and behavior with respect to seeking care in a health institution. They may be divided into two groups: sociocultural characteristics and perceived benefits/needs, which influence the intention to use care; and economic accessibility (affordability) and physical accessibility, which influence behavior. However, all these factors interact with one another. In this study, we are more specifically interested in the sociocultural characteristics pertaining to the use of assisted childbirth. However, these sociocultural determinants are not the only ones that influence the use of assisted delivery by nomads. They constitute the first part of the results of the doctoral thesis of the lead author (MAAA). The second part of our results will be presented in another publication and will focus on the determinants related to nomads' perceptions of the quality and geographical and financial accessibility of health services.

Methods and study setting

The commune of Gossi (Timbuktu region) was selected as the setting for this research. It encompasses a total surface area of 15,000 km^2 for a population of 24,065 inhabitants, of whom 90% are nomads [46]. It is mainly inhabited by Tamasheq (or Tuareg) and Fulani [47]. The choice of this commune was based on its characteristics (nomadic); the presence of a functional health center (Kaigourou); and the feasibility of research (security conditions for accessing nomads).

Study design, population, and sampling

The research design is qualitative, which is particularly apt for describing, explaining, and analyzing complex phenomena that have been little explored. The approach used is similar to ethnography. However, we did not have sufficient time of immersion and direct observation that requires an ethnographic approach. The study population includes nomadic women living in their camps who have given birth during the last 3 months preceding data collection, in order to minimize memory bias. Tamasheq nomads were chosen due to the fact that they form the largest group in the commune and that we are fluent in the local language, which facilitates interview administration and data analysis. A mixture of purposive and convenience sampling techniques was used. Interviews were conducted with women until saturation [48]. To diversify our sample [49], we included women of all ages and with varying parities, who gave birth in health facilities or elsewhere, and whose camps were located at a limited distance from the closest health center.

In preparation for recruitment, we identified the position and movements of nomadic camps in the commune. Then, during eight field trips to four cardinal points, we reached these camps in their pasture areas for four to seven-day stays. Given our limited financial means and security conditions, all trips were within an 80-km radius of Gossi. Once in a camp, we first contacted the camp leader, introducing ourselves, explaining our goals, and asking if there were women who had given birth in the last 3 months. When a woman was identified, we camped nearby and the recruited assistant contacted the woman to explain our goals and ask her for an interview.

Data collection

The collection of data for this research project took place in three stages. A one-month preparatory stage made it possible to explain the study to the actors (health services, administrative and political authorities), to identify the pasture areas, and to get an insight into the movements of the nomad camps. Logistic means of collection were also identified. Similarly, a local assistant fluent in the Tamasheq language was recruited and trained to conduct the interviews in order to minimize the researcher's gender bias. Interview guides were translated into the Tamasheq language and pre-tested. They were then slightly adjusted before being validated by our research directorate. A second two-month phase allowed us to collect data in nomad camps. Then, after the interviews were transcribed, we returned to check their validity with five participants.

Three collection techniques were used concomitantly:

Semi-structured interviews were conducted individually by a trained research assistant and administered in a quiet place away from family members in order to allow research participants to speak freely and thus prevent possible response biases. After obtaining women's informed consent, all interviews were recorded and lasted between 42 and 76 min each. An internal validation process was undertaken after each interview by compiling information that was not clear under a list of topics, which were pursued more extensively in the next interviews. This technique was suggested as a means of improving the quality and rigor of the interview guide [50].

The guide consisted of open questions based on the conceptual framework provided by Gabrysch and Campbell [43] as well as our review of the literature and was designed to identify the factors determining use of assisted childbirth by the nomads. The guide was flexible and provided the relevant points to be addressed. The questions of the first part of the interview guide focused on the socio-demographic characteristics of the participants. Then, the other sections discussed the representations and experiences of women during pregnancy and delivery, their use of care, their access to information, their knowledge about health services and the decision-making process for assisted childbirth.

Non-participant observation helped us to get an insight into the context while not being directly involved, thus maintaining an external perspective. In order to carry out these observation procedures, we designed an observation grid [51]. The observation sites were nomadic camps. Although the observation sites and procedures were not hidden, we tried to remain as discreet as possible, while taking notes so as not to miss anything. We noted the different stages of the fieldwork (dates, people met, etc.) along with the situations encountered (what the nomads do and the nature of their interactions, etc.), and developed a preliminary interpretation of the phenomena observed as a prelude to data analysis.

We also kept *a logbook* aimed at minimizing our influence on the collection and analysis of data by stimulating our reflexivity and capacity to become aware of our own feelings and biases [52]. The logbook thus helped clarify our positions and ensure greater transparency in the process by recording the way we made decisions throughout the research project.

Data analysis

Thematic content analysis was used as it is particularly indicated for exploratory and explicative approaches [53]. It describes the material collected and explores its meaning to reflect what the participants said in the most objective and reliable way possible. The analysis started during data translation and transcription. Interviews were first translated in French (language of the thesis) by us, and then in English (for this article) thanks to the services of a professional translator. To ensure that we accurately reported what our participants said, we went back to the field to check the accuracy of the transcripts with five of them.

The verbatim reports were then re-read using the audio recordings in order to validate them and thus ensure the reliability of opinions. This also made it possible to better understand and become familiar with the content of the interviews and separate substantial information from anecdotal elements [54]. This step enabled us to identify the first themes [53] in order to design a draft analysis grid. Next, we began to codify and categorize the data based on inter-coder agreements concerning four interviews, reached with our research supervisor in order to ensure the validity of our analysis.

Initially, verbatim were examined line by line and paragraph by paragraph to generate label codes attached to analysis units of variable size. These codes made it possible to decipher the different sociocultural determinants of the use of assisted childbirth by nomads. This coding step is intended to facilitate the manipulation of the data. Once this coding step was completed, the thematization (or categorization) phase started, which consisted of grouping several close codes under a same sub-theme. This process made it possible to group similar answers under the same generic title. Once all the sub-themes were obtained, they were in turn grouped into themes.

We used QDA Miner analysis software, to which the verbatim report was exported in order to facilitate data management. Data were then categorized favoring a type of sequenced approach [53] using both inductively derived and pre-existing themes. First, using an inductive approach, a reading of the verbatim led to the creation of sub-themes and themes. Then, in a second step, they were put into perspective with those predefined through our conceptual framework to build an analysis grid that took into account the important elements reported by participants.

We created a thematic tree representing the hierarchy of themes and sub-themes according to their main or peripheral role to answer our research questions. Their recurrence allowed to have a synthetic representation of the analyzed content in relation to the different cases identified in our study [53]. Thus, thematic groupings (which may be convergent, divergent or complementary) have emerged as kinds of matrices of meaning that coexist with each other. They made it possible to name the different dimensions of the sociocultural determinants. Relationships were then established to find links between these dimensions, and contrasted to form a universe of meaning that allowed us to describe and understand the different sociocultural determinants of the use of assisted childbirth by nomads.

During this process, several steps have been taken to ensure the validity and reliability of our data and analyses. Our interview guide was pre-tested and then adjusted before being validated by the thesis supervisors to ensure that it met our research objectives. The use of the triangulation technique by juxtaposing collection methods and the diversification of sources of information also ensured the validity of our results. Our good knowledge of the field allowed us to understand participants' language and values in order to minimize interpretative biases that may arise from cultural differences between researchers and participants. Our results have also been compared with those of similar studies on the determinants of health service utilization in SSA. Moreover, we tried to be as transparent as possible throughout the research process. We provided a detailed description of the methods and procedures of our study and continued to improve them as we progressed in our research. Although we are aware that neutrality is impossible in qualitative research, we have undertaken a honest and reflexive approach by reporting in the logbook the different methodological approaches on the ground and recognizing our biases.

Results

The results are presented in two parts: the sociodemographic characteristics of the participants and the sociocultural determinants of the utilization of assisted childbirth.

Sociodemographic characteristics of participants

We visited 35 nomadic camps and recruited 26 women. These women were found in 24 camps. The sociodemographic profile of these women includes their place of residence, their age, their occupation as well as that of their husband, and their number of pregnancies. We also noted the use or non-use of prenatal consultation (PNC) and assisted childbirth.

The camps visited are within a radius of 16 to 62 km from the nearest health center (Kaigourou). The study participants are 18 to 40 years old. Their age distribution is as follows: 18 to 25 years ($n = 11$); 26 to 35 years ($n = 11$); and 36 years and older ($n = 4$). Of the 26 participants, 19 (73.1%) claim to have received prenatal care (PNC) at least once at the health center, while only 11 (42.3%) have given birth there during their lifetime. Women in the youngest group report less use of assisted childbirth (7 out of 11 have not had recourse to assisted childbirth).

All the participants are married housewives, and their spouses are breeders. No woman has been to school. The distribution of the number of pregnancies ranges from one to nine pregnancies per woman. Two were primiparous, eight had two or three pregnancies, and 16 had four or more pregnancies. Most of them started to have children at a very young age (11 of the women before the age of 25).

In addition, during 3 months of non-participant observation, we were able to appreciate the social and living environment of the nomads. In the camps we visited, nomads usually live in family (couple and children) under a single tent of leather or cotton of about 20 square meters. The distribution of work within the family seems well codified. The animals are at the center and punctuate nomads' life. In the daytime, men tend the livestock in the pasture and at night, the whole family gets involved in animal care. When milking is finished and the milk is distributed, families meet to exchange information around a fire. We participated in these exchanges, which, for the occasion, concerned the

difficulties of resorting to health services. On the other hand, the life of nomads seems well organized. Their socioeconomic level is function of their social status but also the number of livestock they have. The elderly and the women are highly respected, which gives them several privileges. Also, their way of life allows nomads to be quite autonomous to the extent that they produce most of what they need to live (milk, meat, butter). Other food is often considered as a supplement or luxury that not everyone can afford. In case of illness, self-medication is used first, sometimes with modern medicines brought from the city. However, nomads seem very open to modern health. On the other hand, nomads perceive themselves as quite vulnerable because their whole economy is dependent on unpredictable rainfall. At the same time, they demonstrate resilience capacities under extreme conditions. These observations allowed us to better understand the sociocultural dimensions that directly or indirectly influenced their use of assisted childbirth.

Body representations and experiences of pregnancy and childbirth

Our findings show that the use of assisted childbirth is influenced by some dominant representations of their body that women develop during pregnancy, at the beginning of labor, and during childbirth.

During pregnancy

For many participants, pregnancy is a normal, even unavoidable process. All eyes in the community are turned toward married women waiting for pregnancy: "Pregnancy is a normal phenomenon for us women. All women are supposed to get pregnant." (Aicha, 22).

According to them, the femininity of women and their status as wives are confirmed only through their ability to get pregnant. But beyond that, the fact of not being able to get pregnant could even create problems within the couple: "Pregnancies are part of our life as a woman even if they make us tired. Married woman are expected to give birth. The opposite would be very frowned upon and could even be problematic." (Ami, 38).

Paradoxically, the participants affirm that their pregnancy is often hidden, especially during the first months, because they feel ashamed of having gotten pregnant insofar as this implies the performance of a sexual act, which is a taboo topic of conversation, even with one's husband:

Even if I am pregnant, I cannot talk to people; it is a source of shame otherwise. They must understand by themselves ... I do not tell my husband because I do not know what he may think. I do not know if he is aware of what happened to me; we do not talk about it. (Lalla, 20)

Several participants admit that the neighbors can imagine that a woman is pregnant when she shows some signs, but this will only be confirmed when there is a change in the parturient's body (visible belly). Typical subterfuge includes keeping the pregnancy secret for several months, which can delay recourse to maternal care.

Once considered pregnant, the woman is viewed as fragile and vulnerable. As such, she receives special attention and measures including the use of healthcare facilities to protect her and enable completion of pregnancy: "*Once she becomes pregnant, a woman is considered a fragile human being. People pay close attention to her so that the pregnancy will succeed. If we feel that she needs something, we must give it to her very quickly; otherwise she risks aborting.*" (Mariama, 33).

However, women recognize the capacity and limits of their bodies to cope with pregnancy and childbirth, a recognition which determines their use of healthcare. Thus, some participants refer to knowledge or experiences related to their bodies, enabling them to deal with any pregnancy without seeking healthcare. They refer to a body that practices, learns, gets used to, and acquires its own abilities to take on pregnancy and childbirth without any assistance: "*With each pregnancy and childbirth, you learn, and your body gets used to dealing with them.*" (Tahouskat, 23).

In addition, other parturients, without questioning their abilities, recognize the limits of this body, especially when obstetric complications appear. In these cases, using healthcare is envisaged or desired by most participants to lessen their suffering: "*You can suffer from illness at such a level that you cannot stand it anymore. One should then consider going to the health center to receive healthcare.*" (Rokiatou, 30).

The beginning of labor

The beginning of labor is also an important moment for the participants. It is marked by several representations that tend to delay the use of care. When labor begins, some participants said they would hide the pains to make sure that this was indeed the beginning of the labor and thus avoid conveying false information to neighboring people: "*I had pain for a day and felt that I should give birth, but I did not want to tell anyone about it until I was sure.*" (Fadimatou, 30) Furthermore, to show their bravery, other women hide the beginning of childbirth as long as possible: "*Our tradition is to hide the birth until the last minute so that the woman shows that she is strong.*" (Fatimata, 27).

Once labor begins and the neighbors are informed, a small group of women come to stay with the parturient woman to support her. These women pray at a distance, but the parturient gives birth without any direct assistance: "*I gave birth on my own. The women were there, but they did not help me. They cannot do anything, nor do they care to do so.*" (Safietou, 20) A woman, more often than not the mother of the parturient, will intervene only to cut the umbilical cord: "*I have always given birth at home with the help of my mother. Her assistance involves waiting until I give birth to cut the cord of the child and that's all.*" (Zeinabou, 32).

Childbirth

Childbirth is feared by nomadic women and their neighbors, as this proverb illustrates: "*Before giving birth, every woman has her two feet hung in her grave until delivery.*" (Zeinabou, 32) Indeed, childbirth is unanimously perceived by our participants as a period of danger, and the outcome is uncertain, entailing a high risk of dying: "*The biggest fear for we women is the sinking of the genitals* (genital prolapses).... *In addition, we can have miscarriages or even die.*" (Tafa, 22) Furthermore, delivery is sometimes feared because of the pain associated with it, although there are different perceptions of this pain among pregnant women. For many participants, giving birth in pain is natural, self-evident, and transient, making health services less relevant: "*Women give birth every week, and deliveries are naturally painful, but it happens anyway and without the presence of health workers.*" (Mamata, 22) Facing the magnitude of these pains, others have recognized their own limits when it comes to bearing pregnancy and thus say they are more favorable to using healthcare services, of which they recognize the effectiveness: "*Delivery is very painful. Even if it is normal, we need help, and health services are very effective.*" (Mariama, 33).

On the other hand, several emotions, combined with their personal experiences, also seem crucial for these women in deciding whether or not to use assisted childbirth. Women talk about their worries and their fears when they refer to the various consequences of a delivery that went wrong and could affect their womanhood and compromise their union. "*I am always afraid because at each delivery, I can end up with a tedafé* (vesico-vaginal fistula in Tamasheq) *or other problems that can make me infertile.*" (Taliat, 22) Also, experiences of anxiety or stress are conveyed when women recount cases of abnormal childbirth. "*Imagine, when childbirth is impeded, you lose hope of living. You tell yourself it's all over for you.*" (Ami, 38) Facing these emotions, several participants prefer to turn to assisted childbirth.

Home delivery is the most common recourse for pregnant women, although it is not necessarily the first choice of the majority of participants. It is however a deliberate and assumed choice for some parturient women, who for the most part only know this type of childbirth: *"I prefer to give birth at home."* (Taliat, 22) Their preference for home deliveries will only change if their lives are threatened or when they are no longer able to make a decision. *"Personally, I would go to the health center only when I have no hope left, when people decide for me."* (Fatimata, 27) Some justify their preferences with a concern for adhering to a social standard or tradition that recommends giving birth at home: *"For home deliveries, we found our parents doing so and we followed in their footsteps."* (Lalla, 20).

Assisted childbirth is of interest for the majority of participants, although some women gave birth at home:

> I think it would have been better to give birth at the health center according to what I hear. Personally, I always gave birth at home, but that's because I had no other choice. People here are afraid to give birth at the health center; they do not know how it will happen. It is easier for me and my family to give birth at home. (Safietou, 20)

Women have found several benefits to assisted childbirth, including shorter labor hours and the lessening of pain: *"When you give birth at the health center, with the drugs, the labor time is shortened, and you suffer less."* (Khadou, 35) Also, parturient women have confessed that health services are also very effective postpartum: *"Since I gave birth at the health center, I'm doing everything to come back because the conditions are better there. You're cared for and your child too."* (Mariama, 33) For these reasons, many women no longer consider giving birth outside of health centers: *"Since I discovered delivery at the health center, I try to come back even when I am living far away."* (Khadou, 35).

Risks during pregnancy and childbirth
During our interviews, the women insisted on a vast array of simple and complicated risks to which they are exposed during pregnancy and childbirth and which determine their use of healthcare. They represent these risks in different ways according to their own criteria, with a great variability of interpretations. Almost all parturient women acknowledge having experienced various diseases/risks during their pregnancy and childbirth periods: *"As soon as I get pregnant, I get sick. Abdominal pain with constant vomiting. I have to lie down all the time. During pregnancy and childbirth, we face a lot of risks."* (Lawal, 38) Others also refer to the ultimate risk, which could be death: *"Risks during childbirth are many and various and may lead to death."* (Tahousket, 23) They report that age and a high number of pregnancies (multiparity) add to these risks.

Given this strong perception of risk and the perceived effectiveness of assisted childbirth, the majority of women seek healthcare services: *"I gave birth at home, but more and more women tend to seek care and to give birth at the health center because it seems really helpful for a quick recovery."* (Fatimata, 27) However, they turn to healthcare services only when they are facing complications.

The autonomy of nomadic women
Our findings also highlight three dimensions related to the low autonomy of nomadic women, all three constraining their use of assisted childbirth. These are autonomy of movement, of decision-making, and of economic agency.

Autonomy of movement
Most participants admitted that they did not have freedom of movement and that their movements were governed by rules. In this regard, a woman traveling alone would not be well perceived, and the authorization of the husband or a family member (father or brother) would be required for the use of assisted childbirth. Indeed, the Muslim woman owes obedience and respect to her husband, and as such, challenging his authority is perceived as a religious transgression: *"We are Muslims; the woman cannot challenge instructions from her husband and travel to the center without his authorization as well."* (Rokiatou, 30) Moreover, for other participants, this is part of the education received from their parents that should be maintained: *"We have always been taught that this is how it is and how our mothers behaved. We must get these authorizations and follow their example."* (Assietou, 29).

In addition, for most participants, a second requirement for assisted childbirth is that the parturient women be accompanied by a man. The reasons given are primarily pragmatic. The ailing woman needs sturdy arms to cope with the unsuitable mode of transport on damaged roads: *"To go to the health center, you need to find companions first. How can I travel sick in a transport vehicle without being accompanied by a man, a member of my family? It's not acceptable."* (Leila, 24) The company of a man during their evacuation was very much appreciated by the participants. However, men are not always available to accompany them, which sometimes makes it impossible to use assisted childbirth: *"I was sick (childbirth), while no man was available to bring me to the health center. They were all busy with the animals."* (Salka, 30).

Also, once at the health center, the presence of a man would also be required to make decisions regarding expenses and hospitalization, or act as an intermediary between the woman and the health workers: *"I have spoken very little with health workers. They talk to the man (husband) and give him the papers (prescriptions).*

Then he pays for the drugs." (Fatimata, 27) For the participants, all these are elements that limit their mobility as regards recourse to assisted delivery.

Decision-making autonomy as regards the use of assisted childbirth

Participants explained a complex decision-making process that follows several stages in which various interactions between different people occur. This process highlights the low autonomy of women as regards decision-making.

A network of actors controlling the decision-making process

For the participants, decision-making is controlled by a network of actors essentially made up of men. For these women, it is primarily the husbands who would be at the forefront when it comes to making decisions: *"I did not see how I could go to the health center while my husband was on a trip."* (Taliat, 22) Moreover, the parturient woman's parents, in whose house she gives birth, would preferably be other important actors: *"When the woman gives birth at her parents' house, they are the ones who decide. This case is the most common one, especially for young people."* (Fadimata, 40) Sometimes, decision-making is extended to the community, particularly to the notables and especially to the head of the camp, who manages the problem and proposes solutions to the husband. Indeed, at an advanced stage of complications, it is often badly perceived for the husband to decide alone for his wife without referring to the notables: *"It is the notables of the camp who decide ... it is sometimes badly seen for a man to decide alone for his wife."* (Leila, 24).

This interdependence among husbands, parents, and relatives is recognized by participants as being very valuable in facilitating decision-making.

In addition, some participants negotiated with their spouses to await their delivery in a family near the health center a few weeks before the pregnancy reached full term: *"For deliveries at the health center, if I'm not too stuck by that time, I will live and wait with a family near the center."*(Khadou, 35) In these cases, the woman asks permission of the husband, who evaluates the suitability of the request, and the decision is made by mutual agreement of the two spouses. This decision is also facilitated by the presence of host families (parents, acquaintances, or friends).

In other cases, this process of negotiation between the spouses did not result in the use of assisted childbirth because the decision was made late, either due to issues of modesty or because the communication between them was incomplete. Despite the insistence of some parturient women, their husbands felt that there were not enough reasons for them to give birth at the health center, which led to their not using the services:

> *Once I tried to talk to my husband about going to the village and giving birth at the health center. But he thinks that I am in a good shape and that my deliveries have always gone well at home. So he did not want me to, and I gave birth at home.* (Safietou, 20)

In most cases, the decision of the husband or parents is final, which limits the power of women to use assisted childbirth.

When there are complications, the decision is made without the parturient woman's input

For many participants, the decision-making process is different, and for them childbirth entails other steps when there are obstetric complications. In such cases, their decision is determined by the seriousness of the parturient woman's state of health, which is itself judged on the basis of two criteria. On the one hand, there is the duration of her extended labor: *"The decision is made when the woman spends several days of labor, and the family realizes that she cannot give birth at home."* (Fadimatou, 26) On the other hand, there is damage relating to the physical health of the parturient woman (fainting, labor stoppage, etc.):

> *I had to pass out before my mother would ask my father to take me to the health center. I do not remember anything. My mother later told me how it went. Fortunately, I arrived at the health center in time.* (Khadou, 35)

This decision-making process is subject to a series of negotiations and consultations and requires consensus among family members: *"The decision is made in a concerted manner. There should be mutual agreement before the decision is reached."* (Fadimata, 40) As a first step, the parturient's female assistants assess the seriousness and urgency of the situation and provide guidance for the use of the healthcare center. They then inform the men, who make the decision for her evacuation: *"The women around you will recognize the complications. Then they will go to the men to find solutions."* (Fatimata, 27) For many participants, decision-making would depend heavily on the values and opinions of their husband or parents (father or brothers).

The majority of parturient women mentioned not having participated in this decision-making process, a reflection of their weak autonomy as regards their recourse to assisted childbirth.

Economic autonomy: Control of financial resources by men

Our interviews show that all the participants are housewives. They do not perform any paid work, which limits their autonomy to seek care. *"We do not perform any paid work to earn money. We take care of the family, children, and old people. It's already a lot of work. But how can we have money in our bush here? There is no trade or income-generating activity."* (Lawal, 36) In addition, participants acknowledged that men control family resources and decide on all financial issues. As such, they are responsible for the health of the family and it is up to them, regardless of their wealth, to cope with the expense of caring for their wives: *"When I'm at my husband's house, he's the one who decides and gives me the means to go to the health center for care."* (Khadou, 35) The payment of expenses related to the care of women is therefore an obligation for men. As a result, the costs of care would sometimes discourage them from sending their women to the health center: *"It is the men who decide about everything. Even if a woman has her property, she cannot decide for herself. Their authorization is therefore required to give birth at the health center."* (Lalla, 20) Women thus acknowledge that they have limited access to family resources and that their control by men would affect their decision-making power to seek care: *"Maybe if women had their own means, they could decide on their own!"* (Lalla, 20).

Discussion

This study provides important contextual information on a complex combination of determinants, the result of which is the use or non-use of assisted childbirth by Tamasheq nomads in matters of health in the commune of Gossi in Mali. Most participants indicated that they prefer to give birth in health centers, but this is often impossible due to many constraints related to their sociocultural, health, and economic context. In this difficult environment, the use of assisted childbirth is more often an expression of pragmatic choices by nomads and its limitation is related to several determinants.

In fact, the relationship that nomadic women have with their bodies seems to be one of the important elements in explaining their use of assisted childbirth. It appears that this recourse is largely influenced by certain dominant representations that women have of their bodies, risks, pain, and emotions during pregnancy and childbirth. In this regard, our study is in line with several others in SSA that have achieved similar results [55–65]. These studies emphasize, and sometimes differ on, the links between sociocultural determinants and the use of maternal healthcare. However, for the most part, their findings support the contention that these determinants would deter women from using obstetric care [60].

Also, the results of some studies in nomadic areas in SSA mainly match those of our study, namely how pregnancy is detected, the modesty that it entails, and the hiding of the women's condition which limits their use of maternal healthcare [31, 35–42]. According to these authors, pregnancy gives women a fragile and vulnerable status, more attention, and privileges. On the other hand, the women of Gossi seem to refer less to traditional healers, marabouts, and birth attendants than others in SSA. However, childbirth is also dreaded by all these women, and the rules regarding delivery in particular are similar. Recourse to healthcare is seen as useful only in the case of complications. These sociocultural barriers to the use of maternal healthcare sometimes seem more ingrained than other obstacles, such as those of a geographical or financial nature [36].

Apart from these studies on nomads, several authors in SSA have shown that the representations that women and the communities in which they live make in relation to pregnancy and childbirth largely guide their behavior in the use of healthcare. For most participants, pregnancy and childbirth are seen as "normal phenomena," giving them the feeling that their bodies are competent to deal with whatever might arise. As such, they do not need to be provided with healthcare [66]. Therefore, this dominant perception of "normal" pregnancy prevents many women from seeking care for routine deliveries [67]. This is why in many contexts, paradoxically, women with access to care give birth at home. In line with our results, some authors conclude that it is not enough to have accessible care for the use of assisted delivery to be effective [67]. They consider that this recourse would instead depend to a greater extent on the relevance to and appropriation of services by the communities in question. On the other hand, if childbirth is often considered as not requiring the use of healthcare, this is not the case when obstetric complications appear. For many nomadic women in our study, only complications would warrant assisted childbirth. On the other hand, the impact of this late recourse on maternal mortality in obstetric emergencies is questionable given the time required to intervene and save women in distress. Some authors even associate it with a high maternal mortality [67].

In addition, the use of assisted childbirth in the Hausa area (Nigeria), for example, is also limited by the fact that unaided childbirth is seen as an act of bravery and pride [56]. Likewise, it is seen in Uganda as an endurance test to which the woman must submit, and maternal death is seen as an act of fate [62]. However, there seems to be an evolution in these beliefs. Presumably, many of our study participants, including those who have never used assisted childbirth, are increasingly recognizing its benefits, particularly to shorten labor hours and postpartum care. Also, the risks and pain associated with childbirth generate a number of emotions that may trigger a preference for assisted childbirth. On the other hand, nomadic women hide their pregnancy, but not for the same reasons mentioned in some studies in SSA. For the nomads, their condition is hidden because acknowledging the pregnancy would suggest the sexual act, which is a taboo topic of conversation. This is not the case, for example, in Cameroon or Zimbabwe, where women apparently hide their pregnancies to protect themselves from "evil spirits," including witchcraft, to which they believe themselves more vulnerable [61, 66]. Similarly, in Nigeria, it is because of a belief called "Kunya" (meaning modesty) that the primigravida in particular would hide her pregnancy [56].

In several SSA countries, as in the case of nomadic women in our study, childbirth is often perceived as very risky, and this element of risk would justify going to the health center [68]. Indeed, the combination of fear of suffering or of dying during childbirth would largely justify women's preferences for assisted childbirth. On the other hand, the happiness related to this process seems better expressed in other countries in SSA [69] than among the nomadic women we met.

Moreover, the analysis of participants' discourse in our study also revealed a low autonomy of nomadic women, which seems to limit their use of assisted childbirth. This is in line with several other studies in SSA that identify three dimensions to judge the level of autonomy of women with respect to using maternal care [70–74].

These authors evaluated the autonomy of women though their level of mobility, participation in decision-making, and finally their access and control of financial resources. Also, they defined autonomy as the ability of women to take control of resources and decisions that affect them and to act independently from the men or the society in which they live [75]. They agree that in SSA, more independent women are more likely to use maternal care [71]. For some authors, women in SSA do not always have freedom of movement [70], as we have observed with the nomads of Gossi. In fact, the consent of their mothers-in-law or their husbands appears to be required before they can seek care [70]. Without the consent of these agents, recourse to medical care is seen as a lack of respect. Furthermore, since the woman has to pay at the health center, she must discuss this matter with her husband or mother-in-law, which is badly perceived locally. On the other hand, when women have greater freedom of movement, they are more likely to use maternal care [70, 74].

Our results are also consistent with other studies having highlighted the low participation of women in decision-making related to assisted childbirth in SSA [70, 73]. As seen in our study, their lack of decision-making power would largely contribute to late recourse or non-use of healthcare [38]. For example, in Ethiopia, when women ultimately decide where to deliver, they are more likely to give birth in a health center than is the case where others make this decision for them [39, 73]. The same is true in Niger, Burkina Faso, or Zambia, where women with some decision-making autonomy are more likely to give birth in a health facility than women who do not have such power [70, 71, 74]. In these countries, women with a greater degree of autonomy are free to make the decision to seek care and are also better equipped to face the imposed constraints.

Another study in Malawi shows that decision-making processes for the use of maternal healthcare are dominated by the men who make the final decision, especially when it comes to obstetric complications [76]. Thus, faced with the opposition of their relatives, some women could not assert themselves and were unable to force their relations to take measures in favor of seeking care [76]. Moreover, the nomadic women in our study have no source of income, and family resources are controlled by men, which seems to limit their use of assisted childbirth. Studies in SSA indicate that maternal care is less important when expenditures are controlled by other household members [72]. In addition, when women have better control over their financial resources, they can then decide how to use them to pay for care.

Our results also match those of Hampshire [36] who found that most of the nomadic women in her study had limited economic power that did not allow them to cope with health costs without the help of others. Their use of healthcare depends on the availability and the good will of men. Furthermore, achieving access to the husband's resources is different or variable depending on a woman's marital status (single, geographically single, or married). However, this individualistic and atomistic conception of the origin of autonomy is subject to a certain degree of criticism [77, 78]. According to this conception, individuals are supposed to be sufficiently independent and rational to make their own decisions [77, 79]. It does not recognize people's social character based on their relationships with others, their interdependence, and the mutual support that defines human lives [80].

According to several authors, this conception thus offers a poor or an incomplete vision of autonomy [80, 81]. Conversely, they put forward a more relational form of autonomy which asserts that individuals are never independent enough to make decisions alone. This alternative conception of autonomy places the individual in a socially integrated network [82]. Its attributes are relationships with the family, the community, and society, and thus mutual responsibility and interdependence are recognized as playing a major role in any decision-making process.

Indeed, for any decision-making, including recourse to maternal care, the mutual responsibility and cooperation of women with spouses, parents, and relatives therefore play a determining role, as noted in our study. As a result, women's social environment and their relationships are recognized as continually contributing to their autonomy [82].

To illustrate the importance of the social network, Gage said in the same vein that in rural Mali, it is not only where you live that is crucial for the use of maternal care, but also who your neighbors are [83]. This suggests that living close to women who have used maternal care is likely to mean more help offered by neighbors. As such, autonomy analyzed from an "individualistic" angle by several authors in SSA has limitations, particularly for the evaluation of the decision-making power of nomadic women encountered in the commune of Gossi regarding the use of assisted childbirth. Indeed, these nomads are organized within their camp and with their neighbors in a supportive community environment. This interdependence within a social network is crucial for their survival in often hostile environments far from urban centers where health services are located. For these nomadic women, the use of assisted childbirth can be seen as a collective process involving multiple actors who interact and share roles according to certain social standards and at different points in the decision-making process. In analyzing the discourse of our participants, we note that the logic of solidarity and mutual aid seems to have determined their use of assisted childbirth given the inaccessibility of health services for them. They described many roles in their social networks that allow them to seek care and, in particular, to exchange information on the services available, as well as to support and help each other and thus to facilitate such use. This information seems to be well appreciated and often considered as a priority for rapid decision-making as regards the use of assisted childbirth. In addition, studies in other contexts have shown the importance of these social networks and their links to the use of healthcare [84–86]. Some authors argue that social networks are an important source of information [86]. For the nomadic women of our study, their social network, including friends or relatives, seems to play an important role in motivating them to seek care. Pregnant women were able to receive emotional support, counseling, or help with housework to enable them to visit health centers.

Our participants consider that recourse to assisted childbirth depends to a greater extent on the suitability of services provided and their appropriation by the communities. On the other hand, if childbirth is often considered as not requiring the use of healthcare, it is not so when obstetric complications ensue. For many participants, it is not enough to have accessible care for

the use of assisted childbirth to be effective [67]. Similarly, other authors show that women are more likely to seek care when their networks are broader and more homogenous, and when the level of solidarity is more important [85]. In other words, a network made up of people who are closely related and with homogeneous family ties is stronger and more reliable, as is the case for the participants in our study. Nomadic women seem to appreciate the fact that they do not feel alone in dealing with complex and difficult decisions that require important means, community mobilization, and, above all, knowledge and initiative, to be shown while they are suffering and not always able to cope. They seem to perceive this solidarity and interdependence as a source of strength, an integral part of their identity, and a component of a strategy of support upon which they can rely in a hostile environment. Therefore, we can question the ability of nomadic women with little education to make decisions alone with respect to seeking care in this difficult environment.

Limitations

This study is one of the first in Mali to address the determinants of the use of assisted childbirth by nomads. It was conducted in a challenging research environment and with limited resources. However, we have sought to mitigate or minimize the impact of these constraints by applying a suitable and rigorous methodology. We decided to provide space for nomadic women, who are not very accessible, to express their views. However, the views of other family members or health professionals could have enriched the data by providing a more complete picture of the different sociocultural determinants. Moreover, it is not possible to generalize or extrapolate the results of this type of qualitative study beyond the commune of Gossi where the data were collected. Nevertheless, what we uncovered was remarkably similar to the findings of other authors in SSA and reflected the difficulties they too noted in nomadic environments.

Another possible limitation is that the assistant who conducted the interviews is from this area, and despite our explanations and instructions, there is a potential bias of social desirability, that is to say that participants have expressed what they perceive as appropriate or socially desired responses. Similarly, a misinterpretation of the French translations of Tamasheq interviews may lead to a distortion of original meanings or a less nuanced understanding of participants' perceptions as to why they are or are not using assisted childbirth. To mitigate these risks, we returned to the field to check the validity of our data with some participants. The transcripts were also often cross-referenced with our field notes and any discrepancies were discussed and clarified.

Sociocultural determinants of nomadic women's utilization of assisted childbirth...

117

Conclusion

This study helped to identify and understand a set of sociocultural determinants whose interaction influences the use of assisted childbirth by Tamasheq nomadic women in the health area of the commune of Gossi, Mali. It shows that despite a certain evolution, this recourse stems from pragmatic choices and perceived needs, which themselves are determined, on the one hand, by representations and experiences from pregnancy and childbirth, and on the other, by their lack of decision-making autonomy. Moreover, despite the preference of the majority of participants for assisted childbirth, which is recognized as being effective, many of them continue to give birth at home.

Furthermore, interventions aimed at promoting the use of assisted childbirth by nomads should target these different sociocultural determinants. Such interventions should take into account the relationship that nomadic women have with their bodies and their capacity and limits to cope with pregnancy and childbirth. In addition, they would take into account women's perceptions of the multiple risks recognized as punctuating their experiences of pregnancy and childbirth, as well as the unpredictable complications that strongly motivate demand for healthcare.

Similarly, the study describes the mobilization of a social capital that must be recognized to the extent that it seems a very valuable component in this decision-making process. Therefore, potential interventions should capitalize on the social network of nomadic women to support decision-making where the use of assisted childbirth is being promoted.

Abbreviations

DCs: Developing countries; DHS: Demographic Health Survey; Km: Kilometer; MMR: Maternal mortality ratio; PNC: Prenatal consultation; SSA: Sub-Saharan Africa; WHO: World Health Organization

Funding

We would like to thank the team members of the research project entitled *"des interventions innovantes et réalistes pour améliorer la santé des mères, des nouveau-nés et des enfants en Afrique de l'Ouest"* - "Innovative and Realistic Interventions for Improving the Health of Mothers, Newborns, and Children in West Africa" headed by Prof. Slim Haddad.
The authors thank the Quebec Population Health Research Network (QPHRN) for its contribution to the funding of this publication.
Project sponsors had no influence on the study design, data collection and analysis, decision to publish, or preparation of the manuscript.

Authors' contributions

MAAA (doctoral researcher), LHB, and MPG (both supervisors and professor-researchers, Université Laval) contributed to the study design. MAAA was involved in data collection; data analysis was conducted by MAAA, and LHB. MAAA drafted the manuscript with significant input from LHB and MPG, and all authors critically reviewed and contributed to the manuscript. All authors read and approved the final manuscript.

Competing interests

The authors declare that they have no competing interests.

Author details

[1]Université Laval, 1050 Avenue de la Médecine, room 3696, Québec G1V 0A6, Canada. [2]Faculty of Nursing Sciences, Université Laval, 1050 Avenue de la Médecine, room 3447, Québec G1V 0A6, Canada. [3]Faculty of Nursing Sciences, Université Laval, 1050 Avenue de la Médecine, room 1426, Québec G1V 0A6, Canada.

References

1. Lawn JE, Cousens S, Darmstadt GL, Paul V, Martines J. Why are 4 million newborn babies dying every year? Lancet. 2004;364:2020.
2. Lawn JE, Cousens S, Zupan J. 4 million neonatal deaths: when? where? why? Lancet. 2005;365:891–900.
3. WHO, UNICEF, UNFPA, The World Bank, The United Nations Population Division. Trends in Maternal Mortality: 1990 to 2015. Geneva: WHO; 2015.
4. Sarah P, Say ES, Wilmoth J. Comprendre les tendances mondiales de la mortalité maternelle. Perspectives Internationales sur la Santé Sexuelle et Génésique, numéro spécial 2014 : 2–11, https://doi.org/10.1363/FR00214
5. WHO, UNICEF, UNFPA, the World Bank, United Nations population division. Trends in maternal mortality: 1990 to 2013: WHO; 2014. http://apps.who.int/iris/handle/10665/112697.
6. WHO U. UNFPA and The World Bank. Trends in Maternal Mortality: 1990 To 2008. In: Estimates developed by WHO, UNICEF. UNFPA and the World Bank. Geneva: WHO; 2010.
7. OMS. Tendances de la mortalité maternelle: 1991-2015: estimations de l'OMS, l'UNICEF, l'UNFPA. In: le Groupe de la Banque mondiale et la Division de la population des Nations Unies: résumé d'orientation; 2015.
8. Ronsmans C, Graham WJ. Maternal mortality: who, when, where, and why. Lancet. 2006;368(9542):1189–200.
9. Say L, Raine R. A systematic review of inequalities in the use of maternal health care in developing countries: examining the scale of the problem and the importance of context. Bull World Health Organ. 2007;85(10):812–9.
10. Schelling E, Weibel D, Bonfoh B. Apprendre de l' offre de services sociaux aux pasteurs: Elements de bonne pratique. 2008. https://www.iucn.org/sites/dev/files/import/downloads/social_services_to_pastoralists__french_.pdf.
11. Maine D. Programme pour la maternité sans danger: options et problèmes. Nueva York: Center for Population and Family Health Faculty of Medicine Columbia University; 1992.
12. Patton GC, Coffey C, Sawyer SM, Viner RM, Haller DM, Bose K, et al. Global patterns of mortality in young people: a systematic analysis of population health data. Lancet. 2009;374:881–92.
13. WHO. 10 Facts on Maternal Health. 2015 (http://www.who.int/features/factfiles/maternal_health/en/).
14. Prual A. La réduction de la mortalité maternelle dans les pays en voie de développement: théorie et pratique. Med Trop. 2004;64(6):569.
15. Say L, Chou D, Gemmill A, Tuncalp O, Moller AB, Daniels J, et al. Global causes of maternal death: a WHO systematic analysis. Lancet Glob Health. 2014;2(6):323–33.

16. Prual A, Bouvier-Colle M-H, Bernis L, Breart G. Severe maternal morbidity from direct obstetric causes in West Africa: incidence and case fatality rates. Bull World Health Organ. 2000;78(5):593–602.

17. Bang AT, Bang RA, Baitule SB, Reddy MH, Deshmukh MD. Effect of home-based neonatal care and management of sepsis on neonatal mortality: field trial in rural India. Lancet. 1999;354(9194):1955–61.

18. Baqui A, Williams EK, Rosecrans AM, Agrawal PK, Ahmed S, Darmstadt GL, et al. Impact of an integrated nutrition and health programme on neonatal mortality in rural northern India. Bull World Health Organ 2008;86(10):796-804A.

19. Graham WJ, Bell JS, Bullough CH. Can skilled attendance at delivery reduce maternal mortality in developing countries? Safe motherhood strategies: a review of the evidence. Brussels, Belgium: Paper presented at: European Commission expert meeting on safer motherhood; 2000. p. 27–8.

20. WHO. MDG 5: Improve Maternal Health. 2013. http://www.who.int/topics/millennium_development_goals/maternal_health/en/.

21. OMS. Rapport sur la santé dans le monde, 2005-donnons sa chance à chaque mère et à chaque enfant. Genève: OMS; 2005. p. 21–2.

22. Campbell OM, Graham WJ. And lancet maternal survival series steering group. Strategies for reducing maternal mortality: getting on with what works. Lancet. 2006;368(9543):1284–99.

23. UNICEF. Statistics by Area - Delivery Care - The Challenge. 2013. https://data.unicef.org/.

24. WHO. Global Health Observatory data repository. 2013. http://www.who.int/gho/en/.

25. Montavon A, Jean-Richard V, Bechir M, Daugla D, Abdoulaye M, Naré B, et al. Health of mobile pastoralists in the Sahel–assessment of 15 years of research and development. Tropical Med Int Health. 2013;18(9):1044–52.

26. Randall S. Visibilité et invisibilité statistique en Afrique. Adapter les méthodes de collecte de données aux populations ciblées. Afrique contemporaine. 2016;258(2):41–57.

27. Wiese M. La vulnérabilité des éleveurs nomades face aux problèmes de santé humaine au Tchad. Réflexions pour une meilleure prise en charge de la santé en milieu nomades au Tchad; 2000. p. 14–29.

28. OMS. Résultats de l'Enquête rapide sur la disponibilité de services de santé au Mali avec l'outil HeRAMS de l'OMS. 2016.

29. Ministère de la santé du Mali. Annuaire 2012. Système National d'Information sanitaire (SNIS). 2013. http://www.sante.gov.ml/index.php/annuaires/send/2-annuaires-statistiques/1-snis-2012.

30. Kruger C, Olsen OE, Mighay E, Ali M. Where do women give birth in rural Tanzania? Rural Remote Health. 2011;11(3):1791.

31. Mekonnen MG, Yalew KN, Umer JY, Melese M. Determinants of delivery practices among Afar pastoralists of Ethiopia. Pan African medical journal. 2012;13(Suppl 1). Published online 2012 Dec 26. PMCID: PMC3587020. https://www.ncbi.nlm.nih.gov/pmc/articles/PMC3587020/pdf/PAMJ-SUPP-13-1-17.pdf.

32. Wyss K, Bechir M, Schelling E, Daugla D, Zinsstag J. Quels types de services de sante pour les populations nomades? Apprentissages des activites de recherche et d'action au Tchad. Revue de Médecine Tropicale. 2004;64:493–6.

33. Ould Taleb M. Santé, vulnérabilité, et tuberculose en milieu nomade Sahélien: Contribution à l'étude des représentations sociales de la tuberculose chez les populations nomades de la Mauritanie et du Tchad: Dissertation, University of Cocody, Abidjan, Côte d'Ivoire; 2004.

34. Wiese M, Donnat M, Wyss K. Utilisation d'un centre de santé par des pasteurs nomades arabes–une étude de cas au Kanem, Tchad. Médecine tropicale. 2004;64:486–92.

35. Ag EM. La grossesse et le suivi de l'accouchement chez les Touaregs Kel-Adagh (Kidal, Mali). Paris: Harmattan; 2010. p. 400.

36. Hampshire K. Networks of nomads: negotiating access to health resources among pastoralist women in Chad. Soc Sci Med. 2002;54(7):1025–37.

37. Wako WG, Kassa DH. Institutional delivery service utilization and associated factors among women of reproductive age in the mobile pastoral community of the Liban District in Guji Zone, Oromia, Southern Ethiopia: a cross sectional study. BMC Pregnancy Childbirth. 2017;17(1):144.

38. Jackson R, Tesfay FH, Gebrehiwot TG, Godefay H. Factors that hinder or enable maternal health strategies to reduce delays in rural and pastoralist areas in Ethiopia. Tropical Med Int Health. 2017;22(2):148–60.

39. King R, Jackson R, Dietsch E, Hailemariam A. Utilisation of maternal health services in Ethiopia: a key informant research project. Dev Pract. 2016;26(2):158–69.

40. Zepro NB, Ahmed AT. Determinants of institutional delivery service utilization among pastorals of Liben Zone, Somali Regional State, Ethiopia, 2015. Int J Women's Health. 2016;8:705.

41. Caulfield T, Onyo P, Byrne A, Nduba J, Nyagero J, Morgan A, et al. Factors influencing place of delivery for pastoralist women in Kenya: a qualitative study. BMC Womens Health. 2016;16(1):52.

42. El Shiekh B, van der Kwaak A. Factors influencing the utilization of maternal health care services by nomads in Sudan. Pastoralism. 2015;5(1):23.

43. Gabrysch S, Campbell OM. Still too far to walk: literature review of the determinants of delivery service use. BMC Pregnancy Childbirth. 2009;9(1):34.

44. Thaddeus S, Maine D. Too far to walk: maternal mortality in context. Soc Sci Med. 1994;38(8):1091–110.

45. Lee AC, Lawn JE, Cousens S, Kumar V, Osrin D, Bhutta ZA, et al. Linking families and facilities for care at birth: what works to avert intrapartum-related deaths? Int J Gynecol Obstet. 2009;107:S65–88.

46. CSA. Plan de sécurité alimentaire de la commune rurale de Gossi 2006-2010. 2006.

47. Wateraid. Plan sectoriel de developpement de la commune de Gossi dans la région de Tombouctou. 2007.

48. Savoie-Zajc L. Comment peut-on construire un échantillonnage scientifiquement valide. Recherches qualitatives. Hors série. 2007;5:99–111.

49. Pires A. De quelques enjeux épistémologiques d'une méthodologie générale pour les sciences sociales. In: La recherche qualitative Enjeux épistémologiques et méthodologiques Montréal: Gaëtan Morin Éditeur; 1997. p. 3–54.

50. Ouellet F, Mayer R. Méthodologie de recherche pour les intervenants sociaux: Boucherville. Québec: G. Morin; 1991.

51. Martineau S. L'observation en situation: enjeux, possibilités et limites. Recherches qualitatives. 2005;2:5–17.

52. Gauthier B. Recherche sociale: de la problématique à la collecte des données: Puq; 2003.

53. Paillé P, Mucchielli A. L'analyse qualitative en sciences humaines et sociales. 3e éd éd. Paris: A. Colin; 2012. p. 423.

54. Pope C, Mays N. Qualitative research in health care. 3rd ed ed. Malden, Mass: Blackwell Pub; 2006. p. 156.

55. Okafor I, Sekoni A, Ezeiru S, Ugboaja J, Inem V. Orthodox versus unorthodox care: a qualitative study on where rural women seek healthcare during pregnancy and childbirth in Southwest, Nigeria. Malawi Med J. 2014;26(2):45–9.

56. Babalola S, Fatusi A. Determinants of use of maternal health services in Nigeria-looking beyond individual and household factors. BMC Pregnancy Childbirth. 2009;9(1):43.

57. Brieger WR, Luchok KJ, Eng E, Earp JA. Use of maternity services by pregnant women in a small Nigerian community. Health Care Women Int. 1994;15(2):101–10.

58. Iyoke C, Ifeadike C, Nnebue C, Onah H, Ezugwu F. Perception and care-seeking behaviour for post partum morbidity among mothers in Enugu south east, Nigeria. Niger J Med. 2010;20(2):260–5.

59. Mwangome F, Holding P, Songola K, Bomu G. Barriers to hospital delivery in a rural setting in Coast Province, Kenya: community attitude and behaviours. Rural Remote Health. 2012;12(2):1852.

60. Magadi MA, Madise NJ, Rodrigues RN. Frequency and timing of antenatal care in Kenya: explaining the variations between women of different communities. Soc Sci Med. 2000;51(4):551–61.

61. Mathole T, Lindmark G, Majoko F, Ahlberg BM. A qualitative study of women's perspectives of antenatal care in a rural area of Zimbabwe. Midwifery. 2004;20(2):122–32.

62. Kyomuhendo GB. Low use of rural maternity services in Uganda: impact of women's status, traditional beliefs and limited resources. Reprod Health Matters. 2003;11(21):16–26.

63. Rwenge MJ-R, Tchamgoue-Nguemaleu HB. Facteurs sociaux de l'utilisation des services de soins obstétricaux parmi les adolescentes camerounaises. Afr J Reprod Health. 2011;15(3):81–92.

64. Adjamagbo A, Guillaume A. La santé de la reproduction en milieu rural ivoirien. Autrepart. 2001;(3):11–27.

65. Abel Ntambue ML, Malonga F, Dramaix-Wilmet M, Donnen P. Determinants of maternal health services utilization in urban settings of the Democratic Republic of Congo–a case study of Lubumbashi City. BMC Pregnancy Childbirth. 2012;12(1):66.

66. Beninguissé G. Entre tradition et modernité: fondements sociaux de la prise en charge de la grossesse et de l'accouchement au Cameroun. Editions L'Harmattan ed 2003.

67. Bedford J, Gandhi M, Admassu M, Girma A. 'A normal delivery takes place at home': a qualitative study of the location of childbirth in rural Ethiopia. Matern Child Health J. 2013;17(2):230–9.

68. Myer L, Harrison A. Why do women seek antenatal care late? Perspectives from rural South Africa. J Midwifery Womens Health. 2003;48(4):268–72.

69. Ganle JK, Parker M, Fitzpatrick R, Otupiri E. A qualitative study of health system barriers to accessibility and utilization of maternal and newborn healthcare services in Ghana after user-fee abolition. BMC Pregnancy Childbirth. 2014;14(1):425.

70. Niang M, Dupéré S, Bédard E. Le non-recours aux soins prénatals au Burkina Faso. Santé Publique. 2015;27(3):405–14.

71. Gabrysch S, Cousens S, Cox J, Campbell OM. The influence of distance and level of care on delivery place in rural Zambia: a study of linked national data in a geographic information system. PLoS Med. 2011;8(1):1000394.

72. Pembe AB, Urassa DP, Darj E, Carlstedt A. Qualitative study on maternal referrals in rural Tanzania: decision making and acceptance of referral advice. Afr J Reprod Health. 2008;12(2):120–31.

73. Hailu D, Berhe H. Determinants of institutional childbirth service utilisation among women of childbearing age in urban and rural areas of Tsegedie district, Ethiopia. Midwifery. 2014;30(11):1109–17.

74. Rai RK, Singh PK, Singh L, Kumar C. Individual characteristics and use of maternal and child health services by adolescent mothers in Niger. Matern Child Health J. 2014;18(3):592–603.

75. Mason KO. The impact of Women's social position on fertility in developing countries. Sociol Forum. 1987;2(4):718–45.

76. Kumbani L, Bjune G, Chirwa E, Odland JØ. Why some women fail to give birth at health facilities: a qualitative study of women's perceptions of perinatal care from rural southern Malawi. Reprod Health. 2013;10(1):9.

77. Ricard L. L'autonomie relationnelle : un nouveau fondement pour les théories de la justice. Philosophiques. 2013;401:139–69.

78. Dove ES, Kelly SE, Lucivero F, Machirori M, Dheensa S, Prainsack B. Beyond individualism: is there a place for relational autonomy in clinical practice and research? Clin Ethics. 2017;12(3):150–65.

79. Donagan B. The origins of English individualism: the family, property and social transition. Alan Macfarlane. Ethics. 1980;91(1):168–70.

80. Christman J. Relational autonomy, Liberal individualism, and the social constitution of selves. Philos Stud. 2004;117(1/2):143–64.

81. Donchin A. Understanding autonomy relationally: toward a reconfiguration of bioethical principles. J Med Philos. 2001;26(4):365–86.

82. Baylis F, Kenny NP, Sherwin S. A relational account of public health ethics. Public Health Ethics. 2008;1(3):196–209.

83. Gage AJ. Barriers to the utilization of maternal health care in rural Mali. Soc Sci Med. 2007;65(8):1666–82.

84. Edmonds JK, Hruschka D, Bernard HR, Sibley L. Women's Social Networks and Birth Attendant Decisions: application of the network-episode model. Soc Sci Med. 2012;74(3):452–9.

85. St Clair PA, Smeriglio VL, Alexander CS, Celentano DD. Social network structure and prenatal care utilization. Med Care. 1989;27(8):823–32.

86. Helleringer S, Kohler HP. Social networks, perceptions of risk, and changing attitudes towards HIV/AIDS: new evidence from a longitudinal study using fixed-effects analysis. Popul Stud. 2005;59(3):265–82.

11

Obstetrical outcomes after vaginal repair of caesarean scar diverticula in reproductive-aged women

Xingchen Zhou[1], Xiaoqian Yang[2], Huihui Chen[1], Xuhong Fang[1*] and Xipeng Wang[1*] (iD)

Abstract

Background: Although vaginal repair has been conducted to manage caesarean scar diverticula, most studies evaluated only the gynaecological outcomes post-surgery, and their obstetrical outcomes were unknown. This study aimed to evaluate the obstetrical outcomes in vaginal repair-treated caesarean scar diverticula patients.

Methods: A series of 51 symptomatic women with caesarean scar defects or a thickness of the remaining muscular layer of less than 3 mm according to transvaginal ultrasound were included. We retrospectively evaluated the gynaecological and obstetrical outcomes after vaginal repair and histologically analysed the defect.

Results: Transvaginal ultrasound revealed that the thickness of the remaining muscular layer significantly increased from 2.24 ± 0.81 mm to 6.10 ± 1.43 mm 3 months after vaginal repair. The duration of menstruation significantly decreased from 14.29 ± 3.13 days to 8.31 ± 2.14 days post-vaginal repair. Notably, 26 of the 51 (50.98%) women who were followed for more than 15.04 months post-surgery achieved pregnancy. A total of 6 of the 26 pregnancies (23.08%) resulted in miscarriages, including 5 early miscarriages and 1 late miscarriage. Among the 20 women who achieved pregnancy without miscarriage, 18 had term deliveries, 2 had preterm birth, and none reported uterine rupture. Histological analysis was performed in all 51 cases. Muscle fibre density was significantly lower in the scar than in the myometrium adjacent to the scar and collagen expression was markedly increased in the scar tissue.

Conclusion: Satisfactory gynaecological and subsequent obstetrical outcomes can be achieved in vaginal repair-treated caesarean scar diverticula patients.

Keywords: Caesarean scar defect, Vaginal repair, Prolonged menstrual bleeding, The thickness of the remaining muscular layer, Obstetrical outcomes

Background

In China, the proportion of caesarean sections (CSs) performed in 2010 was 35–58%, which has attracted significant concern regarding the development of caesarean scar diverticula (CSD) [1]. CSD are reservoir-like pouch defects at the site of a previous caesarean incision and result from incomplete scar healing on the anterior wall of the uterine isthmus (Fig. 1) [2]. It has been suggested that the incidence of CSD is as high as 61% after one CS and reaches 100% after at least three CSs [3]. With the increasing CS rate and the two-child policy implemented in China, the complications of CSD, such as prolonged menstrual bleeding, secondary infertility, and even uterine rupture during a subsequent pregnancy, have emerged as important clinical problems [4]. The prevalence of CSD-associated prolonged menstrual bleeding ranges from 63.6 to 88% [5]. The exact pathogenesis responsible for CSD has not been fully elucidated. Multiple CS procedures, a retroflexed uterus, cervical dilation, the type and technique of uterine closure, and maternal age at the time of caesarean section were suggested to contribute to the potential risk for CSD [2, 6–8].

Clinical guidelines have yet to be established for the management of CSD. CSD can be treated using a

* Correspondence: fangxuhong@xinhuamed.com.cn;
wangxipeng@xinhuamed.com.cn
Xingchen Zhou and Xiaoqian Yang are co-first authors.
[1]Department of Gynecology, Xinhua Hospital affiliated with Shanghai Jiaotong University, 1665 Kong Jiang Rd, Yang Pu District, Shanghai 200092, China
Full list of author information is available at the end of the article

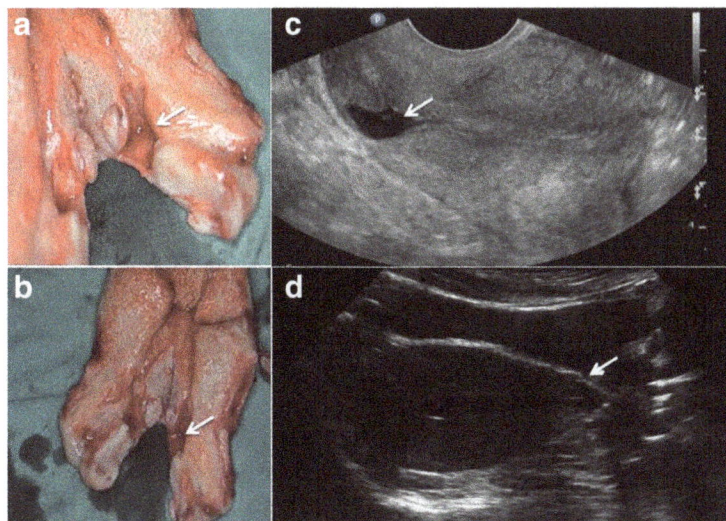

Fig. 1 The shape of CSD. **a, b**: A section view of a hysterectomy specimen. A deep anterior defect covered with a thin layer of myometrium (white arrow) can be observed at the level of the supposed site of CS. **c, d**: The white arrows indicate the shape of CSD under transabdominal and transvaginal ultrasonography

hysteroscopy transcervical approach, laparoscopic abdominal approach, and transvaginal surgical repair. Above all, vaginal repair has been identified by our group and other researchers as a less invasive, safe and effective surgical procedure to treat CSD [9–11]. Vaginal repair can not only resolve CSD-associated prolonged menstrual bleeding but can also restore the anatomical structure in patients with CSD. A retrospective review reported that the improvement in menstruation can reach 93.5% (43/46) in CSD patients who received vaginal repair [9]. Since April 2013, our team has performed vaginal repair to treat CSD. Our previous studies reported that 80.3% (94/117) of CSD patients experienced a duration of menstruation ≤ 10 days, and the thickness of the remaining muscular layer (TRM) exhibited significant improvements $(2.56 \pm 1.32$ vs 8.65 ± 3.11, $P < 0.001)$ at 6 months post-surgery [10]. The results of our other study revealed that 60.0% (48/80) of the patients with CSD that resolved after surgery achieved a duration of menstruation ≤ 7 days at the median follow-up (11.28 months) [11]. Therefore, we believe that vaginal repair can benefit women who experienced CSD and want to achieve pregnancy again.

However, the subsequent pregnancy outcome in vaginal repair-treated women was not included in our previous studies. To address this deficiency, women who had undergone vaginal repair of CSD, whose TRM was less than 3 mm and who attempted pregnancy were followed long term in our institution. Their clinical characteristics were analysed, and obstetrical outcomes were recorded.

Methods

Patient population

A total of 340 CSD patients were managed using vaginal repair between April 2013 and May 2016 at Shanghai First Maternity and Infant Hospital, Tongji University. he presence of remaining myometrium (TRM) was determined by transvaginal ultrasound (TVU), which was clearly described in our previous studies [10, 11] To measure the thickness of the residual muscle layer of the diverticulum, the patient's should be a cursor was placed at the interface between the uterine and the bladder wall, and another cursor was positioned at the bottom of the CSD. Three different measurements of length, width, height, depth and TRM were obtained. All of the patients underwent TVU to evaluate the parameters of the CSD preoperatively and postoperatively, namely, CSD length, width, depth and TRM. Among the enrolled participants, 51 patients attempted to become pregnant; their clinical characteristics are summarized in Table 1. Our present retrospective study was approved by the Ethics Committee of Shanghai First Maternity and Infant Hospital (KS1512). Informed written consent was obtained from all participants after they received clear information about the procedure and possible surgical outcomes of vaginal repair.

Surgical technique

The complete surgical technique was described in detail in our previous studies and has been recognized as an effective approach for anatomic correction of CSD as well as symptomatic relief of prolonged menstrual duration [11]. The most important steps of vaginal repair of CSD are summarized again here. Briefly, the bladder was carefully dissected away from the uterus towards the abdominal cavity to open the vesicovaginal space and reach the peritoneum. CSD tissue was easily found once the abdominal cavity was entered, and the lower uterine

Table 1 Clinical characteristics of the patients with CSD

Characteristic	CSD patients (n = 51)
Age, y	31.25 ± 3.36 (24–42)
Menstruation, d	
Before VR	14.29 ± 3.13 (8–25)
After VR	8.31 ± 2.14 (5–14)
Uterus position, %	
Anteflexion	37.3% (19/51)
Retroflexion	62.7% (32/51)
Number of previous caesarean sections	1.04 ± 0.20
One, %	96.1% (49/51)
More than one, %	3.9% (2/51)
CSD parameters before VR, mm	
CSD length	7.77 ± 3.39 (2–16)
CSD width	12.00 ± 5.42 (4–27)
CSD depth	6.32 ± 2.45 (2–12)
TRM, mm	2.24 ± 0.81 (0.7–4.6)
Postoperative TRM, mm	8.36 ± 2.96 (3.0–13.9)
CSD resolved after VR, %	68.63% (35/51)
Persistent CSD after VR, %	31.37% (16/51)
Persistent CSD parameters, mm	
CSD length	5.78 ± 2.64 (2–11)
CSD width	9.00 ± 5.32 (3–20)
CSD depth	4.33 ± 1.00 (3–6)
TRM, mm	6.10 ± 1.43 (3.8–8.1)
Pregnancy rate, %	50.98% (26/51)
Spontaneous abortion rate, %	23.08% (6/26)
Median follow-up time, months	28.42 ± 9.74 (15.04–50.46)

Data are presented as the means ± SD or percentages
Note: CSD = caesarean scar diverticula; VR = vaginal repair of CSD; TRM = thickness of the remaining muscular layer

segment was completely exposed. The CSD tissue was then thoroughly removed. All surgical procedures reported in the current series were performed by the same surgeon. All patients were discharged from the hospital on postoperative day 3. After the subsequent TVU at 3 months post-surgery, the women were told they could attempt pregnancy starting 1 year post-surgery if their TRM had reached a thickness of more than 3 mm.

Data collection and follow-up

Preoperative and postoperative clinical information was gathered, including age; uterus position; reproductive history; menstrual duration; CSD length, width, and depth; and TRM. The follow-up was scheduled at 3 months after surgery for all patients, at which time a TVU was performed. The patients with a postoperative TRM more than 3 mm and a subsequent pregnancy attempt were recorded, and long-term follow-up was conducted. Their gestational

age, pregnancy complications, interval from vaginal repair to pregnancy, neonatal birth weight, and infant sex were collected.

Histology

Histology was performed on tissues from all patients, and histochemical and Masson's staining were performed on the tissues of the 51 patients who attempted to become pregnant post-surgery to evaluate the muscle or collagen density of the remaining myometrium. Two areas were evaluated: the myometrium covering the scar and the myometrium directly adjacent to the scar. Haematoxylin-eosin staining was used for histology. Masson's staining was used to detect collagen. Panoramic viewer software was applied for histochemical quantification and morphological analysis.

Statistical analysis

Data are presented as the means ± SD or percentage when appropriate. A paired t-test was used to analyse preoperative and postoperative data. Statistical analysis was performed using SPSS software (version 22, IBM Co., Armonk, NY, USA). Statistical significance was set at $P < 0.05$.

Results
Gynaecological outcomes

The background characteristics of the women with CSD who attempted pregnancy after vaginal repair are shown in Table 1. Three months after the surgical procedure, the TRM dramatically ($P < 0.001$) recovered from 2.24 ± 0.81 mm (range, 0.7–4.6) to 8.36 ± 2.96 mm (range, 3.0–13.9) on TVU. The menstrual duration significantly decreased ($P < 0.001$) from 14.29 ± 3.13 days to 8.31 ± 2.14 days 3 months after vaginal repair. CSD disappeared in 68.63% of patients (35/51) at the 3-month follow-up. We present the clinical characteristics of the women with vaginal repair-treated CSD who achieved pregnancy without miscarriage in Table 2. A total of 19 women underwent one CS, and one woman underwent two CSs before vaginal repair of the CSD. The uterine positions were anteflexion in 11 women and retroflexion in 9 women. TVU revealed that the TRM significantly ($P < 0.001$) increased from 2.42 ± 1.04 mm (range, 1.0–4.6) to 8.36 ± 3.11 mm (range, 3.8–12.0) after the vaginal surgical procedure at the 3-month follow-up. The duration of menstruation significantly decreased ($P < 0.001$) from 14.20 ± 2.76 days to 8.00 ± 2.19 days post-vaginal repair. At the 3-month follow-up, 14 of the 20 (70.0%) women had no evidence of CSD as measured by TVU. The interval from vaginal repair to pregnancy was 32.06 ± 10.09 months (range, 16.88–50.36).

Obstetrical outcomes

The obstetrical outcome of pregnancy was assessed in 26 of the 51 women (50.98%) who were followed for

Table 2 Clinical characteristics of the women who achieved pregnancy without miscarriage

Characteristic	CSD patients (n = 20)
Age, y	31.00 ± 3.06 (26–38)
Menstruation, d	
Before VR	14.2 ± 2.76 (8–20)
After VR	8.00 ± 2.19 (5–13)
Uterus position, %	
Anteflexion	55.0% (11/20)
Retroflexion	45.0% (9/20)
Number of C-section deliveries	1.05 ± 0.22
One, %	95.0% (19/20)
More than one, %	5.0% (1/20)
CSD parameters before VR, mm	
CSD length	7.21 ± 3.14 (2–13)
CSD width	11.74 ± 5.61 (4–20)
CSD depth	6.53 ± 2.65 (2–11)
TRM, mm	2.42 ± 1.04 (1.0–4.6)
Postoperative TRM, mm	8.36 ± 3.11 (3.8–12.0)
CSD resolved after VR, %	70.0% (14/20)
Persistent CSD after VR, %	30.0% (6/20)
Persistent CSD parameters, mm	
CSD length	5.5 ± 2.12 (4–7)
CSD width	6.5 ± 4.95 (3–10)
CSD depth	4.5 ± 0.71 (4–5)
TRM, mm	4.95 ± 1.48 (3.9–6.0)
Interval from VR to pregnancy, months	32.06 ± 10.09 (16.88–50.36)
Gestational age (days)	266.03 ± 6.44 (245–273)
Preterm birth rate, %	10% (2/20)
Neonatal birth weight, g	3149.75 ± 308.24 (2500–3850)
Apgar score (5 min)	10
Pregnancy complication rate, %	20.0% (4/20)
Follow-up time, months	32.06 ± 10.09 (16.88–50.36)

Data are presented as the means ± SD or number (percentage)
Note: CSD caesarean scar diverticula, C-section caesarean section, VR vaginal repair of CSD, TRM thickness of the remaining muscular layer, M male, F female

more than 15.04 months post-surgery. Unfortunately, 6 of 26 pregnancies (23.08%) resulted in miscarriages, which included 5 early miscarriages and 1 late miscarriage (Tables 1 and 2). None of the women attempted to deliver vaginally, and no cases of threatened uterine rupture or uterine rupture were detected in women who had successful births. As shown in Table 2, the mean gestational age was 266.03 ± 6.44 days, and the mean neonatal birth weight was 3149.75 ± 308.24 g among the women who gave birth (Table 2). The detailed outcomes

after vaginal repair of CSD in reproductive-aged women are shown in Table 3. Among the 20 women who achieved pregnancy without miscarriage, 18 had term deliveries, and 2 had preterm deliveries during the long-term follow-up period (32.06 ± 10.09 months). In the women who had preterm deliveries, one woman gave birth at 35 weeks of gestation because of foetal heart rate decelerations on a non-stress test at a routine pregnancy check-up and threatened preterm labour. Another woman gave birth at 36 + 6 weeks of gestation due to preterm premature rupture of the membranes. This woman haemorrhaged 945 ml during the caesarean section. Four women who achieved term deliveries experienced pregnancy complications, including 2 women with gestational diabetes mellitus (GDM), 1 woman with placenta previa, and 1 woman with GDM as well as hypothyroidism during pregnancy (Table 3). However, all 20 women delivered healthy babies (Fig. 2).

Histology

Histological analysis was performed in all 51 cases. The muscular density of the residual myometrium covering the scar (Fig. 3a and b) was found to be significantly lower ($P < 0.005$) than that directly adjacent to the scar. Moreover, Masson's staining showed that the expression of collagen in CSD was 71.37 ± 19.82% compared to 52.75 ± 17.33% in healthy myometrium (Fig.3b). The collagen expression significantly increased in the scar defect (Fig. 3c and d).

Discussion

The most important clinical problems related to CSD are prolonged menstrual bleeding and adverse events that may affect subsequent pregnancies, including infertility, miscarriage, and uterine rupture. The prevalence of CSD-associated prolonged menstrual bleeding ranges from 63.6 to 88% [5]. Although the risk with CSD remains unclear, there is an obvious association between TRM and uterine rupture or dehiscence in subsequent pregnancies [12, 13]. Therefore, repairing the CSD, especially rebuilding the muscular layer of the scar site, might control the symptoms of prolonged menstrual bleeding and decrease the risk of uterine rupture caused by CSD. Hysteroscopy niche resection, laparoscopic repair, laparoscopic-assisted vaginal repair, and vaginal repair are currently employed to treat CSD-related symptoms [1, 14].

Vaginal repair is effective for improving the menstrual duration in patients with CSD. An improvement in uterine bleeding after vaginal repair occurs in 80.3% to 93.5% of cases. A retrospective review reported that the improvements in menstruation can reach 93.5% (43/46) in CSD patients who undergo vaginal repair [9]. Another study revealed that 92.9% (39/42) of vaginal repair-treated CSD

Table 3 Detailed gynaecological and obstetrical outcomes in vaginal repair-treated CSD patients who achieved pregnancy

Number	Interval form VR to pregnancy, months	Gestational weeks	Preoperative TRM, mm	Postoperative TRM, mm	Preoperative menstruation, d	Postoperative menstruation, d	Time from last cesarean section to menstruation	Neonatal birth weight, g	Apgar score (5 min)	Pregnancy complication	Supplementary information
1	50.36	38 + 5	2.2	6.0	14	12	5	3650	10	GDM, Hypothyroidism in pregnancy	
2	48.06	38	2.0	10.0	15	8	12	2500	10		
3	44.38	38 + 1	1.2	10.5	12	8		3320	10	Placenta previa	Amenorrhoea
4	39.72	37	3.0	10.0	12	7		3000	10		Amenorrhoea
5	39.09	38	3.5	9.5	14	9.5		2945	10	GDM	Amenorrhoea
6	36.50	39	1.6	11.5	15	6	10	3250	10		
7	36.10	38 + 3	2.2	11.0	13	6	13	3200	10		
8	26.22		2.7	10.0	15	7				Spontaneous abortion	
9	35.28	37 + 5	1.4	10.0	20	8	10	3280	10	GDM	
10	34.82	38 + 3	2.9	12.0	17	13	12	2900	10		
11	32.42	38 + 2	1.0	11.0	11	5		3850	10		Amenorrhoea
12	31.96	38	4.5	12.0	15	7.5	7	3500	10		
13	31.83	38	2.0	3.9	14	8.5	7	3150	10		
14	13.34		2.6	10.0	12	6				Spontaneous abortion	
15	31.21	39	2.0	8.0	13	11		3300	10		
16	30.75	38 + 5	2.8	3.8	12	10		3000	10		Amenorrhoea
17	29.70	38 + 6	3.0	4.0	15	8.5		3150	10		Amenorrhoea
18	11.63		1.8	3.0	20	13				Spontaneous abortion	
19	19.64	38 + 4	4.6	9.0	14	7		3200	10		
20	16.39		1.5	6.0	15	8				Spontaneous abortion	
21	18.33	36 + 6	3.1	11.3	15	7		3090	10	preterm premature rupture of the membranes, haemorrhage	Amenorrhoea
22	17.25	38 + 6	1.0	3.9	20	7		3080	10		
23	16.95	35	2.9	5.0	8	5	5	2650	10	Non-reassuring foetal status, Threatened preterm labour	
24	9.10		2.9	4.8	10	4				Spontaneous abortion	
25	16.88	38 + 5	1.5	4.7	15	6		2980	10		
26	3.29		0.7	13.2	17	13				Spontaneous abortion	

Note: VR vaginal repair of CSD, *TRM* thickness of the remaining muscular layer, *GDM* gestational diabetes mellitus

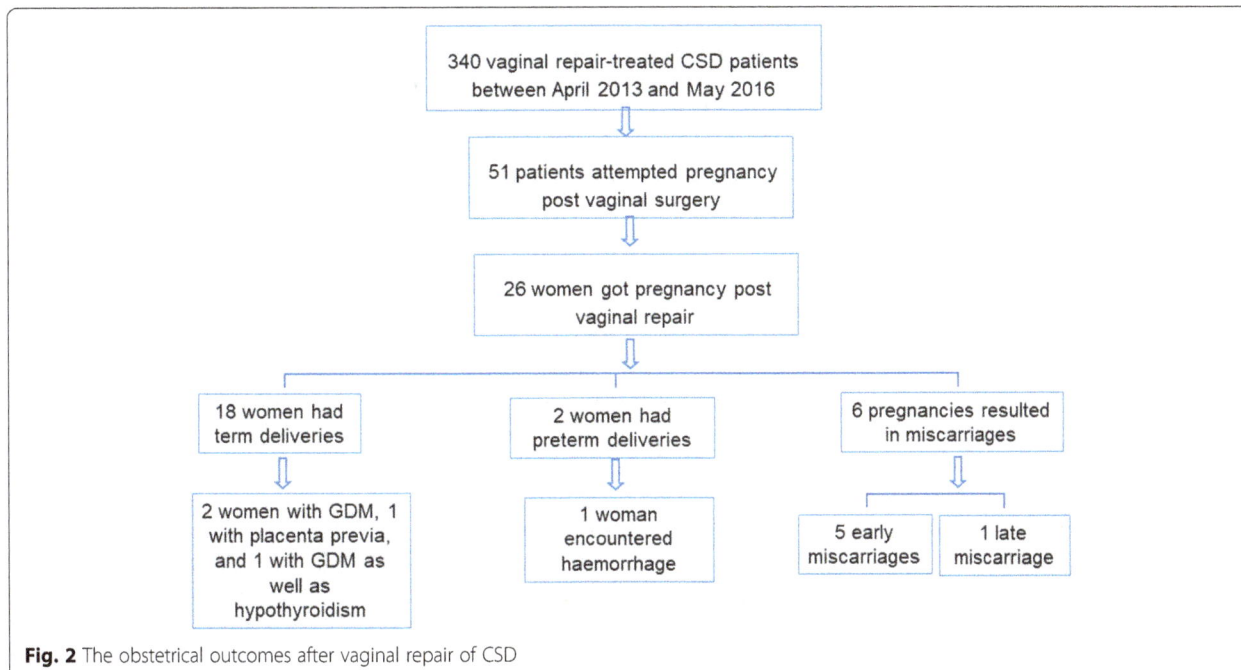

Fig. 2 The obstetrical outcomes after vaginal repair of CSD

patients reported significant improvements in menstruation at follow-up [15]. Our previous studies showed that 80.3% (94/117) of vaginal repair-treated CSD patients experienced a menstrual duration ≤10 days [10]. We also reported that the defect width of the preoperative CSD was the best prognostic index of the CSD anatomical repair effect post-vaginal repair [11]. The prognostic factors for the recovery of normal menstrual duration in CSD vaginal repair-treated CSD patients were assessed in the following study.

Although a series of studies have been conducted to investigate the management of CSD, most of the studies evaluated only the gynaecological outcomes post-surgery, and their obstetrical outcomes were unknown. Moreover, to date, no studies have compared obstetrical outcomes of laparoscopic repair and vaginal repair, and there are no guidelines for the selection of operative strategies for women with CSD who desire to become pregnant post-surgery. It has been reported that pregnancies occurred in 14 of 27 (51.9%) women who underwent

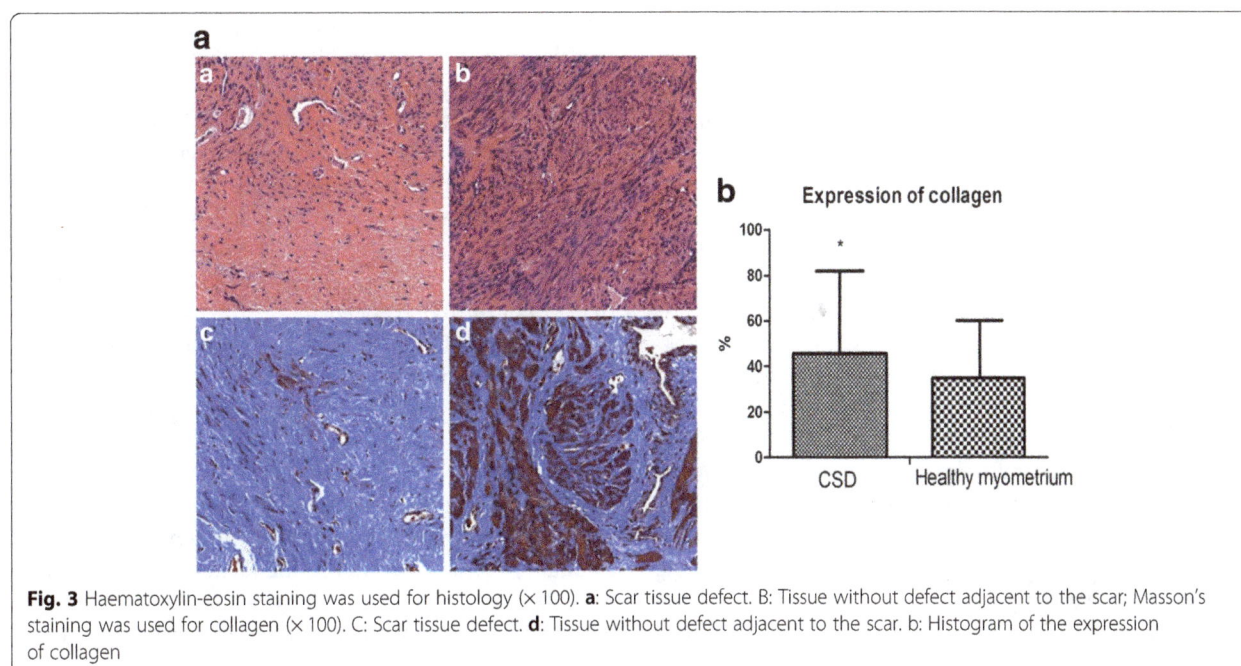

Fig. 3 Haematoxylin-eosin staining was used for histology (× 100). **a**: Scar tissue defect. B: Tissue without defect adjacent to the scar; Masson's staining was used for collagen (× 100). C: Scar tissue defect. **d**: Tissue without defect adjacent to the scar. b: Histogram of the expression of collagen

laparoscopic surgery [16, 17]. In another study, 10 of 18 (55.6%) women who were treated by laparoscopic repair achieved pregnancy following surgery [18]. The findings from an observational study showed that 44.4% (8/18) of women with infertility conceived and subsequently delivered their new-borns via CS after laparoscopic repair [1]. A total of 50.98% of the women in our study achieved pregnancy after vaginal repair, which indicates that vaginal repair is effective for improving fertility in patients with CSD. CS may lead to reduced fertility and prolonged inter-pregnancy intervals compared with vaginal deliveries. A meta-analysis conducted by Gurol-Urganci et al. suggests that the probability of future pregnancy and birth in women who have had a CS was 9% lower and 11% lower, respectively, than that in women who delivered vaginally [19]. The median inter-pregnancy intervals after CS were 2–6 months longer than those after vaginal delivery [19]. A meta-analysis that included 85,728 women in whom CS was previously performed found the rate of subsequent pregnancy to be reduced by 10% compared with that in women who had vaginal deliveries [20]. Even if the precise pathophysiology remains unclear, incomplete uterine healing and postoperative infection may contribute to the pathophysiological reasons underlying the above phenomenon [21]. The rate of infertility caused by CSD has not been elucidated. It is reasonable to speculate that the rate of infertility in women with CSD was higher than that in women who had undergone CS. The accumulation of mucus or blood in the defect, which leads to the presence of intrauterine fluid, could prevent the penetration of sperm cells, endometrial receptivity, or embryo implantation, which may be responsible for the infertility caused by CSD [1, 18]. In our study, 49.02% of women still did not achieve pregnancy.

Miscarriage was the most common adverse pregnancy outcome in 26 women with recognized pregnancy and previous CSD. Six women (6/26) suffered miscarriage in different stages of pregnancy. The underlying mechanisms of the association between CSD and miscarriage are unclear, and this adverse event may occur with no obvious underlying cause. Some studies report that the rate of spontaneous miscarriage ranges between 10 and 15% of recognized pregnancies [22]. Another study showed that miscarriage occurred in one in five pregnancies in women aged 31–36 years [21]. This number is greater in vaginal repair-treated CSD patients, with a rate of 23.08% reported in the current study. We believe that the miscarriage rate was correlated with age, and the relationship among CSD, miscarriage, and subsequent fertility warrants further investigation.

Uterine rupture is the most feared complication during pregnancy and labour in women who had previous deliveries via CS. TRM in the lower uterine segment (LUS) is a widely accepted indicator for the prediction of uterine rupture during labour. A full thickness of 3.0 mm determined via LUS can be considered a cutoff value to identify women at risk of uterine rupture, with a specificity of 85% and sensitivity of 100% in an observational case-control study [23]. Another study indicated that a full LUS thickness of < 2.3 mm measured between 35 and 38 weeks of gestation is associated with a higher risk of complete uterine rupture [20]. No uterine dehiscence occurred when the full LUS thickness was more than 4.5 mm [24]. In the current study, TRM measured using LUS significantly increased from $2.42 \pm 0.1.04$ mm to 8.36 ± 3.11 mm, and no cases of threatened uterine rupture or uterine rupture were detected in women who had successful deliveries. This result further demonstrated that vaginal repair has the ability not only to resolve the symptom of prolonged menstrual bleeding but also to rebuild the muscular layer of the scar site.

As reported by Vervoort [25], a number of factors may explain the development of a caesarean scar defect: [1] a very low incision through the cervical tissue; [2] inadequate suturing or incomplete closure of the uterine wall due to a single-layer endometrial-saving closure technique or use of locking sutures; and [3] surgical interventions that encourage adhesion formation (namely, non-closure of the peritoneum, inadequate haemostasis, visible sutures, and others). Our research is the first of its type to detect residual myometrium under the microscope. We found that the collagen density of the residual myometrium covering the scar was significantly higher than that of healthy myometrium directly adjacent to the scar. We believe that the excessive expression of collagen may be an important factor in the formation of diverticula. Thus, the formation of the diverticula may be associated with an imbalance between the ratio of muscle fibres to collagen fibres. Further research will be needed to clarify these issues.

In the current study, 6 of the 20 (30.0%) women who achieved pregnancy without miscarriage experienced pregnancy complications, including 2 women with preterm births, 2 women with GDM, 1 woman with placenta previa, and 1 woman with GDM as well as hypothyroidism during pregnancy. Notably, haemorrhage (945 ml blood) occurred in the patient who had a preterm birth. The ages of the women and the intervals from vaginal repair to pregnancy may be responsible for the relatively high rate of pregnancy complications.

Conclusion

The current study demonstrated that vaginal repair can not only resolve CSD-associated prolonged menstrual bleeding but can also restore the anatomical structure in patients with CSD. Furthermore, subsequent satisfactory obstetrical outcomes can be achieved in vaginal repair-treated CSD patients.

Abbreviations
CS: Caesarean section; CSD: Caesarean scar diverticula (defect);
GDM: Gestational diabetes mellitus; LUS: Lower uterine segment;
TRM: Thickness of the remaining muscular layer; TVU: Transvaginal ultrasound

Acknowledgements
We thank all of the patients, doctors and nurses who participated in this study.

Funding
This study was supported by a Key grant from the Shanghai Scientific and Technology Commission (15411961600) and a action plan from Shenkang(16CR4028A). Key grant from the Shanghai Scientific and Technology Commission (15411961600): design of the study, collection, analysis. Action plan from Shenkang(16CR4028A): interpretation of data, and in writing the manuscript.

Authors' contributions
XZ: Manuscript writing,data analysis. HC: Data collection. XY: Data collection or management. XF: Manuscript revision,data analysis. XW: Project development, manuscript editing. All authors read and approved the final manuscript.

Competing interests
The results and writing of this study was supported by a Key grant from the Shanghai Scientific and Technology Commission (15411961600) and a action plan from Shenkang(16CR4028A), the authors have no conflicts of interest.

Author details
[1]Department of Gynecology, Xinhua Hospital affiliated with Shanghai Jiaotong University, 1665 Kong Jiang Rd, Yang Pu District, Shanghai 200092, China. [2]Department of Gynecology, Shanghai First Maternity and Infant Hospital, Affiliated to Tongji University, Shanghai, China.

References
1. Donnez O, Donnez J, Orellana R, Dolmans MM. Gynecological and obstetrical outcomes after laparoscopic repair of a cesarean scar defect in a series of 38 women. Fertil Steril. 2017;107(1):289–96 e282.
2. Vikhareva Osser O, Valentin L. Risk factors for incomplete healing of the uterine incision after caesarean section. BJOG : an international journal of obstetrics and gynaecology. 2010;117(9):1119–26.
3. Osser OV, Jokubkiene L, Valentin L. High prevalence of defects in cesarean section scars at transvaginal ultrasound examination. Ultrasound in obstetrics & gynecology : the official journal of the International Society of Ultrasound in Obstetrics and Gynecology. 2009;34(1):90–7.
4. van der Voet LF, Vervoort AJ, Veersema S, BijdeVaate AJ, Brolmann HA, Huirne JA: Minimally invasive therapy for gynaecological symptoms related to a niche in the caesarean scar: a systematic review. BJOG : an international journal of obstetrics and gynaecology 2014; 121(2):145–156.
5. Chang Y, Tsai EM, Long CY, Lee CL, Kay N. Resectoscopic treatment combined with sonohysterographic evaluation of women with postmenstrual bleeding

as a result of previous cesarean delivery scar defects. *American journal of obstetrics and gynecology*. 2009;200(4):370 e371–4.
6. Bij de Vaate AJ, van der Voet LF, Naji O, Witmer M, Veersema S, Brolmann HA, Bourne T, Huirne JA. Prevalence, potential risk factors for development and symptoms related to the presence of uterine niches following cesarean section: systematic review. Ultrasound in obstetrics & gynecology : the official journal of the International Society of Ultrasound in Obstetrics and Gynecology. 2014;43(4):372–82.
7. Hager RM, Daltveit AK, Hofoss D, Nilsen ST, Kolaas T, Oian P, Henriksen T. Complications of cesarean deliveries: rates and risk factors. Am J Obstet Gynecol. 2004;190(2):428–34.
8. Ofili-Yebovi D, Ben-Nagi J, Sawyer E, Yazbek J, Lee C, Gonzalez J, Jurkovic D. Deficient lower-segment cesarean section scars: prevalence and risk factors. Ultrasound in obstetrics & gynecology : the official journal of the International Society of Ultrasound in Obstetrics and Gynecology. 2008;31(1):72–7.
9. Xie H, Wu Y, Yu F, He M, Cao M, Yao S. A comparison of vaginal surgery and operative hysteroscopy for the treatment of cesarean-induced isthmocele: a retrospective review. Gynecol Obstet Investig. 2014;77(2):78–83.
10. Zhou J, Yao M, Wang H, Tan W, Chen P, Wang X. Vaginal repair of cesarean section scar diverticula that resulted in improved postoperative menstruation. J Minim Invasive Gynecol. 2016;23(6):969–78.
11. Zhou X, Yao M, Zhou J, Tan W, Wang H, Wang X. Defect width: the prognostic index for vaginal repair of cesarean section diverticula. Arch Gynecol Obstet. 2017;295(3):623–30.
12. Roberge S, Boutin A, Chaillet N, Moore L, Jastrow N, Demers S, Bujold E. Systematic review of cesarean scar assessment in the nonpregnant state: imaging techniques and uterine scar defect. Am J Perinatol. 2012;29(6):465–71.
13. Vikhareva Osser O, Valentin L. Clinical importance of appearance of cesarean hysterotomy scar at transvaginal ultrasonography in nonpregnant women. Obstet Gynecol. 2011;117(3):525–32.
14. Zhang X, Yang M, Wang Q, Chen J, Ding J, Hua K. Prospective evaluation of five methods used to treat cesarean scar defects. International journal of gynaecology and obstetrics: the official organ of the International Federation of Gynaecology and Obstetrics. 2016;134(3):336–9.
15. Luo L, Niu G, Wang Q, Xie HZ, Yao SZ. Vaginal repair of cesarean section scar diverticula. J Minim Invasive Gynecol. 2012;19(4):454–8.
16. Jeremy B, Bonneau C, Guillo E, Paniel BJ, Le Tohic A, Haddad B, Madelenat P: [uterine ishtmique transmural hernia: results of its repair on symptoms and fertility]. Gynecologie, obstetrique & fertilite 2013; 41(10):588–596.
17. Marotta ML, Donnez J, Squifflet J, Jadoul P, Darii N, Donnez O. Laparoscopic repair of post-cesarean section uterine scar defects diagnosed in nonpregnant women. J Minim Invasive Gynecol. 2013;20(3):386–91.
18. Tanimura S, Funamoto H, Hosono T, Shitano Y, Nakashima M, Ametani Y, Nakano T. New diagnostic criteria and operative strategy for cesarean scar syndrome: endoscopic repair for secondary infertility caused by cesarean scar defect. J Obstet Gynaecol Res. 2015;41(9):1363–9.
19. Gurol-Urganci I, Bou-Antoun S, Lim CP, Cromwell DA, Mahmood TA, Templeton A, van der Meulen JH: Impact of caesarean section on subsequent fertility: a systematic review and meta-analysis. Hum Reprod 2013; 28(7):1943–1952.
20. Bujold E, Jastrow N, Simoneau J, Brunet S, Gauthier RJ. Prediction of complete uterine rupture by sonographic evaluation of the lower uterine segment. *American journal of obstetrics and gynecology*. 2009;201(3):320 e321–6.
21. Giakoumelou S, Wheelhouse N, Cuschieri K, Entrican G, Howie SE, Horne AW. The role of infection in miscarriage. Hum Reprod Update. 2016;22(1):116–33.
22. O'Neill SM, Kearney PM, Kenny LC, Khashan AS, Henriksen TB, Lutomski JE, Greene RA. Caesarean delivery and subsequent stillbirth or miscarriage: systematic review and meta-analysis. PLoS One. 2013;8(1):e54588.
23. Gizzo S, Zambon A, Saccardi C, Patrelli TS, Di Gangi S, Carrozzini M, Bertocco A, Capobianco G, D'Antona D, Nardelli GB. Effective anatomical and functional status of the lower uterine segment at term: estimating the risk of uterine dehiscence by ultrasound. Fertil Steril. 2013;99(2):496–501.
24. Rozenberg P, Goffinet F, Phillippe HJ, Nisand I. Ultrasonographic measurement of lower uterine segment to assess risk of defects of scarred uterus. Lancet. 1996;347(8997):281–4.
25. Vervoort AJ, Uittenbogaard LB, Hehenkamp WJ, Brolmann HA, Mol BW, Huirne JA. Why do niches develop in caesarean uterine scars? Hypotheses on the aetiology of niche development. Hum Reprod. 2015;30(12):2695–702.

12

The association between daily 500 mg calcium supplementation and lower pregnancy-induced hypertension risk in Bangladesh

Fouzia Khanam[1], Belal Hossain[1], Sabuj Kanti Mistry[1], Dipak K. Mitra[2], Wameq Azfar Raza[3], Mahfuza Rifat[4], Kaosar Afsana[4] and Mahfuzar Rahman[1]*

Abstract

Background: Evidence suggests that daily supplementation of 1500 to 2000 mg of calcium during pregnancy reduces pregnancy-induced hypertension (PIH). However, the evidence on the efficacy of low-dose calcium supplementation on PIH is limited. This paper assesses the longitudinal correlation between low-dose calcium intake (500 mg daily) and change in blood pressure during pregnancy among a homogeneous population in terms of hypertension and pre-eclampsia.

Methods: The study followed a retrospective cohort study design, and was carried out among 11,387 pregnant women from 10 rural *upazilas* (sub-districts) of Bangladesh where maternal nutrition initiative (MNI), implemented by Building Resources Across Communities (BRAC), was ongoing. The modified Poisson regression model was used to estimate the association (risk ratio) between consumption of calcium tablets and PIH.

Results: The present research found that women who consumed 500 mg/d calcium tablets for more than 6 months during their pregnancy had a 45% lower risk of developing hypertension compared to those who consumed less calcium (RR = 0.55, 95% CI = 0.33–0.93).

Conclusions: Daily supplementation of 500 mg oral calcium during pregnancy for at least 180 tablets is associated with a considerably reduced risk of PIH, but this study is unable to confirm whether this association is causal. The causal relationship needs to be confirmed through a large scale randomized controlled trial.

Keywords: Pregnancy-induced hypertension, Calcium supplementation, Maternal nutrition initiative (MNI), Global health, Maternal mortality

Background

Pregnancy-induced hypertension (PIH), defined as systolic blood pressure (sBP) > 140 mmHg or diastolic blood pressure (dBP) > 90 mmHg [1], is a major determinant of pre-eclampsia/eclampsia (PE/E). High BP is responsible for approximately 14% of global maternal deaths [2]. Pre-eclampsia affects an estimated 3.2% of all live births - a total of more than four million cases each year -nearly 1.8% of which are fatal [3–5]. First described in 1980 [6], the inverse relationship between calcium

supplementation during pregnancy and the risk of pregnancy-induced high blood pressure (BP) is well documented [7–15].

Based on evidence from a meta-analysis of randomized controlled trials [16], the World Health Organization (WHO) recommends routine prenatal calcium supplementation of 1500 to 2000 mg daily beginning from 20th gestational week for all pregnant women, particularly those residing in low-calcium intake areas which are considered as high risk population [17]. It is notable that the overall calcium intake among the Bangladeshi population is low due to lack of calcium in the regular diet [18]. Although the WHO calcium regimen is

* Correspondence: mahfuzar.rahman@brac.net
[1]Research and Evaluation Division, BRAC Center, Dhaka 1212, Bangladesh
Full list of author information is available at the end of the article

endorsed by the government of Bangladesh, in reality the adoption rate has been lower due to bottlenecks such as poor compliance [19].

However, evidence of the impact of low-dose calcium supplementation (intake of 500 mg/d calcium tablet) on PIH is limited. A systematic review of the effects of low-dose calcium intake on pre-eclampsia has shown significant results [20]. The review included studies from both high-risk and low-risk populations and found a larger effect among high-risk populations accordingly. Since the data for this review came primarily from small studies, the authors called for larger trials to confirm the results.

Previous researchers have also suggested that a lower dose regimen may actually result in a higher cumulative calcium dose consumption through improved adherence [21]. High dose supplementation as recommended by WHO has not been widely adopted, likely because of practical impediments such as the size and number of units of conventional calcium tablets required to deliver the recommended daily dose (3 to 4 tablets). Furthermore, calcium tablets must be ingested separately from iron because of the negative impact of calcium on iron absorption. Therefore, building an evidence base on the effects of a low dose recommendation could have a tremendous impact in developing countries through saved resources. This study aims to assess the effects of different durations of low-dose calcium supplementation (500 mg daily) during pregnancy on the incidence of PIH.

Methods
Study design, sampling and participants
The study followed a retrospective cohort design. Participants were women who gave birth between November 2016 and May 2017. Basic and vital information of the pregnant mothers was extracted from the registrars of *Shashthya Kormis* (SKs) - the community health workers (CHW) working in the maternal nutrition initiative (MNI) program implemented by BRAC. All participating women received calcium tablets during the pregnancy period; therefore, there was no control group in the study.

Sample size for this study was calculated to compare incidence of PIH between women those who consumed daily 500 mg calcium for the optimal duration and women those who consumed calcium for a sub-optimal duration. Considering a 6% incidence of PIH among women with sub-optimal calcium dosing, a 4% incidence among women with optimal dosing, 5% type I error, 90% power, and a design effect of 2, a sample of 10,400 pregnant women were required for the study. We included 11,387 participants in our study. We excluded individuals with completely missing data ($n = 3$), with missing data on ANC timing ($n = 2962$), those diagnosed with hypertension before the first follow-up ($n = 90$), and those missing data on systolic blood pressure (sBP) or diastolic BP (dBP) or calcium distribution and consumption after 5 months of gestation due to lost to follow-up ($n = 485$) (Fig. 1).

The intervention
BRAC has been implementing the maternal nutrition initiative (MNI) program in 10 upazilas (sub-district) i.e., Gafargaon, Dhobaura, Tarakanda, Trishal of Mymensingh, Badarganj and Mithapukur of Rangpur, Aditmari and Patgram of Lalmonirhat, and Rajarhat and Ulipur of Kurigram districts of Bangladesh since July 2015. The program is conducted by community health workers (CHW) which are divided into two groups - *Shashthya Kormis* (SKs) and *Shashthya Sebikas* (SSs). SKs were trained on providing different health care services such as pregnancy identification, antenatal care (ANC) and postnatal care (PNC), while SSs were selected from local communities and were trained on providing essential health care services at the community level. After identification, SKs visited every pregnant woman to provide ANC services on a monthly basis until childbirth. During consultations, SKs discussed dietary diversity, recommended high quality foods, recommended taking iron folic acid (IFA) and calcium, and collected anthropometric data including weight and blood pressure.

SKs were tasked to distributing 500 mg calcium tablets from the first ANC visit. The total number of calcium tablets received by a pregnant woman depended on gestational age at her first ANC visit. Women who began to receive ANC within the first 3 month of pregnancy received 180 tablets or more, those who came around 6 or 7 months received 90 tablets or more, and those who came at 8 or 9 months received fewer than 90 tablets. The comprehensive intervention is comprised of the following four components: (i) counseling about the importance of calcium tablet during pregnancy; (ii) free delivery of 30–35 calcium tablets (500 mg each) per month until the end of term; (iii) recording the compliance of calcium intake by counting strips of calcium tablets provided during earlier visits; and (iv) collecting anthropometric information such as weight and BP measurements.

Women were instructed to take one calcium tablet (500 mg) daily in the morning for 6 months (180 tablets) or until pregnancy termination. The daily dose was determined based on the trials included in the 2010 Cochrane review [16]. Due to concerns that calcium might interfere with IFA absorption [22], the women were instructed to take calcium tablets after their morning meal and not to take it with iron, which was to be taken with the evening meal.

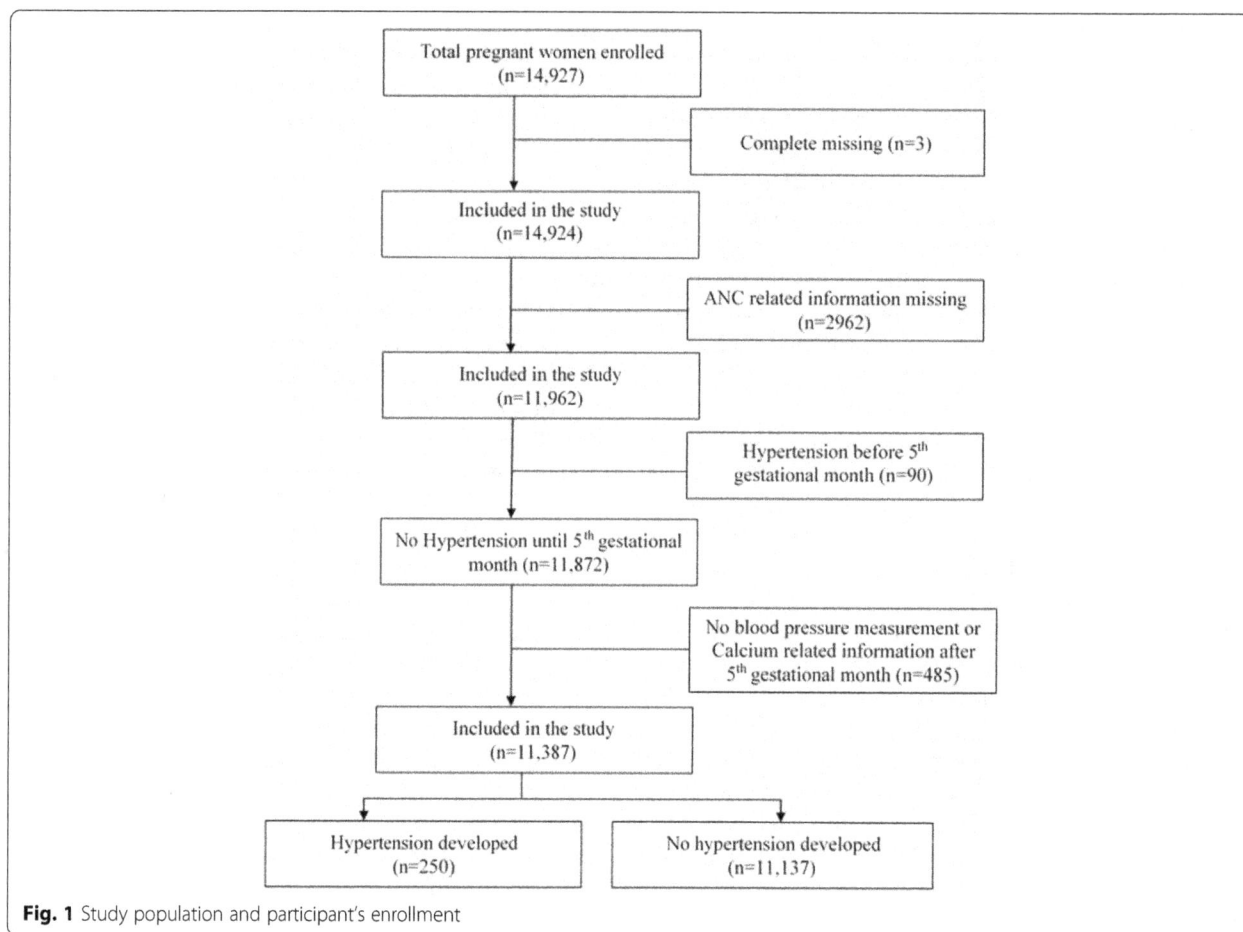

Fig. 1 Study population and participant's enrollment

Measurement of outcome and exposure variables

Blood pressure was the primary outcome variable. BP was measured at enrollment (5th gestational month) and at each follow-up visit (6th through 9th gestational months) by trained field workers using a sphygmomanometer [23]. Measurements were taken with participants in a seated position after 5 min of rest, with the cuff around the upper left arm in accordance with recommended guidelines [24]. Two BP measurements were taken at each follow-up with a minimum 1 h interval [25], and an average of those measurements was recorded. Women were considered to have PIH if sBP ≥140 mmHg and/or dBP ≥90 mmHg in any visit after the 20th week of gestation with previously known normotensive.

Calcium consumption was the primary exposure variable. The level of calcium tablet consumption was classified into three categories: 500 mg/d for more than 6 months, 500 mg/d for 3–6 months, and 500 mg/d for less than 3 months. Weight was measured at every household visit with electronic scales (UNISCALE) accurate to 100 g. The number of living children, household structure, and monthly income were also collected at enrollment.

We validated the main outcome variable through cross-checking by medical professionals. The professionals cross-checked 105 measurements of 105 individuals in a given visit. The reliability of the BP measurements was quantified by using intra-cluster correlation coefficient [26]. We found that the intra-class correlation coefficients were very high for both systolic and diastolic BP measurements (for sBP: 0.91 and for dBP: 0.86).

Statistical analysis

Descriptive statistics were performed to assess the distribution of the exposure variables. A Chi-squared test was conducted to compare calcium consumption groups by other exposure variables. Predicted mean blood pressure (sBP and dBP) was estimated using the mixed-effect linear regression model which accounts for the correlation among BP measurements within subjects and variations across subjects. The dependent variable of the mixed-effect model considers all successive BP measurements of individuals with complete information by considering a random intercept for each subject and BP over time in the population as fixed effect.

Finally, we investigate the unadjusted and adjusted association between calcium intake and PIH using a modified Poisson regression model assuming an uniform risk period and robust standard errors [27]. Our initial goal was to run a log-binomial regression model to assess the effectiveness of the consumption of 500 mg calcium tablets, but this model had a convergence problem with many covariates. To overcome this problem, we ran the modified Poisson regression model which is equivalent to the log-binomial regression model when estimating risk ratio (RR) [27]. The unadjusted analyses were performed for the potential confounders such as enrollment age, weight, occupation, parity, number of living child, number of antenatal care visits, household type, household assets, and administrative district. The variables with $P < 0.25$ in the unadjusted analyses were considered as confounders and included in the final model [28]. The RR and corresponding confidence interval (CI) were estimated with a 5% significance level. All analyses were performed using statistical software package STATA 13.0.

Results

Table 1 shows the distribution of demographic and lifestyle factors among the study population. A total of 57.4% women were aged between 20 and 29 years. Most of the women (99.1%) were housewives and 76.2% women had at least one child. 14.6% women had pacca/semi-pacca households and 46.8% were from poor households. Of the total 11,387 participants 9358 had four sBP measurements and 9356 had four dBP measurements; 10,376 had three sBP and 10,377 had three dBP measurements (Table 1).

Table 2 shows the calcium consumption during pregnancy by demographic and socio-economic variables. A total of 19.8% women consumed < 90 tablets (i.e. 500 mg/d calcium tablets for less than 3 months), while 66.0% consumed 90–179 tablets (i.e. 500 mg/d calcium tablets for 3–6 months) and 14.2% consumed 180 or more tablets (i.e. 500 mg/d calcium tablets for more than 6 months).Women between 20 and 29 years consumed more calcium tablets than women aged < 20 or > 30 years ($P < 0.001$). Low body-weight women (< 45 kg at enrollment) consumed a higher number of calcium tablets than higher body-weight women ($P = 0.105$). Women living in pacca/semi-pacca households consumed more tablets ($P = 0.047$), while consumption was similar between poor and non-poor households ($P = 0.794$). Moreover, calcium consumption largely depended on the number of ANC visits. Women who had four or more ANC check-ups consumed more calcium tablets than those who did not ($P < 0.001$). However, among all 11,387 study women, all had at least one ANC visit while 86% had four or more (Additional file 1: Table S1).

Table 3 shows the predicted mean sBPs and dBPs at baseline and four follow up visits by calcium intake

Table 1 Background characteristics of study participants ($n = 11,387$)

Characteristics	n	% or Mean ± SD
District		
Mymensingh	5649	49.61
Rangpur	2270	19.94
Lalmonirhat	1613	14.17
Kurigram	1855	16.29
Age (years)		
< 20	2733	24.00
20–24	3237	28.43
25–29	3297	28.95
≥ 30	2120	18.62
Occupation		
Housewife	11,286	99.11
Working outside	101	0.89
Parity		
1	2803	24.62
2	4452	39.10
≥ 3	4132	36.29
Number of living children		
None	2715	23.84
1	5098	44.77
≥ 2	3574	31.39
Household type		
Pacca/semi-pacca	1666	14.63
Tin and others	9721	85.37
Household asset		
Poor	5321	46.73
Non-poor	6066	53.27
Systolic blood pressure		
Baseline	11,387	99.27 ± 7.27
Follow up 1	10,151	99.94 ± 8.31
Follow up 2	10,376	100.75 ± 8.57
Follow up 3	9358	101.59 ± 9.15
Follow up 4	5224	102.41 ± 9.63
Diastolic blood pressure		
Baseline	11,387	62.50 ± 6.99
Follow up 1	10,151	63.77 ± 7.76
Follow up 2	10,377	64.52 ± 7.97
Follow up 3	9356	65.43 ± 8.48
Follow up 4	5225	66.06 ± 8.80
Weight (kg)		
Baseline	11,387	49.02 ± 8.03
Follow up 1	10,111	50.46 ± 7.99
Follow up 2	10,369	51.98 ± 8.04
Follow up 3	9363	53.58 ± 8.20
Follow up 4	5221	54.93 ± 8.28

Baseline = 5th gestational month, Follow up 1–4 = 6th – 9th gestational month

Table 2 Background characteristics of women by calcium consumption level during pregnancy (n = 11,387)

Characteristics	n	500 mg/d calcium intake (%)			P
		< 3 months	3–6 months	≥6 months	
Age (years)					< 0.001
< 20	2733	21.08	66.26	12.66	
20–24	3237	19.56	64.94	15.51	
25–29	3297	17.26	67.52	15.23	
≥ 30	2120	22.36	65.09	12.55	
Occupation					0.006
Housewife	11,286	19.68	66.16	14.16	
Working outside	101	30.69	51.49	17.82	
Baseline weight (kg)					0.105
< 45	3585	20.00	64.44	15.56	
45–50	3571	19.46	67.04	13.50	
51–60	3171	19.55	66.98	13.47	
> 60	1060	20.75	65.19	14.06	
Parity					0.006
1	2803	20.91	65.93	13.16	
2	4452	18.60	65.90	15.50	
≥ 3	4132	20.28	66.24	13.48	
Number of living children					< 0.001
None	2715	21.22	66.08	12.71	
1	5098	18.24	66.40	15.36	
≥ 2	3574	20.87	65.47	13.65	
Number of antenatal care visits					< 0.001
< 4	1295	86.64	13.36	0.00	
4+	10,092	11.20	72.79	16.01	
Household type					0.047
Pacca/semi-pacca	1666	21.49	65.85	12.67	
Tin and others	9721	19.48	66.06	14.45	
Household asset					0.794
Poor	5321	19.51	66.23	14.26	
Non-poor	6066	20.01	65.86	14.13	
Total	11,387	19.78	66.03	14.19	

categories. It also presents the absolute change in mean blood pressures from baseline to the last follow up visit. For both sBP and dBP, we observed a slower increase over time among those who consumed 500 mg/d calcium tablets for more than 6 months during the pregnancy period compared to those who consumed 500 mg/calcium tablets for fewer than 6 months.

We further compared the incidence of PIH after the 5th gestational month between calcium intake groups using log-binomial or modified Poisson regression model. Both unadjusted and adjusted models were implemented and results are presented in Table 4. The final model was adjusted by age and weight at enrollment,

number of antenatal care visits, household asset, and administrative district. The overall incidence of PIH was 2.2% (250 out of 11,387). We found that women who consumed 500 mg/d calcium tablets for more than 6 months during the antenatal period had a significantly lower risk (46%) of developing hypertension than those who consumed 500 mg/d calcium tablets for fewer than 3 months (RR: 0.56, 95% CI: 0.33–0.93).

Discussion

To our knowledge, this large-scale study is the first to examine the effectiveness of low dose supplemental calcium (500 mg) on the risk of PIH. We found that

Table 3 Relation between number of calcium tablets intake and monthly changes in systolic blood pressure (sBP) and diastolic blood pressure (dBP) over 4 months of follow-up (5th to 9th gestational months) of the same individuals

Characteristics	Baseline	F1	F 2	F3	F4	BP increase
sBP (mmHg)						
Calcium intake						
500 mg/d for < 3 months	96.7	98.2	99.2	100.4	102.4	5.7
500 mg/d for 3–6 months	98.9	99.6	100.4	101.1	102.2	3.4
500 mg/d for ≥6 months	99.6	100.5	101.1	101.5	102.7	3.1
dBP (mmHg)						
Calcium intake						
500 mg/d for < 3 months	62.0	62.6	63.0	64.7	67.0	5.0
500 mg/d for 3–6 months	62.5	63.0	63.9	64.7	65.9	3.4
500 mg/d for ≥6 months	63.2	63.9	64.3	65.1	65.8	2.7

Baseline = 5th gestational month, F1 to F4 = Follow up 1 to 4 (6th to 9th gestational month)

women had a 45% lower risk of developing hypertension when they took 500 mg/d calcium tablets for more than 6 months during pregnancy relative to those who consumed 500 mg/d calcium tablets for fewer than 3 months. The association of calcium consumption during pregnancy with decreased PIH is well documented in earlier studies [20, 29], yet the evidence of the use of low-dose calcium in a maternal health and nutrition intervention is scarce in low-income settings. We begin to fill this gap in the literature.

The World Health Organization (WHO) has recommended antenatal calcium supplementation of 1500–2000 mg daily for pregnant women with low dietary calcium intake who are thus at a higher risk for pre-eclampsia [16, 30]. However, a large proportion of Bangladeshi pregnant women are at high risk for multiple micronutrient deficiencies including antioxidants [18, 31]. While much research has focused on malnutrition among children, recent reports indicate a high prevalence of micronutrient deficiency among women as well [32]. Under these conditions, BRAC initiated the MNI program which includes the 500 mg daily calcium supplement.

Our study found that women living in the Rangpur and Lalmonirhat districts are at higher risk of PIH compared to Mymensingh district when adjusting for other factors including calcium intake. This result is consistent with the fact that Rangpur division has a higher prevalence calcium deficiency compared to the Dhaka division [18]. We also found that older age and higher weight significantly increased the risk of PIH which is consistent with findings from other studies [33].

Nevertheless, cross-sectional assessments of the association between calcium exposure and BP are limited by a) possible selection bias in capturing only individuals who have lived long enough to participate in the study, and b) weak detection of the latent effects of calcium

exposure on BP. In contrast, longitudinal analyses mitigate some of these problems and may be a robust method for examining the effect of calcium consumption on blood pressure change over time.

In the present study, we found that 500 mg/d calcium tablets consumption for 180 days or more during pregnancy was associated with lower increase in mean BP. Also, the risk of hypertension was 45% lower among those women. While the observed reduction is significant, it does not point directly to clinical outcomes at the individual level. A majority of the women were lost from the sample before receiving ANC visits and calcium tablets, thus resulting in a type of survival bias. Subsequent loss at follow up resulted in missing outcome data. However, as our study population is very homogenous in nature, we expect very little bias from this loss. One major strength of our study is that any biases were minimized by combining individual calcium consumption and outcome data from registry. Moreover, loss at follow-up or missing data is a problem regardless of any possible assuring comparisons. We simply do not know how dropped observations could have affected risk ratios were they not missed. Moreover, most of the previous research which has been undertaken to assess the effectiveness of low-dose calcium was carried out among populations at high risk for calcium deficiency. In contrast, the present research was more robust in the sense that the data were collected from a general group of population, i.e. there was no particular low or high risk population.

The study is not without limitations. First, the conclusions are drawn in the absence of full-fledged randomized control trial. Due to lack of a true comparison group - especially the absence of a high dose supplementation group - we are unable to attribute the effectiveness with greater strength. We also did not collect the information through a questionnaire; rather information

Table 4 Relation between amount of calcium intake and pregnancy-induced hypertension

Characteristics	Unadjusted			Adjusted		
	RR	P	95% CI	RR	P	95% CI
Calcium intake						
500 mg/d for < 3 months	1.0			1.0		
500 mg/d for 3–6 months	0.78	0.089	0.59–1.04	0.83	0.273	0.59–1.16
500 mg/d for ≥6 months	0.51	0.005	0.32–0.82	0.56	0.026	0.33–0.93
Age (years)	1.04	0.001	1.02–1.06	1.02	0.065	1.00–1.05
Weight (kg)	1.07	< 0.001	1.06–1.08	1.06	< 0.001	1.05–1.07
Occupation						
Housewife	1.0			Not retained in the final model		
Working outside	0.74	0.594	0.24–2.26			
Parity						
1	0.96	0.802	0.70–1.32	Not retained in the final model		
2	1.0					
≥ 3	1.08	0.601	0.81–1.43			
Number of living children						
None	1.0			Not retained in the final model		
1	1.05	0.781	0.76–1.44			
≥ 2	1.14	0.444	0.82–1.59			
Number of antenatal care visits						
< 4	1.0			1.0		
4+	0.72	0.054	0.51–1.01	0.91	0.646	0.60–1.37
Household type						
Pacca/semi-pacca	1.0			Not retained in the final model		
Tin and others	0.87	0.423	0.63–1.22			
Household asset						
Poor	1.0			1.0		
Non-poor	1.36	0.016	1.06–1.75	1.14	0.307	0.88–1.48
District						
Mymensingh	1.0			1.0		
Rangpur	2.05	< 0.001	1.52–2.77	1.84	0.000	1.36–2.50
Lalmonirhat	1.69	0.004	1.19–2.42	1.56	0.013	1.10–2.23
Kurigram	1.34	0.121	0.93–1.93	1.18	0.378	0.82–1.70

RR Risk ratio, *CI* Confidence interval

was extracted from the registrars of the SKs who were already working in the MNI areas. The registrars did not contain much relevant information which may influence both the calcium intake and blood pressure level among the women. Therefore, the study result should be used with caution as the information of few confounders such as body mass index, diabetes, family history of PIH and previous incident of PIH were missing [34, 35]. We are also unable to account for measurement errors as only one method of measurement was employed throughout the study duration.

Also, because the MNI initiative included the improvement of the dietary practices of pregnant and lactating mothers, the observed reduction in PIH could be due to an increase in calcium intake resulting from a generally improved diet. We did not assess the role of specific nutrients or nutritional intake in the present study. Future studies are needed to investigate whether the association of calcium intake and the rate of BP change differ by nutritional status.

Conclusion
The study demonstrated a positive association between low dose calcium supplementation and reduction in risk of BP among a large cohort of pregnant women who were homogeneous with respect to disease risk. The

findings have several policy implications. These findings are consistent with other studies about reducing the risk of PIH which could have implications for current guidelines and their global implementation. Currently, the high cost of implementing the WHO recommended daily dose of calcium is regarded as prohibitive in low income settings. Moreover, this dose has not been widely adopted due to implementation bottlenecks, such as the difficulty of multiple (3–4 tablets) administrations per day. Therefore, the dilemma facing health policy-makers in these settings is often whether supplementation with a lower-dose would be better than no supplementation at all. The findings of this research are a step towards addressing the issue.

Currently, the introduction of calcium supplementation in maternal health program is strongly recommended by WHO especially among populations with low dietary intake of calcium. So farm knowledge is inadequate concerning adherence, motivation, costing and logistics to implement the scaling-up of public health program. Therefore, larger well-designed RCTs are still required to determine the efficacy of low dose calcium of 500 mg/d and to determine the optimal duration of supplementation. Future research should focus on the causal impact of these interventions as well as implementation research to find out optimal program strategies including cost-effectiveness.

Abbreviations
ANC: antenatal care; BP: blood pressure; BRAC: Building Resources Across Communities; CHW: community health worker; dBP: diastolic blood pressure; IFA: iron folic acid; MNI: maternal nutrition initiative; PE/E: pre-eclampsia/eclampsia; PIH: pregnancy-induced hypertension; PNC: post natal care; sBP: systolic blood pressure; SK: shashthya kormi; SS: shashthya sebika; WHO: world health organization

Acknowledgements
We would like to thank Fakir Md Yunus, Susan Whitening (*University of Saskatchewan) and Lars Ake Persson (LSHTM)* for reviewing the draft manuscript and helping with preliminary analysis, and John Thiemel for editing assistance.

Funding
The research was funded by the Alive and Thrive of FHI360. The study sponsors had no role in the design, data gathering, data analysis, data interpretation, or writing of the report. The corresponding author had full access to all the data in the study, and takes responsibility for the integrity of the data and the accuracy of the data analysis.

Authors' contributions
FK and SKM participated in all phases of the study and were responsible for analysis of data and drafted the manuscript. KA, DM and MR2 participated with designing, analytical planning, and writing. FK, MR1, BH was responsible for field supervision, DK and BH participated in analyzing data and writing manuscript. KA, WR and MR2 contributed in the analysis plan and critical review of manuscript. All authors read and approved the final manuscript.

Competing interests
The authors declare that they have no competing interest.

Author details
[1]Research and Evaluation Division, BRAC Center, Dhaka 1212, Bangladesh. [2]Department of Public Health, North South University, Dhaka, Bangladesh. [3]Poverty and Equity, The World Bank, Dhaka, Bangladesh. [4]Health, Nutrition and Population Program, BRAC Center, Dhaka, Bangladesh.

References
1. Kintiraki E, Papakatsika S, Kotronis G, Goulis DG, Kotsis V. Pregnancy-induced hypertension. Hormones (Athens). 2015;14(2):211–23.
2. Say L, Chou D, Gemmill A, Tunçalp Ö, Moller A-B, Daniels J, Gülmezoglu AM, Temmerman M, Alkema L. Global causes of maternal death: a WHO systematic analysis. Lancet Glob Health. 2014;2(6):e323–33.
3. AbouZahr C. Global burden of maternal death and disability. Br Med Bull. 2003;67(1):1–11.
4. Mosha D, Liu E, Hertzmark E, Chan G, Sudfeld C, Masanja H, Fawzi W. Dietary iron and calcium intakes during pregnancy are associated with lower risk of prematurity, stillbirth and neonatal mortality among women in Tanzania. Public Health Nutr. 2017;20(4):678–86.
5. Lawn JE, Blencowe H, Waiswa P, Amouzou A, Mathers C, Hogan D, Flenady V, Frøen JF, Qureshi ZU, Calderwood C. Stillbirths: rates, risk factors, and acceleration towards 2030. Lancet. 2016;387(10018):587–603.
6. Belizan J, Villar J. The relationship between calcium intake and edema-, proteinuria-, and hypertension-gestosis: an hypothesis. Am J Clin Nutr. 1980;33(10):2202–10.
7. Lassi ZS, Mansoor T, Salam RA, Das JK, Bhutta ZA. Essential pre-pregnancy and pregnancy interventions for improved maternal, newborn and child health. Reprod Health. 2014;11(1):S2.
8. Imdad A, Bhutta ZA. Effects of calcium supplementation during pregnancy on maternal, fetal and birth outcomes. Paediatr Perinat Epidemiol. 2012;26(s1):138–52.
9. Belizán JM, Villar J, Zalazar A, Rojas L, Chan D, Bryce GF. Preliminary evidence of the effect of calcium supplementation on blood pressure in normal pregnant women. Am J Obstet Gynecol. 1983;146(2):175–80.
10. Belizán JM, Villar J, Gonzalez L, Campodonico L, Bergel E. Calcium supplementation to prevent hypertensive disorders of pregnancy. N Engl J Med. 1991;325(20):1399–405.
11. Payne R, Evans R. Dietary calcium supplementation and prevention of pregnancy hypertension. Lancet. 1990;335(8693):861.
12. Asayehu TT, Lachat C, Henauw SD, Gebreyesus SH. Dietary behaviour, food and nutrient intake of women do not change during pregnancy in southern Ethiopia. Matern Child Nutr. 2017;13(2):e12343.
13. Lopez-Jaramillo P, Narvaez M, Wetgel R, Yepez R. Calcium supplementation reduces the risk of pregnancy-induced hypertension in an Andes population. J Obstet Gynaecol. 1989;96(6):648–55.
14. Marcoux S, Brisson J, Fabia J. Calcium intake from dairy products and supplements and the risks of preeclampsia and gestational hypertension. Am J Epidemiol. 1991;133(12):1266–72.
15. Villar J, Belizan JM, Fischer PJ. Epidemiologic observations on the relationship between calcium intake and eclampsia. Int J Gynecol Obstet. 1983;21(4):271–8.

16. Hofmeyr GJ, Lawrie TA, Atallah ÁN, Duley L. Calcium supplementation during pregnancy for preventing hypertensive disorders and related problems. Cochrane Libr. 2010;(8):CD001059.

17. WHO. WHO recommendations for prevention and treatment of pre-eclampsia and eclampsia. Geneva: WHO Press; 2011.

18. Bromage S, Ahmed T, Fawzi WW. Calcium deficiency in Bangladesh: burden and proposed solutions for the first 1000 days. Food Nutr Bull. 2016;37(4):475–93.

19. Hallberg L, Brune M, Erlandsson M, Sandberg A-S, Rossander-Hulten L. Calcium: effect of different amounts on nonheme-and heme-iron absorption in humans. Am J Clin Nutr. 1991;53(1):112–9.

20. Hofmeyr G, Belizán J, Dadelszen PV. Low-dose calcium supplementation for preventing pre-eclampsia: a systematic review and commentary. BJOG Int J Obstet Gynaecol. 2014;121(8):951–7.

21. Ingersoll KS, Cohen J. The impact of medication regimen factors on adherence to chronic treatment: a review of literature. J Behav Med. 2008;31(3):213–24.

22. Barton JC, Conrad ME, Parmley RT. Calcium inhibition of inorganic iron absorption in rats. Gastroenterology. 1983;84(1):90–101.

23. O'brien E, Waeber B, Parati G, Staessen J, Myers MG. Blood pressure measuring devices: recommendations of the European Society of Hypertension. BMJ. 2001;322(7285):531.

24. Pickering TG, Hall JE, Appel LJ, Falkner BE, Graves J, Hill MN, Jones DW, Kurtz T, Sheps SG, Roccella EJ. Recommendations for blood pressure measurement in humans and experimental animals. Circulation. 2005;111(5):697–716.

25. Rouse CE, Eckert LO, Wylie BJ, Lyell DJ, Jeyabalan A, Kochhar S, McElrath TF, Group BCPW. Hypertensive disorders of pregnancy: case definitions & guidelines for data collection, analysis, and presentation of immunization safety data. Vaccine. 2016;34(49):6069.

26. Müller R, Büttner P. A critical discussion of intraclass correlation coefficients. Stat Med. 1994;13(23–24):2465–76.

27. Zou G. A modified poisson regression approach to prospective studies with binary data. Am J Epidemiol. 2004;159(7):702–6.

28. Agresti A. Categorical data analysis. Vol. 482. New Jersy: Wiley; 2003.

29. Hofmeyr G, Duley L, Atallah A. Dietary calcium supplementation for prevention of pre-eclampsia and related problems: a systematic review and commentary. BJOG Int J Obstet Gynaecol. 2007;114(8):933–43.

30. Hofmeyr G, Seuc A, Betrán A, Purnat T, Ciganda A, Munjanja S, Manyame S, Singata M, Fawcus S, Frank K. The effect of calcium supplementation on blood pressure in non-pregnant women with previous pre-eclampsia: an exploratory, randomized placebo controlled study. Pregnancy Hypertens. 2015;5(4):273–9.

31. Gernand AD, Schulze KJ, Stewart CP, West KP Jr, Christian P. Micronutrient deficiencies in pregnancy worldwide: health effects and prevention. Nat Rev Endocrinol. 2016;12(5):274.

32. Chowdhury S, Shahabuddin AM, Seal AJ, Talukder KK, Hassan Q, Begum RA, Rahman Q, Tomkins A, Costello A, Talukder M. Nutritional status and age at menarche in a rural area of Bangladesh. Ann Hum Biol. 2000;27(3):249–56.

33. Mehta B, Kumar V, Chawla S, Sachdeva S, Mahopatra D. Hypertension in pregnancy: a community-based study. Indian J Commun Med. 2015;40(4):273.

34. Parazzini F, Bortolus R, Chatenoud L, Restelli S, Ricci E, Marozio L, Benedetto C. Risk factors for pregnancy-induced hypertension in women at high risk for the condition. Epidemiology. 1996;7(3):306–8.

35. Ordas AM, Gomez AR, Benito MH, Luis MF-R, Hernandez RS, Cotera FA-U. Gestational hypertension: risk factors, clinical and laboratory findings: PP. 32.294. J Hypertens. 2010;28:e538.

13

Does a maternal history of abuse before pregnancy affect pregnancy outcomes? A systematic review with meta-analysis

Maryam Nesari[1], Joanne K Olson[1], Ben Vandermeer[2], Linda Slater[3] and David M Olson[4*]

Abstract

Background: Evidence relating maternal history of abuse before pregnancy with pregnancy outcomes is controversial. This study aims to examine the association between maternal histories of abuse before pregnancy and the risk of preterm delivery and low birth weight.

Methods: We searched Subject Headings and keywords for exposure and the outcomes through MEDLINE, EMBASE, Cochrane Database of Systematic Reviews, Cochrane Central Register of Controlled Trials, Psycinfo, CINAHL, Scopus, PILOTS, ProQuest Dissertations & Theses Global and Web of Science Core Collection in April 2017. We selected original studies that reported associations between maternal histories of abuse of any type and either preterm delivery or low birth weight. Studies that included interventions during pregnancy to lower maternal stress but reported no control data were excluded. We utilized the Newcastle-Ottawa Quality Assessment Scales for observational studies to assess the risk of bias in the primary studies. Two independent reviewers performed the selection of pertinent studies, assessment of risk of bias, and data extraction. Unadjusted pooled odds ratios (OR) with 95% Confidence Interval (CI) were calculated for the two outcomes of preterm delivery and low birth weight in 16 included studies.

Results: Maternal history of abuse before pregnancy was significantly associated with preterm delivery (OR 1.28, 95% CI: 1.12–1.47) and low birth weight (OR 1.35, 95% CI: 1.14–1.59). A substantial level of heterogeneity was detected within the two groups of studies reporting preterm birth and low birth weight (I^2 = 75% and 69% respectively). Subgroup analysis based on the specific time of abuse before pregnancy indicated that childhood abuse increases the risk of low birth weight by 57% (95% CI: 0.99–2.49). When the included studies were categorized based on study design, cohort studies showed the highest effect estimates on preterm delivery and low birth weight (OR: 1.69, 95%CI: 1.19–2.40, OR: 1.56, 95% CI: 1.06–2.3, respectively).

Conclusions: We recommend that more high quality research studies on this topic are necessary to strengthen the inference. At the practice level, we suggest more attention in detecting maternal history of abuse before pregnancy during antenatal visits and using this information to inform risk assessment for adverse pregnancy outcomes.

Keywords: Maternal, Abuse before pregnancy, Preterm delivery, Low birth weight

* Correspondence: dmolson@ualberta.ca
[4]Departments of Obstetrics and Gynecology, Pediatrics and Physiology, University of Alberta, Edmonton, AB T6G 2S2, Canada
Full list of author information is available at the end of the article

Background

Maternal chronic stress is increasingly recognized as a risk factor for some pregnancy outcomes such as Preterm Delivery (PTD) andLow Birth Weight (LBW). [1–3] PTD, the major perinatal health problem [4] is identified by the World Health Organization (WHO) as the primary cause of death in children less than five years old. [5] It is associated with impaired developmental trajectories [6, 7] and can lead to adult cardiovascular [8, 9] and metabolic diseases. [10–13] Infants born with LBW often experience severe health problems and developmental issues leading to substantial healthcare costs. [14]

In animal models, it is hypothesized that accumulated prenatal maternal stress leads to a high stress load that shortens gestation length or causes other adverse pregnancy and behavioral outcomes. [15, 16] However, if the stressed subject is placed into a supportive environment, many of the adverse effects of stress can be reversed, suggesting that stress is a modifiable risk factor. [17, 18] In human research, prenatal maternal stressors, such as natural disasters [19] adverse life events, and daily perceived stress [20] are associated with adverse pregnancy outcomes. Abuse and in particular, intimate partner violence (IPV), are the widely researched stressors associated with pregnancy outcomes. Abuse is defined as any attempt to control the behavior of another person and encompasses any direct or indirect physical, sexual or emotional maltreatment. [21] IPV refers to any maltreatment within an intimate relationship that leads to physical, psychological or sexual harm to those in the relationship.

Systematic reviews with meta-analyses indicated that IPV *during pregnancy* associates with PTD and low LBW. [21–24] Moreover, in some primary investigations, maternal history of abuse *before pregnancy* has been associated with adverse pregnancy outcomes; however others reported no association in this regard. [3, 25–33] Two recent systematic reviews examining the existing evidence on the relation between childhood sexual abuse and subsequent adult sequelae found that women who had experience of childhood abuse tended to have more problems and complaints during their pregnancy; [34, 35] nevertheless, both studies reported that the results of the associations between maternal history of childhood abuse and PTD and LBW were inconsistent. [34, 35] Therefore, this systematic review aims to examine whether maternal history of life-long abuse *before pregnancy* is associated with PTD and LBW.

Objective

The purpose of this systematic review was to assess the association between maternal history of abuse (physical, emotional, and sexual) at any time in life *before pregnancy* and risk of PTD and LBW. This systematic review is unique as we classified the relevant literature based on time of abuse to have a clear understanding of the effect of the time of abuse on the outcomes of interest. Consequently, three subgroups of childhood abuse (abuse happened before 18 years of age), anytime abuse (history of abuse anytime during married life until 12 months before pregnancy), and recent abuse (abuse occurred during 12 months before pregnancy) were created.

Methods

We followed the Meta-Analysis of Observational Studies in Epidemiology (MOOSE) criteria for reporting this meta-analysis.

Information sources, search strategy, eligibility criteria

We conducted an initial search intended to scope the literature on the association between lifelong stressors (including but not limited to sexual, physical and emotional abuse) and PTD in July 2015. Databases searched were MEDLINE, EMBASE, Psycinfo, Scopus, Web of Science Core Collection, CINAHL, PILOTS, Cochrane Database of Systematic Reviews and Cochrane Central Register of Controlled Trials. The search strategy is presented in Additional file 1. We performed an updated, more focused, search of MEDLINE, EMBASE, Scopus, Web of Science Core Collection, CINAHL, PILOTS, Violence and Abuse Abstracts, ProQuest Dissertations & Theses Global and Cochrane Database of Systematic Reviews and Cochrane Central Register of Controlled Trials in April 2017 to retrieve literature that studied the association between sexual, physical and emotional abuse and PTD as well as LBW. Full strategies for this search are contained in Additional file 2. To ensure comprehensive coverage of the literature, we screened the results of both searches. Search results are available in Fig. 1.

We initially screened citations to identify potentially relevant studies. Then we retrieved full-texts of the selected articles and assessed them further for eligibility according to a structured inclusion/exclusion form used by the two reviewers. The two steps of the selection process were performed by two reviewers independently, apparent discrepancies between them were resolved by consensus. We selected original studies that reported associations between maternal history of abuse of any kind and either PTD or LBW. Studies that included pharmacological or psychosocial intervention during pregnancy to lower maternal stress but report no control data were excluded. When more than one report was published based on the same sample, we included the more comprehensive report in our analysis.

For this review, abuse is defined as an attempt to control the behavior of another person and encompasses any direct or indirect physical, sexual or emotional maltreatment at any age, before pregnancy. [21] The primary outcomes

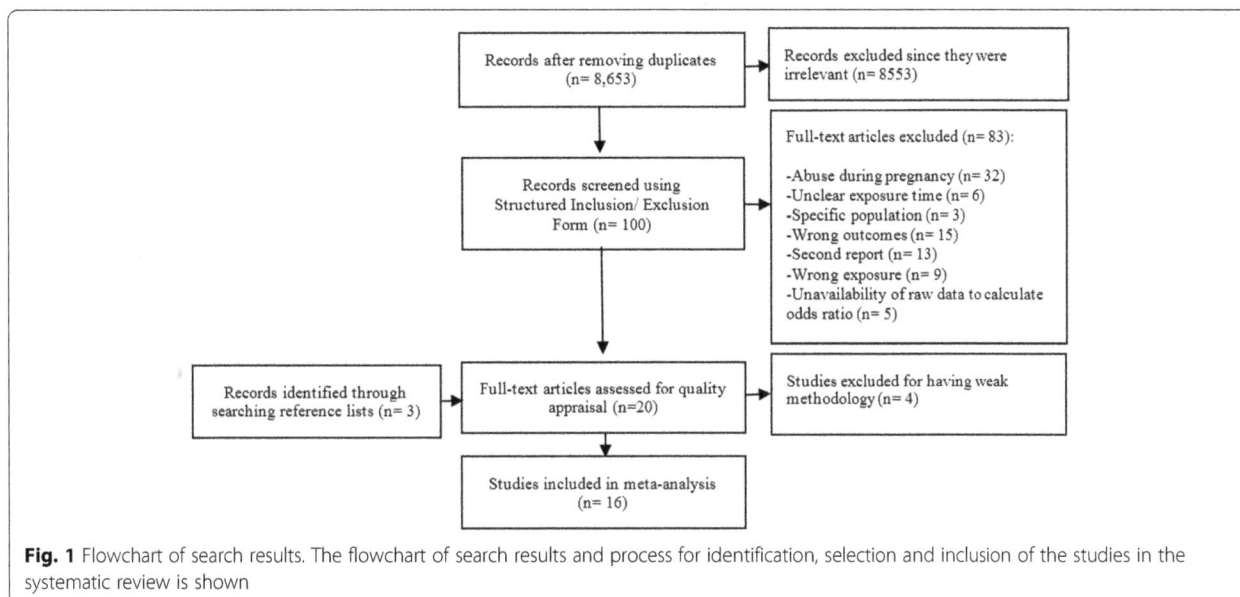

Fig. 1 Flowchart of search results. The flowchart of search results and process for identification, selection and inclusion of the studies in the systematic review is shown

in this review are PTD, defined as giving birth to a singleton at less than 37 weeks of gestation and LBW, defined as a birth weight of a live born infant of less than 2500 g regardless of gestational age.

We searched reference lists in each of the included articles as well as relevant review articles manually. Subsequently, we also examined reference lists of the newly identified articles. Additionally, we e-mailed individual researchers or organizations working on birth outcomes and maternal experience of abuse and violence to determine whether any published or unpublished studies existed that were not retrieved by our search.

Assessment of risk of bias

For the assessment of methodological quality (risk of bias) of the included studies, we utilized the Newcastle-Ottawa Quality Assessment Scales for observational studies. These scales are comprised of seven items that evaluate three domains of quality: sample selection, comparability of cohorts, and assessment of outcomes. A total score of 6 to 8 stars indicated high quality, 4 or 5 stars indicated moderate quality, and 3 or fewer stars related to poor quality. Two researchers from our team conducted the assessment of methodological quality of the included studies independently. Disagreement was discussed among the entire research team. We presented the results of the assessment in Table 1.

Data extraction

We utilized a researcher-constructed data extraction sheet piloted with 10 studies to record data from the included studies. Two researchers from our team extracted the data independently; any inconsistencies between them were resolved by reviewing the full text articles.

Data synthesis

We conducted a Meta-analysis using Review Manager 5.2 (Copenhagen: The Nordic Cochrane Centre, 2012). We calculated odds ratios (OR) with 95% confidence intervals (CI) for those included articles that did not report these measures. Weighting of the studies in this meta-analysis was calculated based on the inverse variance of the study. We assessed the statistical heterogeneity (variability among the studies' results) using the I-squared statistic. We categorized the included studies into three categories according to the time of maternal abuse: childhood abuse, anytime abuse, recent abuse. Pooled OR were computed to estimate the association between maternal experience of abuse and PTD and LBW within each of the subgroups. Despite our expectation, some included articles reported only unadjusted OR for the outcomes variables, and there was not enough data available from these studies to calculate an adjusted OR for them. Also, adjusted confounders were varied among those studies that reported both adjusted and unadjusted OR for the outcome variables. Therefore, we decided to perform the meta-analysis of unadjusted data. We chose a random effects model that accounted for a degree of clinical and statistical heterogeneity that was expected among the included studies. We created funnel plots of the data to assess for the possibility of small study bias. Since all the included studies in the meta-analysis were from high-income countries (United States of America, United Kingdom, Canada, Switzerland, Norway, Australia), we did not conduct subgroup analysis based on study context.

Results
Study selection

After removing duplicates, 8653 records were retained in total. Out of this, we excluded 8553 articles during

Table 1 Characteristics of studies included in the meta-analysis

First Author /Pub Date	Country	Participants	Study Design	Sample size	Type of Abuse	Time of Abuse	Outcomes	Study Quality
Christiaens/2015 [3]	Canada	All ethnic groups	Case-control	622	Childhood abuse	Childhood	PTD	7
Silverman/2006 [29]	USA	All ethnic groups	Case-control	118,579	Intimate partner physical Abuse	Recent	PTD LBW	7
Jagoe/ 2000 [37]	USA	Low risk nonurban population	Cohort	84	Intimate partner physical Abuse	Anytime in married life	PTD LBW	5
Campbell/1999 [27]	USA	All ethnic groups	Case-control	252	Intimate partner emotional physical, and sexual abuse	Anytime in married life	LBW	5
Grimstad/ 1999 & 1997 [25, 36]	Norway	All ethnic groups	Case-control	174	Sexual Abuse Intimate partner sexual abuse	Childhood Anytime in married life	PTD LBW	4
Neggers/ 2004 [28]	USA	Low income/low risk population(82% African-American)	Case-control	3103	Intimate partner physical abuse leading to Injury	Recent	PTD LBW	4
Stevens- Simon/1994 [39]	USA	Low income, African American	Cohort	127	Physical abuse	Childhood	PTD LBW	5
Noll/ 2007 [30]	USA	All ethnic groups	Cohort	186	Sexual abuse	Childhood	PTD	8
Henriksen/ 2014 [42]	Norway	All ethnic groups	Cohort	76,870	Sexual violence (severe, mild, moderate)	Childhood Anytime in married life Recent	PTD LBW	7
Taft/ 2007 [31]	Australia	All ethnic groups	Cohort	9692	Intimate partner violence	Anytime in married life	PTD	5
Leeners/ 2014 [33]	Switzerland	All ethnic groups	Cohort	255	Sexual abuse	Childhood	PTD	8
Curry/ 1998 [26]	USA	All ethnic groups	Cohort	1597	Physical abuse Sexual abuse	Recent	LBW	7
Fried / 2008 [41]	USA	All ethnic groups	Cross-sectional	1555	Emotional, physical, Sexual abuse	Anytime in married life	PTD LBW	8
Selk/2016 [51]	USA	Nurses	Case-control	51,434	Physical abuse Sexual abuse	Childhood	PTD	6
Harville/2010 [32]	UK	All ethnic group	Cohort	4865	Violence	Childhood	LBW PTD	6
Scribano/ 2013 [38]	USA	Low income mothers	Case-control	10,855	Intimate partner violence	Recent	LBW PTD	7

Characteristics of all studies that were included in the meta-analysis are presented

the titles and abstract review, and another 83 articles using the structured inclusion/exclusion form. We summarized the reasons for these exclusions in Fig. 1. Through manually searching the reference lists of the included articles, we added three additional studies. Finally, we emailed 13 researchers who may have had relevant manuscripts submitted or in press. Only one responded and indicated that she did not have a relevant article.

From 20 eligible studies, we excluded four because of weak methodologies. This resulted in 16 studies that were included in the meta-analysis. Some of these studies reported both PTD and LBW as outcome variables, while some reported either PTD or LBW. We divided the 16 studies into two groups based on the outcome variables they reported. We included two reports from

one study. [25, 36] As both reports presented data on different outcomes from one sample, we treated them as one study.

Study characteristics

We presented the characteristics of the included studies in Table 1. The majority (62.5%) of the studies originated from the United States and the remainder were from other high income countries. The study designs are cross-sectional, case-control and cohort studies that assessed the association between abuse and PTD or LBW. Sample size in these studies ranged from 84 to 118,579. These samples encompass non-abused women and women who had experienced abuse during their childhood, anytime during their married life, or during the 12 months before pregnancy.

The sample for the majority of these studies included people from all ethnic groups in the country where the study was conducted; however, only one study examined a low risk nonurban population [37] and three studies assessed low income populations. [28, 38, 39] Abuse for subjects in almost 45% of the included studies was defined as abuse that originated from an intimate partner. Measurement tools for abuse varied across the studies. Data related to maternal history of abuse in the included articles were obtained by self-report and were collected through interviews, self-administered questionnaires, or obtained from databases.

Preterm delivery

Fourteen studies reported an association between maternal history of abuse in different points of life before pregnancy and PTD. Pooled OR for PTD among these 14 studies was 1.28 (95% CI: 1.12–1.47, $p < 0.000$); however, we detected a substantial level of heterogeneity among the studies in this group ($I^2 = 75\%$) (Fig. 2). When we conducted analysis within subgroups, having an experience of sexual abuse during childhood, reported by eight studies, increased the odds of PTD by 25% (OR 1.25, 95% CI: 1.06–1.47, $p = 0.008$) compared to women who did not have that experience. The odds of PTD were 26% higher (OR 1.26, 95% CI: 0.83–1.91, $p = 0.29$) in women who experienced sexual or physical abuse any time during their married life before pregnancy, (reported by four studies), compared to those who did not have such an experience. In addition, when maternal abuse happened within the 12 months before pregnancy (reported by four studies), the odds of PTD increased by 28% (OR 1.28, 95%CI: 1.09–1.49, $p = 0.002$) (Fig. 3). We detected a substantial level of heterogeneity among the studies in the anytime abuse and childhood abuse group ($I^2 = 75\%$). The funnel plot for all studies

included in PTD analysis was asymmetric (Additional file 3). However, as the number of studies included is low (14 studies) the power of the plot to distinguish chance from real asymmetry is low. [40] Hence, we conducted an Egger test that indicated a likely publication bias ($P < 0.003$) among included articles reporting PTD.

Furthermore, we stratified the studies by study design (cohort, case- control, and cross-sectional). The pooled OR for PTD among seven studies with cohort designs was 1.69 (95%CI: 95%, 1.19–2.40, $p = 0.004$), which was higher than the effect estimated for six studies with case-control designs (OR: 1.23, 95% CI: 1.03–1.48, $p < 0.03$). There was only one study with a cross-sectional design in this group [41] (Fig. 4).

Low birth weight

Eleven studies examined the association between maternal histories of abuse at different points of their lives before the pregnancy of interest with LBW. Pooled OR for LBW among these studies was 1.35 (95% CI: 1.14–1.59, $p = 0.0005$) (Fig. 5). We detected a substantial level of heterogeneity in this group ($I^2 = 69\%$). The funnel plot for all studies included in LBW analysis was symmetric (Additional file 4). When we classified the studies by time of abuse, the pooled OR for the four studies that reported maternal history of sexual abuse in childhood was 1.57 (OR 1.57, 95% CI: 0.99–2.49, $p = 0.06$). Nevertheless, when abuse happened at any time during maternal married life (reported by five studies), odds of LBW increased by only 9% (OR 1.09, 95% CI: 0.90–1.31, $p = 0.38$). A history of recent abuse before pregnancy, reported by five studies, increased the odds of LBW by 35% (OR 1.35, 95% CI: 1.14–1.60, $p = 0.0004$) (Fig. 6). We noticed the highest degree of heterogeneity in the childhood abuse group ($I^2 = 84\%$). The four studies in

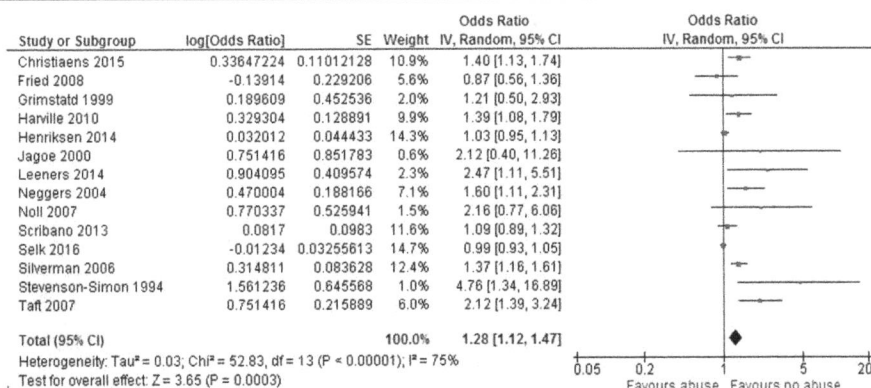

Study or Subgroup	log[Odds Ratio]	SE	Weight	Odds Ratio IV, Random, 95% CI
Christiaens 2015	0.33647224	0.11012128	10.9%	1.40 [1.13, 1.74]
Fried 2008	-0.13914	0.229206	5.6%	0.87 [0.56, 1.36]
Grimstad 1999	0.189609	0.452536	2.0%	1.21 [0.50, 2.93]
Harville 2010	0.329304	0.128891	9.9%	1.39 [1.08, 1.79]
Henriksen 2014	0.032012	0.044433	14.3%	1.03 [0.95, 1.13]
Jagoe 2000	0.751416	0.851783	0.6%	2.12 [0.40, 11.26]
Leeners 2014	0.904095	0.409574	2.3%	2.47 [1.11, 5.51]
Neggers 2004	0.470004	0.188166	7.1%	1.60 [1.11, 2.31]
Noll 2007	0.770337	0.525941	1.5%	2.16 [0.77, 6.06]
Scribano 2013	0.0817	0.0983	11.6%	1.09 [0.89, 1.32]
Selk 2016	-0.01234	0.03255613	14.7%	0.99 [0.93, 1.05]
Silverman 2006	0.314811	0.083628	12.4%	1.37 [1.16, 1.61]
Stevenson-Simon 1994	1.561236	0.645568	1.0%	4.76 [1.34, 16.89]
Taft 2007	0.751416	0.215889	6.0%	2.12 [1.39, 3.24]
Total (95% CI)			**100.0%**	**1.28 [1.12, 1.47]**

Heterogeneity: Tau² = 0.03; Chi² = 52.83, df = 13 (P < 0.00001); I² = 75%
Test for overall effect: Z = 3.65 (P = 0.0003)

SE, standard error; IV, inverse variance; CI, confidence interval; Chi², Chi squared

Fig. 2 Forest plot of overall unadjusted effect estimate for preterm birth. The Forest plot of overall unadjusted effect estimate for preterm birth is shown

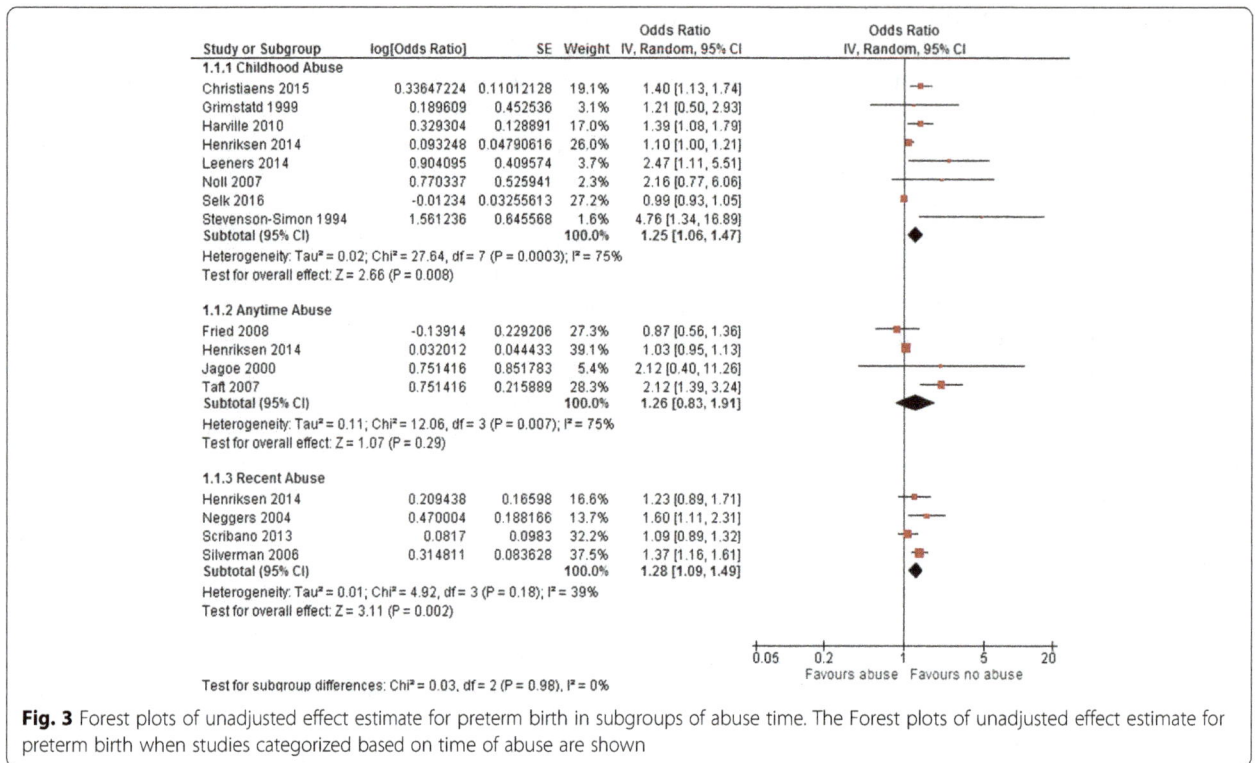

Fig. 3 Forest plots of unadjusted effect estimate for preterm birth in subgroups of abuse time. The Forest plots of unadjusted effect estimate for preterm birth when studies categorized based on time of abuse are shown

this group that examined the association between maternal experience of sexual abuse in childhood and LBW are different in terms of sample size, study design and context of study. [32, 36, 39, 42] The study with the greatest estimated effect is a cohort study that included

low income African/American women living in the United States [39], while the other studies examined women from all ethnic groups.

When we stratified the studies by their design, the highest estimated effect was related to the six cohort

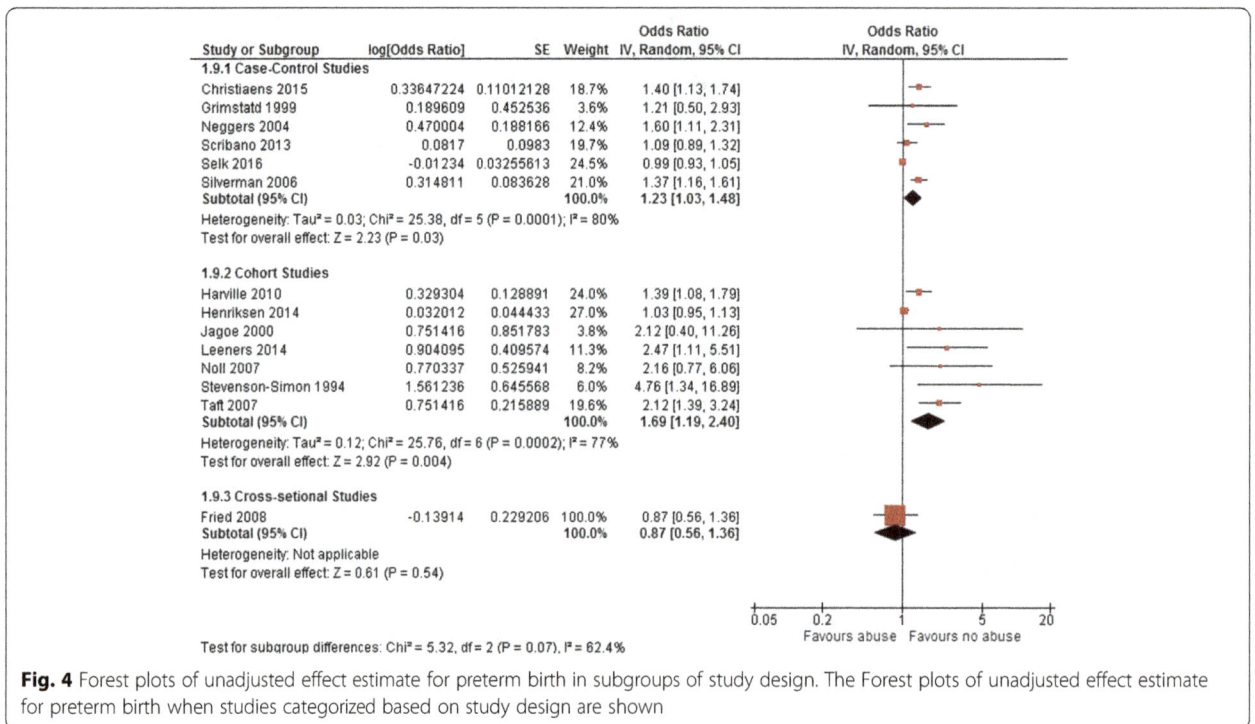

Fig. 4 Forest plots of unadjusted effect estimate for preterm birth in subgroups of study design. The Forest plots of unadjusted effect estimate for preterm birth when studies categorized based on study design are shown

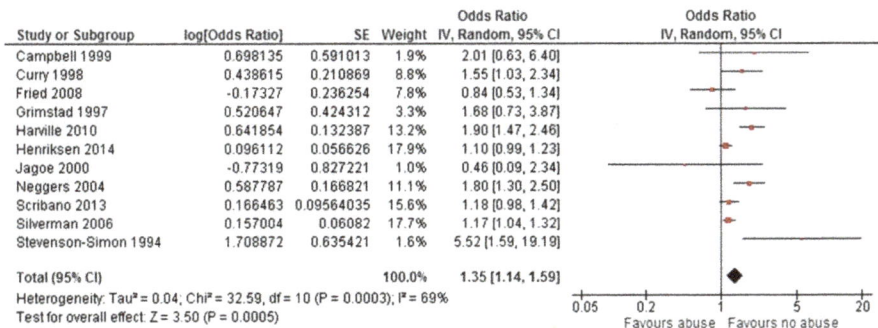

Fig. 5 Forest plot of overall unadjusted effect estimate for low birth weight. The Forest plot of overall unadjusted effect estimate for low birth weight is shown

studies (OR: 1.56, 95% CI: 1.06–2.3, $p = 0.02$), while the pooled OR for the case-control group with five studies was 1.28 (95% CI: 1.08–1.50, $p = 0.004$) (Fig. 7). There was only one study with a cross-sectional design. We did not perform subgroup analysis based on study quality and context, as all the final included studies included in both PTD and LBW categories were high and moderate quality studies originating from high-income countries.

Discussion
Main findings
This study is the first systematic review that examined associations between maternal history of abuse occurring *before*

pregnancy with PTD and LBW. Other reviews have largely explored the associations between abuses *during pregnancy* and the outcomes. Our analysis of 16 qualified articles demonstrated that women who had been abused prior to pregnancy have an increased risk of PTD and LBW compared to those who did not have the experience of abuse. In order to describe the difference in effect estimated, we stratified the included studies based on the time of exposure to abuse. From this, we learned that the subgroup of studies reporting maternal history of childhood abuse showed the highest risk for LBW among the other subgroups of recent abuse and anytime abuse in married life. Further, studies with cohort designs demonstrated the highest pooled OR for both PTD and LBW compared to case control studies.

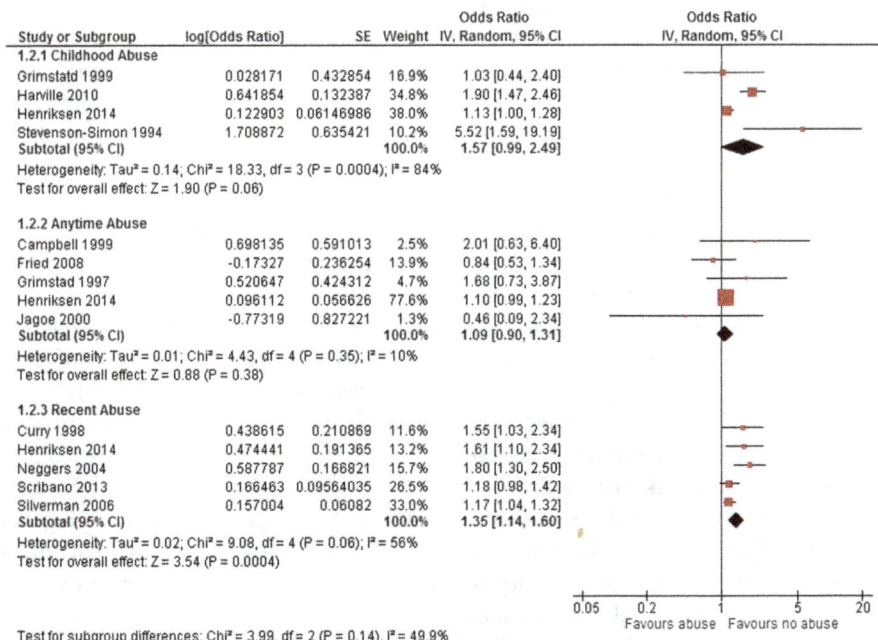

Fig. 6 Forest plots of unadjusted effect estimate for low birth weight in subgroups of abuse time. The Forest plots of unadjusted effect estimate for low birth weight when studies categorized based on time of abuse are shown

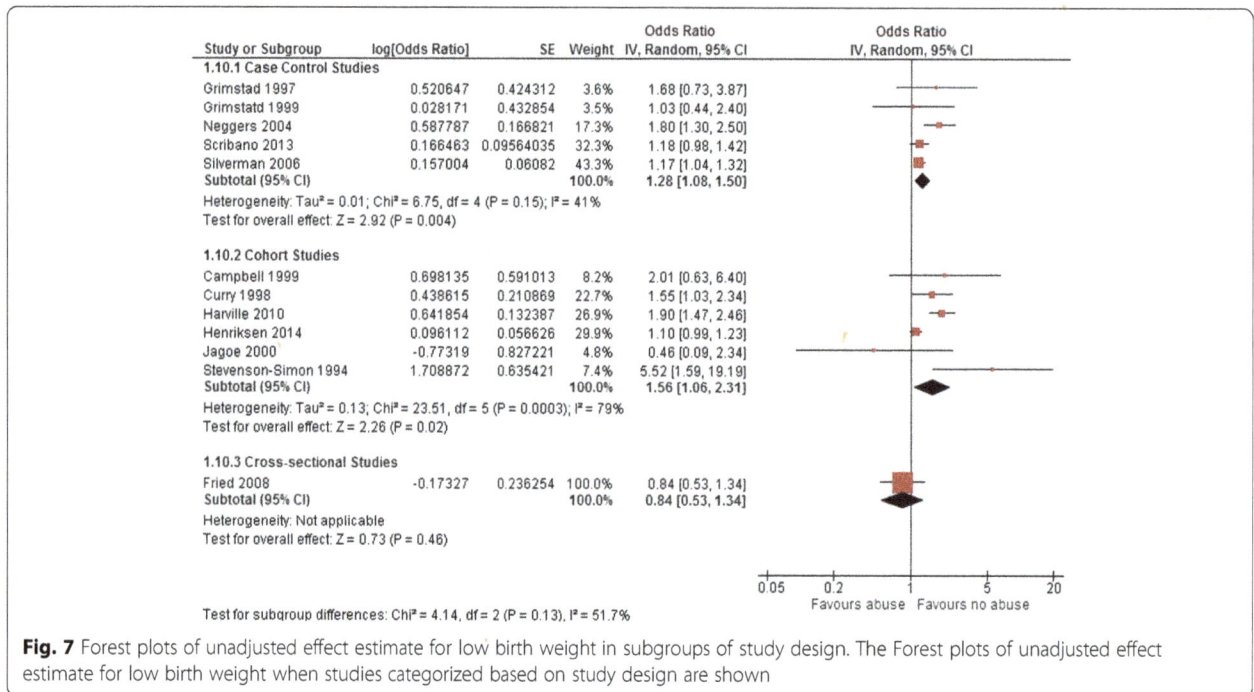

Fig. 7 Forest plots of unadjusted effect estimate for low birth weight in subgroups of study design. The Forest plots of unadjusted effect estimate for low birth weight when studies categorized based on study design are shown

Strengths and limitations

The strengths of this systematic review include an extensive online search using a broad range of keywords and nine databases. We did not confine the search by study context or language. Examination of the reference lists of the included articles and related systematic reviews yielded three studies that our on-line search did not reveal. According to the assessment of risk of bias, we only included primary studies that rated as being moderate and high quality in terms of methodology. We conducted a subgroup analysis according to the time of exposure to abuse, which separates this study from other related systematic reviews examining the association between maternal history of abuse and pregnancy outcomes.

The limitations of this study suggest the results should be interpreted with caution. First, even though we only included moderate and high quality primary studies, they varied in their consideration of confounder variables to calculate adjusted OR for PTD and LBW. We also were limited by the availability of data from these studies to calculate adjusted OR controlling for the important confounders. Subsequently, we pooled unadjusted OR for this systematic review meaning that we were not able to account for other risk factors that can affect PTD and LBW. Second, we detected a substantial heterogeneity among the original studies. Because of a limited number of primary studies in each category of PTD and LBW, we did not explore all the possible sources of heterogeneity such as type of abuse, participants' ethnic group/race, participants' previous gestational experience, and jurisdiction and/or environment.

Third, the three subgroups we created based on time of abuse are not mutually exclusive, as those who experienced childhood abuse might have been abused later. Finally, the funnel plot for the included studies in the PTD category was asymmetric indicating the possibility of publication bias. This could suggest that our computed OR from this analysis is overestimating the true odds ratio for PTD.

Further, the moderate overall effect estimated for the relationship between maternal experience of abuse before pregnancy and the two outcomes of interest in this systematic review may be partly related to the common limitations of the primary studies on abuse. Data on abuse almost always rely on the participants' recall and perceptions. The stigmatization of abuse may prevent participants from expressing their experience. Participants may perceive abuse differently than the researcher; for instance, psychological abuse might be perceived differently across cultures. Some women may use denial as a defense mechanism to avoid painful memories of abuse. [43] The issues with detecting abuse suggest that maternal history of abuse is under reported. In addition, all the included studies in this systematic review were from high-income countries (North America, Europe, and Australia), where social support for abused women and pregnancy health services might be more available than in low-income countries. These conditions can moderate the relationship between abuse and adverse pregnancy outcomes leading to a smaller estimated effect. This is supported by the results of a recently published systematic review by Bussières et al., (2015) on the effect of maternal stress on pregnancy outcomes. They reported a higher effect size for low income countries compared to that of high income countries. [44]

Interpretation

This systematic review showed that maternal history of abuse *before pregnancy*, specifically when abuse happened in childhood, is associated with increased risk of PTD and LBW. The results contrast with the conclusion of the previous systematic reviews. Leeners et al., (2006) and Wosu et al., (2015) applying a narrative analysis, reported that the existing evidence on the link between maternal history of childhood abuse and PTD and LBW was inconsistent. [34, 35] Compared to these systematic reviews, our study had the advantage of a greater number of qualified primary studies since we searched the literature to April 2017. Compared to our results, the most recent systematic review on IPV *during pregnancy* reported higher odds for PTD (OR: 1.91, 95% CI: 1.60–2.29) and LBW (OR: 2.11, 95% CI: 1.68–2.65). For the potential mechanisms, the authors suggested that physical or sexual abuse during pregnancy are associated with placental damage, uterine contractions, premature rupture of membranes, and genitourinary infections which increase the risk PTD and LBW. [24]

One possible explanation for the observed association between maternal history of abuse *before pregnancy* and the two outcome variables is the idea that maternal experience of abuse plus other stressors during a lifetime contribute to an individual's allostatic load. [45, 46] When the allostatic load exceeds a threshold level, the individual becomes vulnerable for diseases [47], or in the case of a pregnant woman, adverse pregnancy outcomes. [16] The findings of this systematic review can support the relationship between early life experiences, accumulation of stressors and risk of LBW and PTD. However, there are alternative explanations for the association between maternal history of abuse and the two outcomes. Having a history of abuse *before pregnancy* is related to high risk behaviors including smoking, drug abuse, and alcohol abuse. [3, 26, 30, 33, 48, 49] Moreover, abused women may not receive adequate family support or prenatal care. A maternal history of abuse can contribute to adverse pregnancy outcomes as a result of these risk factors as well. [34, 50]

Conclusions

In this systematic review we found that women who experienced abuse *before pregnancy* had a higher risk of PTD and LBW; the highest level of risk of LBW was associated with the victims of childhood abuse. Also, the magnitude of the effect estimated by the subgroup of cohort studies for both PTD and LBW was higher than the overall effect estimated for all the included studies in each outcome category. However, respecting our study limitations, we recommend that more high quality research studies on the topic are necessary to strengthen the inference. From our examination of the existing literature, we recommend the following points to be considered when designing primary studies on this topic. First, using an appropriate study design such as a prospective cohort in which researchers have a better control on the confounding factors can lead to a more precise inference compared to other designs. Second, creating a comprehensive list of all known confounding factors related to the outcomes of interest is imperative in reducing risk of bias. Third, the complexity of detecting an abuse experience and the possibility of recall bias demand more attention to assessing history of abuse. We suggest the application of validated tools administered by trained personnel to detect the victims of abuse in research studies.

For practitioners, although the overall effect size we detected was modest, it would be prudent to more carefully examine the maternal history of abuse before pregnancy during antenatal visits in order to use this information to inform their risk assessment for adverse pregnancy outcomes. Detailed assessment of risk factors is a necessary step in order to plan for the effective management of pregnancy.

Abbreviations
LBW: Low Birth Weight; PTD: Preterm Delivery

Acknowledgements
We would like to thank Dr. Bryan F. Mitchell, Department of Obstetrics and Gynecology, University of Alberta and the Alberta SPOR (Strategic Patient Oriented Research) SUPPORT Unit for helpful discussions. We thank Dr. Lisa Hartling, Department of Pediatrics, University of Alberta for offering her expertise to the explanation of the findings in this systematic review.

Funding
Faculty of Nursing, University of Alberta (JKO); the Canadian Institutes of Health Research (DMO); and University of Alberta and the Alberta SPOR (Strategic Patient Oriented Research) SUPPORT Unit.

Authors' contributions
MN developed the study protocol, performed study selection, assessed quality of the articles, extracted the data, contributed to the data analysis, and drafted the manuscript. JKO contributed to the development of the

protocol. BV Analyzed the data. LS conducted the online search. DMO contributed to the development of the protocol and drafted the manuscript. All the authors read and approved the final manuscript

Competing interests
The authors declare that they have no competing interests.

Author details
[1]Faculty of Nursing, University of Alberta, Edmonton, AB, Canada. [2]Alberta Research Centre for Health Evidence, Department of Pediatrics, University of Alberta, Edmonton, AB, Canada. [3]John W. Scott Health Sciences Library, University of Alberta, Edmonton, AB, Canada. [4]Departments of Obstetrics and Gynecology, Pediatrics and Physiology, University of Alberta, Edmonton, AB T6G 2S2, Canada.

References
1. Lilliecreutz C, Larén J, Sydsjö G, Josefsson A. Effect of maternal stress during pregnancy on the risk for preterm birth. BMC Pregnancy Childbirth. 2016;16: 5. https://doi.org/10.1186/s12884-015-0775-x.
2. Seravalli L, Patterson F, Nelson DB. Role of perceived stress in the occurrence of preterm labor and preterm birth among urban women. J Midwifery Womens Health. 2014;59(4):374–9. https://doi.org/10.1111/jmwh.12088.
3. Christiaens I, Hegadoren K, Olson DM. Adverse childhood experiences are associated with spontaneous preterm birth: a case–control study. BMC Med. 2015;13(1):124. https://doi.org/10.1186/s12916-015-0353-0.
4. Howson CP, Kinney MV, McDougall L, Lawn EJ, the Born Too Soon Preterm Birth Action Group. Born too soon: preterm birth matters. Reproductive Health. 2013;10(Suppl 1):s1. https://doi.org/10.1186/1742-4755-10-S1-S1.
5. WORLD HEALTH ORGANIZATION. WHO | Children: reducing mortality. World Heal Organ. 2016. http://www.who.int/mediacentre/factsheets/fs178/en/.
6. Galéra C. Early risk factors for hyperactivity-impulsivity and inattention trajectories from age 17 months to 8 years. Arch Gen Psychiatry. 2011; 68(12):1267. https://doi.org/10.1001/archgenpsychiatry.2011.138.
7. Heinonen K, Eriksson JG, Lahti J, et al. Late preterm birth and neurocognitive performance in late adulthood: a birth cohort study. Pediatrics. 2015;135(4):e818–25. https://doi.org/10.1542/peds.2014-3556.
8. Bensley JG, De Matteo R, Harding R, Black MJ. The effects of preterm birth and its antecedents on the cardiovascular system. Acta Obstet Gynecol Scand. 2016;95(6):652–63. https://doi.org/10.1111/aogs.12880.
9. Robbins CL, Hutchings Y, Dietz PM, Kukina E, Callaghan WM. History of preterm birth and subsequent cardiovascular disease: a systematic review. Am J Obs Gynecol. 2014;210(4):2–23. https://doi.org/10.1016/j.ajog.2013.09.020.History.
10. Hofman PL, Regan F, Jackson WE, et al. Premature birth and later insulin resistance. N Engl J Med. 2004;351(21):2179–86. https://doi.org/10.1056/NEJMoa042275.
11. Hovi P, Andersson S, Eriksson JG, et al. Glucose regulation in young adults with very low birth weight. N Engl J Med. 2007;356(20):2053–63. https://doi.org/10.1056/NEJMoa067187.
12. Kaijser M, Bonamy AE, Akre O, et al. Perinatal risk factors for diabetes in later life. Diabetes J. 2009;58:523–6. https://doi.org/10.2337/db08-0558.
13. Li S, Zhang M, Tian H, Liu Z, Yin X, Xi B. Preterm birth and risk of type 1 and type 2 diabetes: systematic review and meta-analysis. Obes Rev. 2014;15(10): 804–11. https://doi.org/10.1111/obr.12214.
14. Almond D, Chay KY, Lee DS. The costs of low birth weight. NBER Work Pap. 2004. https://doi.org/10.1017/CBO9781107415324.004.
15. Ameh S, Gomez-Olive FX, Kahn K, Tollman SM, Klipstein-Grobusch K. Relationships between structure, process and outcome to assess quality of integrated chronic disease management in a rural South African setting: applying a structural equation model. BMC Health Serv Res. 2017;17(1):224–9. https://doi.org/10.1186/s12913-017-2177-4.
16. Olson D, Severson E, Verstraeten B, Ng J, McCreary J, Metz G. Allostatic load and preterm birth. Int J Mol Sci. 2015;16(12):29856–74. https://doi.org/10.3390/ijms161226209.
17. McCreary JK, Erickson ZT, Hao Y, Ilnytskyy Y, Kovalchuk I, Metz GAS. Environmental intervention as a therapy for adverse programming by ancestral stress. Sci Rep. 2016;6(1):37814. https://doi.org/10.1038/srep37814.
18. McCreary JK, Erickson ZT, Metz GA. Environmental enrichment mitigates the impact of ancestral stress on motor skill and corticospinal tract plasticity. Neurosci Lett. 2016;632:181–6. https://doi.org/10.1016/j.neulet.2016.08.059.
19. Dancause KN, Laplante DP, Oremus C, Fraser S, Brunet A, King S. Disaster-related prenatal maternal stress influences birth outcomes: project ice storm. Early Hum Dev. 2011;87(12):813–20. https://doi.org/10.1016/j.earlhumdev.2011.06.007.
20. Sable MR, Wilkinson DS. Impact of perceived stress, major life events and pregnancy attitudes on low birth weight. Fam Plan Perspect. 2000;32(6): 288–94.
21. Hill A, Pallitto C, McCleary-Sills J, Garcia-Moreno C. A systematic review and meta-analysis of intimate partner violence during pregnancy and selected birth outcomes. Int J Gynaecol Obstet. 2016;133(3):269–76. https://doi.org/10.1016/j.ijgo.2015.10.023.
22. Murphy CC, Schei B, Myhr TL, Du Mont J. Abuse: a risk factor for low birth weight? A systematic review and meta-analysis. Can Med Assoc J. 2001; 164(11):1567–72. https://www.ncbi.nlm.nih.gov/pmc/articles/PMC81110/pdf/20010529s00013p1567.pdf.
23. Shah PS, Shah J, Births KSG on D of P. Maternal exposure to domestic violence and pregnancy and birth outcomes: a systematic review and meta-analyses. J Women's Heal. 2010;19(11):2017–31. https://www.liebertpub.com/doi/pdfplus/10.1089/jwh.2010.2051?casa_token=g2QExTli90kAAAAA%3A3gf1aVhKGcdPeFuCEu-00gks9Flhe0fx9DMrd7a-ISe01lahVbm3HRUGR3h5KwKjR0x2hFK-wmDz&.
24. Donovan BM, Spracklen CN, Schweizer ML, Ryckman KK, Saftlas AF. Intimate partner violence during pregnancy and the risk for adverse infant outcomes: a systematic review and meta-analysis. BJOG An Int J Obstet Gynaecol. 2016;123(8):1289–99. https://doi.org/10.1111/1471-0528.13928.
25. Grimstad H, Schei B, Backe B, Jacobsen G. Physical abuse and low birthweight: a case-control study. Br J Obstet Gynaecol. 1997;104(11):1281–7.
26. Curry MA, Perrin N, Wall E. Effects of abuse on maternal complications and birth weight in adult and adolescent women. Obstet Gynecol. 1998;92(4 Pt 1):530–4.
27. Campbell J, Torres S, Ryan J, et al. Physical and nonphysical partner abuse and other risk factors for low birth weight among full term and preterm babies: a multiethnic case-control study. Am J Epidemiol. 1999;150(7):714–26.
28. Neggers Y, Goldenberg R, Cliver S, Hauth J. Effects of domestic violence on preterm birth and low birth weight. Acta Obstet Gynecol Scand. 2004;83(5): 455–60. https://doi.org/10.1111/j.0001-6349.2004.00458.x.
29. Silverman JG, Decker MR, Reed E, Raj A. Intimate partner violence victimization prior to and during pregnancy among women residing in 26 U.S. states: associations with maternal and neonatal health. Am J Obstet Gynecol. 2006;195(1):140–8.
30. Noll JG, Schulkin J, Trickett PK, Susman EJ, Breech L, Putnam FW. Differential pathways to preterm delivery for sexually abused and comparison women. J Pediatr Psychol. 2007;32(10):1238–48.
31. Taft AJ, Watson LF. Termination of pregnancy: associations with partner violence and other factors in a national cohort of young Australian women. Aust N Z J Public Health. 2007;31(2):135–42.
32. Harville EW, Boynton-Jarrett R, Power C, Hypponen E. Childhood hardship, maternal smoking, and birth outcomes: a prospective cohort study. Arch Pediatr Adolesc Med. 2010;164(6):533–9. https://doi.org/10.1001/archpediatrics.2010.61.
33. Leeners B, Rath W, Block E, Gorres G, Tschudin S. Risk factors for unfavorable pregnancy outcome in women with adverse childhood experiences. J Perinat Med. 2014;42(2):171–8. https://doi.org/10.1515/jpm-2013-0003.
34. Leeners B, Richter-Appelt H, Imthurn B, Rath W. Influence of childhood sexual abuse on pregnancy, delivery, and the early postpartum period in adult women. J Psychosom Res. 2006;61(2):139–51.

35. Wosu AC, Gelaye B, Williams MA. Maternal history of childhood sexual abuse and preterm birth: an epidemiologic review. BMC Pregnancy Childbirth. 2015;15:170–4. https://doi.org/10.1186/s12884-015-0606-0.

36. Grimstad H, Schei B. Pregnancy and delivery for women with a history of child sexual abuse. Child Abuse Negl. 1999;23(1):81–90.

37. Jagoe J, Magann EF, Chauhan SP, Morrison JC. The effects of physical abuse on pregnancy outcomes in a low-risk obstetric population. Am J Obstet Gynecol. 2000;182(5):1067–9.

38. Scribano PV, Stevens J, Kaizar E, Team N-IR. The effects of intimate partner violence before, during, and after pregnancy in nurse visited first time mothers. Matern Child Health J. 2013;17(2):307–18. https://doi.org/10.1007/s10995-012-0986-y.

39. Stevens-Simon C, McAnarney ER. Childhood victimization: relationship to adolescent pregnancy outcome. Child Abuse Negl. 1994;18(7):569–75.

40. Sterne JA, Sutton AJ, Ioannidis JP, et al. Recommendations for examining and interpreting funnel plot asymmetry in meta-analyses of randomised controlled trials. BMJ. 2011;343:d4002. https://doi.org/10.1136/bmj.d4002.

41. Fried LE, Cabral H, Amaro H, Aschengrau A. Lifetime and during pregnancy experience of violence and the risk of low birth weight and preterm birth. J Midwifery Womens Health. 2008;53(6):522–8. https://doi.org/10.1016/j.jmwh.2008.07.018.

42. Henriksen L, Schei B, Vangen S, Lukasse M. Sexual violence and neonatal outcomes: a Norwegian population-based cohort study. BMJ Open. 2014;4(10):e005935. 2014-005935. https://doi.org/10.1136/bmjopen-2014-005935.

43. Briere J. Methodological issues in the study of sexual abuse effects. J Consult Clin Psychol. 1992;60(2):196–203.

44. Bussières E-L, Tarabulsy GM, Pearson J, Tessier R, Forest J-C, Giguère Y. Maternal prenatal stress and infant birth weight and gestational age: a meta-analysis of prospective studies. Dev Rev. 2015;36:179–99. https://doi.org/10.1016/j.dr.2015.04.001.

45. Sterling P, Eyer J. Allostasis: a new paradigm to explain arousal pathology. In: Fisher S, Reason J, editors. Handbook of life stress, cognition and health. Oxford: John Wiley; 1988. p. 629–49.

46. McEwen BS. Protective and damaging effects of stress mediators: central role of the brain. Dialogues Clin Neurosci. 2006;8(4):367–81.

47. Felitti VJ, Anda RF, Nordenberg D, et al. Relationship of childhood abuse and household dysfunction to many of the leading causes of death in adults. The Adverse Childhood Experiences (ACE) Study. Am J Prev Med. 1998;14(4):245–58. https://doi.org/10.1016/S0749-3797(98)00017-8.

48. Bohn DK. Lifetime physical and sexual abuse, substance abuse, depression, and suicide attempts among native American women. Issues Ment Health Nurs. 2003;24(3):333–52.

49. Bohn DK. Lifetime and current abuse, pregnancy risks, and outcomes among native American women. J Health Care Poor Underserved. 2002;13(2):184–98.

50. Lockwood CJ. Risk factors for preterm birth and new approaches to its early diagnosis. J Perinat Med. 2015;43(5):499–501. https://doi.org/10.1515/jpm-2015-0261.

51. Selk SC, Rich-Edwards JW, Koenen K, Kubzansky LD. An observational study of type, timing, and severity of childhood maltreatment and preterm birth. J Epidemiol Community Health. 2016;70(6):589–95. https://doi.org/10.1136/jech-2015-206304.

14

"I'm used to doing it by myself": exploring self-reliance in pregnancy

Blair C. McNamara[1]*[iD], Abigail Cutler[2], Lisbet Lundsberg[3], Holly Powell Kennedy[4] and Aileen Gariepy[5]

Abstract

Background: Self-reliance (the need to rely on one's own efforts and abilities) is cited as a potential coping strategy for decreased or absent social support during pregnancy. Little data exists on how women view self-reliance in pregnancy.

Methods: We recruited women from urban, walk-in pregnancy testing clinics from June 2014–June 2015. Women aged 16 to 44 and at less than 24 weeks gestational age were eligible. Participants completed an enrollment survey and in-person, semi-structured interviews. We used framework analysis to identify key concepts and assess thematic relationships.

Results: Eighty-four English-speaking women completed qualitative interviews. Participants averaged 26 years of age and 7 weeks estimated gestational age. Most identified as Black (54%) or Hispanic (20%), were unemployed or homemakers (52%), unmarried (92%), and had at least one child (67%). Most did not intend to get pregnant (61%) and planned to continue their pregnancy and parent (65%). We identified self-reliance as a prevalent concept that almost half (48%) of participants discussed in relationship to their pregnancy. Self-reliance in pregnancy consisted of several subthemes: 1) past experiences, 2) expectations of motherhood, 3) financial independence, 4) decision making, and 5) parenting.

Conclusions: Self-reliance is an important aspect of women's reproductive lives and is threaded through women's past and current thoughts, feelings, experiences and decisions about pregnancy. Women's belief in their own self-reliance as well as a recognition of the limits of self-reliance merits further research, especially as a potential strategy to cope with decreased or absent social support during pregnancy.

Keywords: United States, Pregnancy, Self-reliance, Decision making, Social support

Background

Social support is defined as the receipt of resources, information, or emotional care through personal relationships [1, 2]. Increased social support during pregnancy and the postpartum period has been associated with decreased psychological distress during pregnancy [1, 3], faster progression of labor, higher Apgar scores, higher birthweight [2, 4], and reduced depression among new mothers and women who have abortions [1, 5–7]. Similarly, decreased or absent social support and increased psychological distress are linked to a variety of negative mental and physical health outcomes for pregnant women [1, 8, 9], including low birth weight and preterm delivery [3, 10–13], and postpartum depressive symptoms [14, 15].

When social support is low or absent, some have posited that pregnant women use resilience, optimism, and self-reliance as coping strategies [9, 16–20]. Resilience, defined as an ability to 'bounce back' after adversity, may act as a protective factor against psychologic stress and decreased social support during pregnancy [9, 16]. Optimism – described as a prospective belief that even without social support, a woman will be able to succeed using her own assets and abilities – has been found to be associated with decreased postpartum depression among pregnant women with low social support [17, 18]. Self-reliance is a similar but distinct concept from resilience or optimism and conveys a dependence on personal resources and abilities as opposed to those of

* Correspondence: blair.mcnamara@yale.edu
[1]Yale School of Medicine, 333 Cedar Street, New Haven, CT 06510, USA
Full list of author information is available at the end of the article

others [19, 20]. Women may employ these potential coping strategies at various points in their reproductive lives and these strategies may intersect and overlap. An optimistic attitude can be a component of self-reliance, and resilient women can also be distinctly self-reliant, or intentionally reliant on others. Few studies have specifically examined self-reliance during the perinatal period, and focused on narrow, non-U.S. populations. Self-reliance has been described as a positive coping strategy for life stress and lack of social support among pregnant HIV-positive women in sub-Saharan Africa [19] and for first-time parents' experiencing home-based postnatal care in Sweden [20].

Given the lack of research evaluating self-reliance among pregnant women, we address the concept of self-reliance as described by a diverse urban cohort of women following confirmation of a new pregnancy. Women discussed experiences with self-reliance as it related to previous and current pregnancies, the expectation of motherhood, finances, decision-making about the pregnancy, and parenting experiences.

Methods

We report on qualitative findings from a study conducted to explore the impact of a new pregnancy on women's lives [21]. The overarching study recruited women presenting for pregnancy testing or abortion care at clinics in New Haven, CT, from June 2014 to June 2015. The data presented here were restricted to participants from pregnancy testing sites only, in order to focus on women with new pregnancy diagnoses who had not yet made a decision about how to resolve the pregnancy. Clinical staff referred interested women with positive pregnancy tests to the research team, who screened them for eligibility. Women were eligible if they were Spanish- or English-speaking, at a gestational age of < 24 completed weeks, 16–44 years old, and completed study enrollment within 1 week of their positive pregnancy test. Refer to Fig. 1 for a flow diagram of those participants screened, eligible, and enrolled in the study. Detailed study methods have been previously published [21]. In the state of Connecticut, pregnant women under the age of 18 are able to make all decisions regarding their pregnancy without parental input or consent. As such, our Institutional Review Board waived the need for parental consent for participants under the age of 18. Eighty-four participants completed in-depth qualitative interviews in English and are the basis of this analysis. Women who chose to participate in Spanish were analyzed separately and are not included in this investigation to ensure cross-language credibility [22].

All 84 participants completed an enrollment survey that collected demographic information (including age, race and ethnicity, relationship status, parity), measures

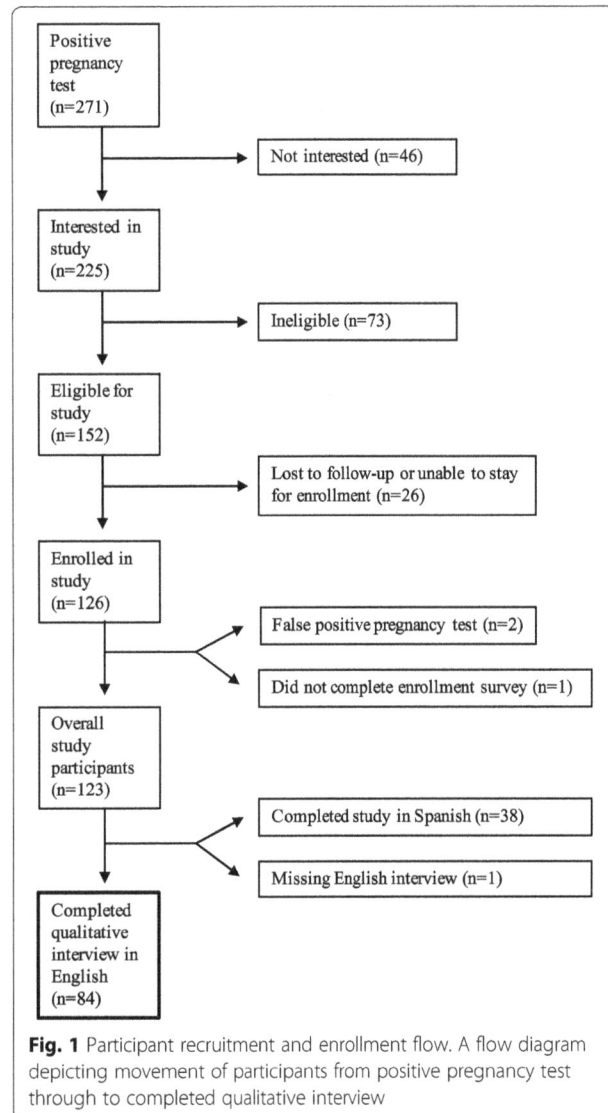

Fig. 1 Participant recruitment and enrollment flow. A flow diagram depicting movement of participants from positive pregnancy test through to completed qualitative interview

of pregnancy intention, and plans for pregnancy termination or continuation. Enrolled participants were offered the opportunity to complete a one-on-one interview or a focus group interview (four women chose a group interview, which occurred as two two-person groups). Interviews were conducted by skilled research team interviewers using a semi-structured interview guide (Additional file 1: Figure S2) to ask participants open-ended questions about pregnancy intentions, initial and current thoughts and feelings after receiving a positive pregnancy test, and how they felt the pregnancy would impact their life, decisions, and relationships. All interviews were audio-recorded and transcribed, while maintaining confidentiality of the participants. We ascertained pregnancy outcome information (e.g. miscarriage, abortion, delivery) for each participant during a follow-up monitoring interview or through medical record review. We categorized pregnancy outcomes as miscarriage, abortion, or delivery. All participants provided written consent and received $50 cash as compensation for participation in the qualitative interviews. The study protocol was reviewed and approved by the Yale University Human Research Protection Program.

We used framework analysis to identify key concepts from our data and to assess thematic relationships [23]. We identified codes to evaluate common and dissimilar conceptual threads among interview transcripts. Four researchers (BM, AC, AG, LL) initially coded the same six interviews and then met to assess inter-coder reliability and generate a shared coding strategy and code list. Two independent coders (BM, AC) then coded the remaining transcripts and met regularly to assess discrepancies in coding. A senior methodologist and software expert (HPK), provided content-checking and guidance on all analysis. We then grouped codes thematically to draw conclusions about interactions and context in the interviews, and then re-evaluated the text using these themes. We used Atlas.ti (Berlin, Germany) to manage and code the transcripts.

Results

At enrollment, participants averaged 26 years of age and 7 weeks estimated gestational age (EGA) (Table 1). Most identified as Black, non-Hispanic (54%) or Hispanic

(20%). The majority reported less than or equal to a high school education (59%), were unemployed or homemakers (52%), were unmarried (92%), and had at least one child (67%). Some reported a previous history of depression (26%) or anxiety (25%). Previous miscarriage was reported by 40% and previous abortion was reported by 41%. When asked about the period just before becoming pregnant (pre-conception perspectives), 61% indicated they did not intend to get pregnant, 32% reported that they did not want to get pregnant and 25% indicated the pregnancy was not planned (Table 2). When asked about how they felt after learning they were pregnant, 29% reported that it was the wrong time to have a baby, 31% said the pregnancy was undesired, and only 13% said they were not happy with the pregnancy news (Table 2). At enrollment,

Table 1 Participant characteristics and sociodemographics, N = 84

Age, mean (SD)	26.1 (6.3)
Estimated gestational age at enrollment, weeks (SD)	7.2 (3.1)
Race-Ethnicity, n (%)	
Black, non-Hispanic	45 (54.2)
White, non-Hispanic	13 (15.7)
Hispanic	17 (20.5)
Multiracial, Other	8 (9.6)
Education, n (%)	
12 years/GED or less	49 (59.0)
Some college or college degree	34 (41.0)
Employment, n (%)	
Unemployed/homemaker	43 (51.8)
Full time/part time	40 (48.2)
Relationship status, n (%)	
Single, never married	42 (50.6)
Married	7 (8.4)
Living with partner, not married	19 (22.9)
Separated/divorced/widowed	15 (18.1)
Previous diagnosis of depression, n (%)	22 (26.2)
Previous diagnosis of anxiety, n (%)	21 (25.0)
Previous abortion, n (%)	34 (41.0)
Previous miscarriage, n (%)	32 (39.5)

Table 2 Measures of pregnancy context among participants, N = 84

Pre-conception perspectives	Intention, n (%)	
	Intended to get pregnant	17 (20.2)
	Intentions changing	16 (19.1)
	Did not intend to get pregnant	51 (60.7)
	Wanted, n (%)	
	Wanted to have a baby	23 (27.4)
	Mixed feelings	34 (40.5)
	Did not want to have a baby	27 (32.1)
	London measure of unplanned pregnancy, n (%)	
	Planned	17 (20.2)
	Ambivalent	46 (54.8)
	Unplanned	21 (25.0)
Post-conception perspectives	Timing, n (%)	
	Right time to have a baby	27 (32.1)
	Ok but not quite right	33 (39.3)
	Wrong time	24 (28.6)
	Desired pregnancy, n (%)	
	Yes	38 (45.2)
	No	26 (31.0)
	Not sure	20 (23.8)
	Happy about pregnancy, n (%)	
	Happy	54 (64.3)
	Neither happy/unhappy, not sure	19 (22.6)
	Unhappy	11 (13.1)
	Pregnancy plans, n (%)	
	Parent	55 (65.5)
	Abortion	15 (17.9)
	Adoption	2 (2.4)
	Unsure	12 (14.3)

65% planned to parent, 18% planned abortion, 2% planned adoption, and 14% were unsure.

We identified self-reliance as a common and complex theme woven throughout women's discussions about their pregnancies. When discussing their reactions, expectations, and decision-making about their pregnancies, approximately half of women ($n = 40$, 48%) spoke of self-reliance (specifically the need to rely on one's own efforts and abilities), rather than those of others. Discussions of self-reliance overlapped with related discussions about prior pregnancy experiences, prior parenting experiences, current children, relationships, social support, decision making about the pregnancy, and maternal health. We found the theme of self-reliance to consist of several intersecting subthemes: 1) past experiences of self-reliance, 2) expectations of motherhood, 3) financial independence, 4) decision making about this pregnancy, and 5) self-reliance in parenting. Social support, or lack thereof, was a pervasive element of all subthemes, and was intimately related to women's discussion of self-reliance.

Past experiences of self-reliance

Many of our participants were already intimately familiar with the notion of self-reliance during pregnancy secondary to the absence of a partner or other social support in previous pregnancies or current experiences as mothers. For some, their previous experience with the reality of self-reliance may have led to decisions to parent, and for others the decision to terminate. For example, several women who were already mothers noted the following.

I'm used to doing it by myself. I'm used to being the parent alone, not having to share, except for doctors' appointments and delivery day. (Age 35)

I mean I [parented other children] by myself, and they're doing good. (Age 38)

Some participants noted both difficulty and gratification as parents who were already self-reliant. One woman who planned to continue her current pregnancy said:

My daughter, her father's not... in her life... as much as he should be... I'm doing everything, everything on my own. With schoolwork and parent teacher night, report card night, family support night, all of that. I mean I don't mind ... I love that she [will] always come to see me, the person that was there. (Age 26)

Participants cited experiences raising children without social support and necessitating self-reliance as reasons why they believed parenting their expected children would be successful. Participants spoke of sacrifice and challenges in being self-reliant parents, but many also described feeling fulfilled by that role.

Similar descriptions were also offered by women planning abortion, perhaps related to their desire to care for and support the children they were already parenting. For example, one woman who planned to terminate (and did) expressed pride in her ability to be self-reliant for her young son:

I do everything I can, for my son to have a good life. So I work...I basically do everything on my own for him... to see him in the morning wake up and smile and say 'Mommy', it's just a good feeling. (Age 21)

Expectations of motherhood

Some participants took as a given that they would have to be self-reliant in both pregnancy and motherhood; for many women, self-reliance was a necessary element of both.

You're the mother... you have a mother and father but at the end of the day if it doesn't work, you're the mother. This is your child. So whether he is excited about it or not, I have to do what I have to do as a mom for my child. (Age 30)

He's the man and I'm the woman. And at the end of the day, when you have a child, all the care for that child is based on the woman. (Age 37)

Some participants described motherhood as a responsibility that required overcoming lack of social supports and embracing self-sacrifice in order to fulfill their duties as mothers.

You're having a baby, it's going to be a struggle sometimes but you have to be able to provide and I'm not the type of person who, who just go and ask somebody, 'hey can you, can you help me' and stuff...I just, you know, feel like I would need to provide for my child. I don't need nobody else to provide. (Age 30)

For some women, the idea that the responsibility of parenting would ultimately (and sometimes inevitably) fall to them stemmed from a social norm that fathers are less duty-bound and reliable than mothers.

And then at the end of the day, it's mommy's baby always. Like, he could get up and say whatever. Men can do whatever they wanna do, he's not obligated to stay here whether we're married, engaged, together or not. (Age 29)

Financial independence

Many women also referred to financial independence as a marker of self-reliance, and the reason why they were making the decision to parent, irrespective of their partners' input on the matter.

> *Yeah, I pay the high rent bill. He pays the cable and the gas and they don't add up, so I got the say. This is how the world works! (Age 20)*

> *I can make my own decisions. I work, I make my own money, pay my own bills, so my decision is my decision. If you're not with it, don't be around.... I don't care. He probably wouldn't be happy, he'd probably be a little discouraged, upset or something. But it's my decision. (Age 21)*

Discussions about financial independence also overlapped with discussions about the influence of family on pregnancy decision-making and lack of social support from family, and sometimes shaped a participant's plans to share (or not) the news of the pregnancy with others.

> *[It's] not that I don't care what anyone has to say, but I don't care what their opinions on it...if they have something negative to say I'm gonna say well...did you take care of any of my other kids? Would you like to pay a bill out of my house? Would you like me to write you a grocery list for us? ... I don't feel the urge to tell everyone cuz I'm like...this isn't their baby. My household isn't their household, I've been on my own since I was eighteen, I've lived in my own place, I've had my own car...if they find out, they find out. If they don't I could care less. (Age 21)*

Conversely, several participants expressed that they did not see themselves as self-reliant because they lacked financial independence and stability. Some women voiced that they did not want to have to rely entirely on themselves in pregnancy or motherhood, which led some to question if continuing the pregnancy was the right decision. Several participants who felt this way also told researchers that they were planning abortion.

> *I don't want to be struggling...out here with two kids and then, you know, who knows? Me and my boyfriend only been together for a couple months... I'm not trying to do it by myself and I'm not trying to struggle and...I want to be more, I want to have a better job and stability. I don't want to be living on food stamps....I'm just trying to be better, like better us, before having another kid. (Age 23)*

> *And if I'm not stable myself, then I'm not gonna bring somebody into this world and have them struggle with me .... Stable, as um, financially having a roof over my head... mostly being prepared for it. I'm not at all. (Age 20)*

Decision-making about this pregnancy

First, women displayed self-reliance simply in discussing decisions about their pregnancy. Many women expressed that they were relying solely on their own counsel to contemplate their decisions.

> *Uh to be honest I could really care less what anyone else thinks because uh I'm 18. I'm gonna be 19 next month, and I mean, I'm an adult. I have to do what I have to do. I feel like [it's] my decision. I mean they can't really have no say, cause it's my decision so. (Age 18)*

> *I can do what I wanna do, I don't have to be pressured into doing anything or listening to somebody. (Age 21)*

Furthermore, conceptualizations of absent or low social support and the need for self-reliance influenced the way some women approached making decisions about their pregnancies. Women cited self-reliance when considering whether or not to continue their pregnancies, including what it would mean to be single parents. For some participants, the knowledge that they would need to be self-reliant and even single-parents (either for the first time or again) influenced their plans to terminate, and for others this same knowledge appeared to factor into and reinforce their plans to parent.

Although a few women stated that their decisions depended in part on their partner's wishes, more women expressed the sentiment that their partners' opinions and roles were more or less irrelevant; in other words, they felt confident in their ability to be self-reliant and make decisions about continuing or terminating the pregnancy whether or not their partners stayed involved.

> *But then I realized that I wanted this child no matter who the father is. So...I was like whatever, either you're gonna be in our lives or not. It's not gonna change anything, I'm gonna keep my baby. (Age 23)*

When asked how the father's feelings about the pregnancy impacted her decision to parent, one participant said:

No, it doesn't influence me in any way cuz I'm a pretty strong-minded person...I don't have to be with everyone, I can do my own thing. I don't mind being alone. So it's kinda like, whether he was OK with it or not, a baby is still gonna be here. (Age 21)

The physical reality of pregnancy also shaped women's perspectives on self-reliance and their pregnancy decision-making. Women saw their pregnancies as ultimately belonging to them, and so all decisions would be made accordingly. Two women who planned to parent expressed this sentiment:

Men tend to be, you know, like (soft laugh), they don't know. We're the ones that carry [the pregnancy], that do all the work. (Age 24)

Self-reliance in parenting

Some women acknowledged that although a possibility, being self-reliant as a single mother without social support was not ideal. Many participants who planned either abortion or adoption pointed to the value of having a partner in parenthood.

Right now I'm single, I don't have anybody... you know I'm not ready for that (e.g. being a single mother) yet. (Age 21)

To be a good mother I think it takes a partnership. Of course single mothers do it, but I think a man and a woman should raise a child, not just a man or a woman. (Age 25)

I know a lot of families don't stay together. But for me myself, to be able to provide for the child on my own... And if I'm not stable myself, then I'm not gonna bring somebody else into this world and have them struggle with me. (Age 20)

Similarly, a few participants expressed that their previous experience as single parents influenced their strong preference for having partner support in the current pregnancy.

I was by myself, had the baby by myself, took care of him by myself, until now... So, I just, kinda don't want to go through that again, but I know that I'm with him now, that it might be different and that he might actually be there for me, but I don't want to like have the baby thinking that. Oh, he's there now and he'll be with me and this will be a better pregnancy and stuff. (Age 25)

One participant who planned to parent expressed that while her preference would be to have partner support, she was prepared to parent by herself if necessary.

I see women do it all the time where you know they go through everything by their self... I just feel like... what mother doesn't want a father there for her child?...And so I feel like that's a big part for me. But I mean either way I'm going to do what I have to do. (Age 30)

Discussion

In this analysis of a racially and ethnically diverse urban population of women with new pregnancies, we identified self-reliance as a prevalent theme that emerged in discussions with women about how they felt the pregnancy would impact their lives, decisions, and relationships. Our findings suggest that both self-reliance and an awareness of the limits of self-reliance can have a substantial impact on a woman's thoughts, feelings, and decision-making about a pregnancy. Experiences with and examination of self-reliance as it related to social support, previous pregnancies and experiences, expectations of motherhood, financial independence, decision making about the current pregnancy, and self-reliance in parenting, all contributed to a woman's assessment of her new pregnancy.

Our findings advance understanding of self-reliance, especially as a potential response to lack of social support, in several ways. To our knowledge, this study is the first evaluation of women's thoughts and expressions regarding self-reliance at the time of pregnancy diagnosis. We identified two previous studies that specifically report on self-reliance related to pregnancy [19, 20]. However, both studies were conducted in the postpartum period, and may be subject to recall bias. Ashaba et al. report on coping strategies used during pregnancy and childbirth by women living with HIV in Uganda ($n = 20$). They conducted postpartum qualitative interviews and identified self-reliance, mostly as it relates to financial independence and parenting, as one of five coping strategies these women used to navigate challenges during pregnancy and beyond [19]. In the second study we identified, Johansson et al. identified self-reliance as one of three main themes that emerged with first-time Swedish parents following same-day discharge from the hospital after childbirth ($n = 21$). In this study, the concept of self-reliance pertained to parents who needed to rely on their own instincts about newborn care at home, as opposed to asking for help or receiving assistance from healthcare professionals [20]. While helpful in defining some aspects of self-reliance and identifying it as an important theme among postpartum women, these two studies are limited to non-U.S. populations and are retrospective in nature. Our findings build on these smaller studies and clarify how self-reliance may function in a larger, urban, U.S. population of women in early pregnancy, prospectively contemplating pregnancy and parenting. We believe that characterizing self-reliance among pregnant women, often in the presence of limited or absent social support, is novel and an area that warrants further inquiry and analysis.

Strengths of our study include employing a qualitative approach using semi-structured interview questions, which allowed participants to express varied and at times contradictory emotions, thoughts, and feelings, which added complexity and richness to our data. The diverse racial and ethnic representation of our participants is also a strength, given prior research that has shown that the effects of social support and self-reliance vary across ethnic and cultural groups [24, 25]. Additionally, this study includes women in early pregnancy with varying pregnancy contexts (intention, wantedness, planning, timing, desirability, happiness) and outcomes (miscarriage, abortion, delivery), and therefore provides important perspectives not often captured in research about pregnancy. Our study may be limited by the lack of specific questions designed to evaluate self-reliance. Instead, the theme of self-reliance emerged from women's discussions about their thoughts and feelings towards a new pregnancy. Another limitation of our study may be that our participants were recruited from a single geographic area; however, this region is diverse and generally representative of demographics in the United States [26].

Additional research is needed to explore self-reliance during pregnancy as there may be different and more complex sub-themes. It remains unclear whether self-reliance is a fixed character trait or rather a transient state of being that can be learned or cultivated over time. Future investigations into self-reliance in pregnancy could aid understanding of whether self-reliance is associated with a woman's decision to continue or abort her pregnancy, if self-reliance can diminish the effects of low or absent social support, or if it positively or negatively affects different maternal and neonatal outcomes, such as postpartum depression or birthweight among women who decide to continue their pregnancy. Although there is evidence that interventions aiming to increase social support during the prenatal and postpartum period lead to better maternal and neonatal outcomes, findings are mixed [6, 27, 28]. Moreover, we do not know whether these same interventions would have any impact on women's self-reliance, or if interventions aimed to increase self-reliance would lead to better outcomes as well, particularly in the absence of increased social support. Additionally, further evaluation regarding which types of social support and self-reliance effect these outcomes and for which ethnic and cultural communities, is warranted.

Conclusion

Our findings suggest that self-reliance is an important aspect of women's reproductive lives and choices. It's a prevalent concept that is threaded through women's thoughts about pregnancy, and may be an important coping strategy women employ to buffer the negative effects of diminished or absent social support. In the end, self-reliance may only take women so far in the absence of social support and financial resources. While healthcare providers can try to cultivate individual patient factors (self-reliance) that may be protective against negative maternal and neonatal outcomes, we must also consider the environment and supports that our healthcare systems and government provide for vulnerable women. As of 2015, 13% of all women aged 15–44 in the United States remain uninsured [29], and over 15 million women living below 250% of the federal poverty level are in need of publicly funded contraceptive services and supplies [30]. The current political climate poses further threats to family planning and preventive healthcare for underserved women [31–33], as well as to maternity and newborn care [34, 35]. Systems can either support or chip away at self-reliance, and in the face of shrinking benefits and worn safety nets, a woman's self-reliance simply may be not enough.

Acknowledgements
The authors would like to thank Yale School of Medicine, Department of Obstetrics, Gynecology, and Reproductive Sciences for their support, as well as all of our research subjects for their candor and participation.

Funding
Dr. Gariepy was supported by funding from NIH CTSA UL1 TR000142, NIDA Yale Drug Abuse Addiction and HIV Research Scholars 5K12DA033312, and the Albert McKern Scholar Awards for Perinatal Research, which also supported Dr. Lundsberg, during the conduct of the study. Funding sources had no involvement in the study or manuscript.

Authors' contributions
All authors have contributed significantly to the development of the manuscript as well as to the analysis of the data described. BM and AC transcribed the qualitative interivews and were responsible for generating a code and theme list. LL and AG coded a small set of interviews to ensure inter-coder reliability. HPK served as an advisor and instructed the group in using Atlas.ti. The manuscript was primarily written by BM, with significant editing contributions from all authors. All authors read and approved the final manuscript.

Authors' information

Blair McNamara, BS. Medical student MS4, Yale School of Medicine.
Abigail Cutler, MD. Clinical Instructor, Department of Obstetrics, Gynecology, and Reproductive Sciences, Yale School of Medicine.
Lisbet Lundsberg, PhD. Associate Research Scientist in Obstetrics, Gynecology, and Reproductive Sciences, Yale School of Medicine.
Holly Powell Kennedy, PhD, CNM, FACNM, FAAN. Executive Deputy Dean & Helen Varney Professor of Midwifery, Yale School of Nursing.
Aileen Gariepy, MD, MPH, FACOG. Assistant Professor of Obstetrics, Gynecology, and Reproductive Sciences and Assistant Clinical Professor of Nursing, Yale School of Medicine.

Competing interests

The authors declare that they have no competing interests.

Author details

[1]Yale School of Medicine, 333 Cedar Street, New Haven, CT 06510, USA. [2]Department of Obstetrics, Gynecology and Reproductive Sciences, Yale School of Medicine, New Haven, CT, USA. [3]Department of Obstetrics, Gynecology and Reproductive Sciences, Yale School of Medicine, New Haven, CT, USA. [4]Yale School of Nursing, West Haven, CT, USA. [5]Department of Obstetrics, Gynecology and Reproductive Sciences, Yale School of Medicine, New Haven, CT, USA.

References

1. Harris LF, Roberts SCM, Biggs MA, Rocca CH, Foster DG. Perceived stress and emotional social support among women who are denied or receive abortions in the United States: a prospective cohort study. BMC Womens Health. 2014;14:76.
2. Feldman PJ, Dunkel-Schetter C, Sandman CA, Wadhwa PD. Maternal social support predicts birth weight and fetal growth in human pregnancy. Psychosom Med. 2000;62:715–25.
3. Dunkel Schetter C. Psychological science on pregnancy: stress processes, biopsychosocial models, and emerging research issues. Annu Rev Psychol. 2011;62:531–58.
4. Turner RJ, Grindstaff CF, Phillips N. Social support and outcome in teenage pregnancy. J Health Soc Behav. 1990;31:43–57.
5. Collins NL, Dunkel-Schetter C, Lobel M, Scrimshaw SC. Social support in pregnancy: psychosocial correlates of birth outcomes and postpartum depression. J Pers Soc Psychol. 1993;65:1243–58.
6. Negron R, Martin A, Almog M, Balbierz A, Howell EA. Social support during the postpartum period: mothers' views on needs, expectations, and mobilization of support. Matern Child Health J. 2013;17:616–23.
7. Major B, Cozzarelli C, Sciacchitano AM, Cooper ML, Testa M, Mueller PM. Perceived social support, self-efficacy, and adjustment to abortion. J Pers Soc Psychol. 1990;59:452–63.
8. Lamarca GA, do C Leal M, Sheiham A, Vettore MV. The association of neighbourhood and individual social capital with consistent self-rated health: a longitudinal study in Brazilian pregnant and postpartum women. BMC Pregnancy Childbirth. 2013;13(1).
9. Keating-Lefler R, Wilson ME. The experience of becoming a mother for single, Unpartnered, Medicaid-eligible, first-time mothers. J Nurs Scholarsh. 2004;36:23–9.
10. Norbeck JS, Anderson NJ. Psychosocial predictors of pregnancy outcomes in low-income black, Hispanic, and white women. Nurs Res. 1989;38:204–9.
11. Dejin-Karlsson E, Hanson BS, Östergren P-O, Lindgren A, Sjöberg N-O, Marsal K. Association of a lack of psychosocial resources and the risk of giving birth to small for gestational age infants: a stress hypothesis. BJOG Int J Obstet Gynaecol. 2000;107:89–100.
12. Pryor JE, Thompson JMD, Robinson E, Clark PM, Becroft DMO, Pattison NS, et al. Stress and lack of social support as risk factors for small-for-gestational-age birth. Acta Paediatr Oslo Nor 1992. 2003;92:62–4.
13. Borders AEB, Grobman WA, Amsden LB, Holl JL. Chronic stress and low birth weight neonates in a low-income population of women. Obstet Gynecol. 2007;109(2 Pt 1):331–8.
14. Razurel C, Kaiser B, Sellenet C, Epiney M. Relation between perceived stress, social support, and coping strategies and maternal well-being: a review of the literature. Women Health. 2013;53:74–99.
15. Howell EA, Mora P, Leventhal H. Correlates of early postpartum depressive symptoms. Matern Child Health J. 2006;10:149.
16. Mautner E, Stern C, Deutsch M, Nagele E, Greimel E, Lang U, et al. The impact of resilience on psychological outcomes in women after preeclampsia: an observational cohort study. Health Qual Life Outcomes. 2013;11:194.
17. Grote NK, Bledsoe SE. Predicting postpartum depressive symptoms in new mothers: the role of optimism and stress frequency during pregnancy. Health Soc Work. 2007;32:107–18.
18. Lobel M, DeVincent CJ, Kaminer A, Meyer BA. The impact of prenatal maternal stress and optimistic disposition on birth outcomes in medically high-risk women. Health Psychol. 2000;19:544–53.
19. Ashaba S, Kaida A, Burns BF, O'Neil K, Dunkley E, Psaros C, et al. Understanding coping strategies during pregnancy and the postpartum period: a qualitative study of women living with HIV in rural Uganda. BMC Pregnancy Childbirth. 2017;17. https://doi.org/10.1186/s12884-017-1321-9.
20. Johansson K, Aarts C, Darj E. First-time parents' experiences of home-based postnatal care in Sweden. Ups J Med Sci. 2010;115:131–7.
21. Gariepy A, Lundsberg LS, Vilardo N, Stanwood N, Yonkers K, Schwarz EB. Pregnancy context and women's health-related quality of life. Contraception. 2017;95:491–9.
22. Squires A. Methodological challenges in cross-language qualitative research: a research review. Int J Nurs Stud. 2009;46:277–87.
23. Gale NK, Heath G, Cameron E, Rashid S, Redwood S. Using the framework method for the analysis of qualitative data in multi-disciplinary health research. BMC Med Res Methodol. 2013;13:117.
24. D'Anna-Hernandez KL, Aleman B, Flores A-M. Acculturative stress negatively impacts maternal depressive symptoms in Mexican-American women during pregnancy. J Affect Disord. 2015;176:35–42.
25. Guendelman S, Malin C, Herr-Harthorn B, Noemi Vargas P. Orientations to motherhood and male partner support among women in Mexico and Mexican-origin women in the United States. Soc Sci Med. 2001;52:1805–13.
26. Kolko J. Normal America. In: Is not a small town of white people. FiveThirtyEight; 2016. https://fivethirtyeight.com/features/normal-america-is-not-a-small-town-of-white-people/. Accessed 8 Jan 2018.
27. Hodnett ED, Fredericks S, Weston J. Support during pregnancy for women at increased risk of low birthweight babies. Cochrane Database Syst Rev. 2010:CD000198.
28. Ickovics JR, Kershaw TS, Westdahl C, Magriples U, Massey Z, Reynolds H, et al. Group prenatal care and perinatal outcomes: a randomized controlled trial. Obstet Gynecol. 2007;110(2 Pt 1):330–9.
29. Jones RK, Jerman J. Abortion incidence and service availability in the United States, 2014. Perspect Sex Reprod Health. 2017;49(1)17-27.
30. Contraceptive Needs and Services, 2014 Update Guttmacher Institute 2016. https://www.guttmacher.org/report/contraceptive-needs-and-services-2014-update. Accessed 8 Jan 2018.
31. Why We Cannot Afford to Undercut the Title X National Family Planning Program. Guttmacher Institute. 2017. https://www.guttmacher.org/gpr/2017/01/why-we-cannot-afford-undercut-title-x-national-family-planning-program. Accessed 8 Jan 2018.
32. Recent Funding Restrictions on the U.S. Family planning safety net may foreshadow what is to come. In: Guttmacher Institute; 2016. https://www.guttmacher.org/gpr/2016/12/recent-funding-restrictions-us-family-planning-safety-net-may-foreshadow-what-come. Accessed 8 Jan 2018.

33. Grossman D. Sexual and reproductive health under the trump presidency: policy change threatens women in the USA and worldwide. J Fam Plann Reprod Health Care. 2017;43:89–91.

34. Carroll AE. Why is US maternal mortality rising? JAMA 2017;318:321–321.

35. No One Benefits If Women Lose Coverage for Maternity Care. Guttmacher Institute. 2017. https://www.guttmacher.org/gpr/2017/06/no-one-benefits-if-women-lose-coverage-maternity-care. Accessed 8 Jan 2018.

15

Not now but later – a qualitative study of non-exercising pregnant women's views and experiences of exercise

Maria Ekelin[1]*, Mette Langeland Iversen[3], Mette Grønbæk Backhausen[2,3,5] and Hanne Kristine Hegaard[1,2,3,4]

Abstract

Background: Evidence has shown that there are several physical and mental advantages of exercise during pregnancy. Despite this, the recommendations for exercise during pregnancy are poorly fulfilled. The aim of this study was to illuminate non-exercising pregnant women's views and experiences concerning exercise before and during pregnancy.

Method: The study had a qualitative design with an inductive approach and was analysed by content analysis. A total of 16 individual and face-to-face interviews were conducted with healthy pregnant women, mainly in the third trimester and living in Sweden. The participating women had not been exercising 3 months before pregnancy or during pregnancy.

Results: The main category "Insurmountable now, but possible in the future" was based on the four categories: "Lost and lack of routines", "Feelings of inadequacy", "Having a different focus" and "Need for support". The women experienced that their lack of routines was a major barrier that prevented them from exercising. Other factors that contributed were, for example, pregnancy-related problems, long working days and prioritizing family life. The women described it as difficult to combine exercise with their focus on the pregnancy and they missed continuous support from the antenatal care provider. The women expressed a need for suggestions concerning exercise during pregnancy and follow-up on previous counselling, especially when pregnancy-related issues arose. Information about easily accessible alternatives or simple home exercises was requested. They felt immobile and were not satisfied with their inactivity and tried to partly compensate with everyday activities. The women identified the postpartum period as an important possibility for becoming more active, for their own sake, but also because they wanted to become role models for their children.

Conclusion: Continuous support during pregnancy is needed concerning exercise. Pregnancy is mostly a barrier that prevents exercise for this group of women but, at the same time, may be a motivator and a possibility for better health. As the result showed that these women were highly motivated to a life-style change post-pregnancy, it may be crucial to support previously non-exercising women postpartum.

Keywords: Pregnancy, Exercise, Sedentary lifestyle, Experience, Health behaviour

* Correspondence: maria.ekelin@med.lu.se
[1]Department of Health Sciences, Lund University, PO Box 157, S-22100 Lund, Sweden
Full list of author information is available at the end of the article

Background

The focus on the importance of exercise during pregnancy has been consistent since the American Congress of Obstetricians and Gynecologists published the recommendation for exercise in 2002 [1]. Today ACOG recommends exercise of moderate intensity for at least 20–30 min on most or all days of the week during pregnancy and the postpartum period [2]. In the years since then, many countries have published similar recommendations [3]. Exercise has been defined as physical activity consisting of planned, structured and repetitive bodily movements done to improve and/or maintain one or more components of physical fitness [4]. However, recent studies have shown that recommendations for exercise during pregnancy are poorly fulfilled [5–9].

This is a concern as it is well documented that exercise during pregnancy is associated with a lower risk of adverse pregnancy outcomes such as gestational diabetes mellitus [10], preeclampsia [11], infants with excessive birth weight (> 4000 g) [7], low back pain [12] and caesarean section [13]. Exercise may also be effective in reducing symptoms of depression during pregnancy among healthy women and women at risk of depression [14, 15].

Pre-pregnancy exercise has shown to be a strong predictor for physical activity during pregnancy [5, 7, 16, 17] and women who exercise before pregnancy have been characterized by having a higher level of income and education, more often being married or living with a partner compared to non-exercising women [18]. Furthermore, lower education level, smoking, overweight, and not speaking the native language have been identified as predictors for not meeting the recommendations for exercise during pregnancy [5]. This may reflect a social inequality concerning exercise during pregnancy, which can lead to social differences in health [19].

In Sweden, midwives have the responsibility for the antenatal care of healthy women. In early pregnancy, the midwife has an informative dialogue with the woman concerning health and lifestyle [20].The Swedish recommendations [20] for exercise during pregnancy are in line with the international recommendations [2, 3] and it was recently shown in a large Swedish study population that 47% of the women met the recommendation for exercise in early pregnancy [21].

Non-exercising pregnant women seem to be particularly in need of advice and support from health professionals concerning exercise and healthy lifestyle. However, Hegaard et al. [17] showed that among women mainly having a sedentary level of leisure-time physical activity before pregnancy, only one in four increased their activity during pregnancy.

Previous quantitative and qualitative studies have explored the reasons why women who exercise before pregnancy reduced their engagement in exercise during pregnancy [22–24]. However, less is known concerning healthy pregnant women who do not engage in physical exercise both before and during pregnancy. More knowledge is needed in order to support exercise and health in these women during pregnancy and in the postpartum period.

Aim

The aim of this study was to illuminate non-exercising pregnant women's views and experiences concerning exercise before and during pregnancy.

Method

This study had a qualitative design with an inductive approach.

Participants

From January 2015 to June 2016 16 face-to-face interviews were performed with pregnant women. The inclusion criteria were Swedish- or English-speaking non-exercising women, and 18 years of age or older. For the purpose of this study non-exercising women were defined as those neither exercising in the last 3 months before pregnancy nor during pregnancy. Women with conditions that contra-indicated exercise were excluded, as well as women diagnosed with gestational diabetes, as they receive special information from the health professionals concerning physical activity.

In line with other studies, we exemplified exercise as swimming, training in water, dancing, yoga, jogging, ball games, fitness, cycling, horseback riding, and other types of similar exercise [5, 25]. The sampling strategy was purposeful sampling with consecutive recruitment. The participating women were enrolled at three different antenatal care centres in the south of Sweden, two situated in a larger city, and one in a rural area. Pregnant women were recruited by their midwife when undergoing a routine glucose tolerance test offered to all pregnant women around gestational week 28, or earlier if the woman has risk factors for diabetes, after having been given verbal and written information about the study. Women who agreed to participate were contacted by the researchers. Initially 21 women agreed to be contacted and 16 finally agreed to take part. Written informed consent was obtained from all participants.

Data collection

One woman was interviewed in the first trimester, all the other women in the third trimester. The interviews took place where the participants preferred, two at the University of Lund and the remainder elsewhere: the antenatal care centre, a café, a library and at the woman's home. The interviews were all conducted by the first author, individually and face to face. Each interview lasted approximately 30 min.

The interviews all started by asking the same overall question: "What are your views and experiences concerning exercise before and during pregnancy?" This was followed by clarifying questions, such as "What do you mean?" or "Can you explain further?". Please see Additional file 1.

The interviews were audio taped and transcribed verbatim by the first author.

Analysis

Data were analysed using content analysis [26, 27] as it is considered a suitable method widely used for developing and extending knowledge in health sciences by interpreting the meaning of text data [27, 28]. Firstly, the interviews were read through to get a sense of the whole. Then, open inductive coding was performed by writing notes consisting of short sentences or single words in the text margin, which summed up what was being said. The initial coding process started after the first interview. Throughout the whole process, memos were made about the topics and categorization of data. The codes, and the text sections belonging to them, were then read, re-read and compared. In this process similar or overlapping codes were grouped together into sub-categories. Subsequently the sub-categories were compared and merged, thereby reducing them in number. The sub-categories were finally sorted into categories until consensus was reached between the authors. Throughout the process of analysis, the transcripts were re-read to verify the emerging findings. All authors were involved in the process of analysis.

Ethics and consent statement

Informed written consent was obtained prior to interviews. The study was approved by the Regional Research Ethics Board (Reg. no. 2014/733). All of the data were treated confidentially.

Results

The women were 23–41 years old and eight were expecting their first child, while the remaining eight women were expecting their second or third baby. The characteristics of the women are presented in Table 1. One women was not Swedish-speaking and was therefore interviewed in English.

The main category "Insurmountable now, but possible in the future" emerged during analysis, and was based on four categories and nine subcategories presented in Fig. 1.

Insurmountable now, but possible in the future

The women had a positive attitude towards exercise in general, but did not find it possible to exercise during pregnancy, at least not without active support from antenatal care providers or significant others. Some women viewed physical activity as impossible, even with support, while

Table 1 Characteristics of the women

Age range:	23–41 years
Education:	
High school	6
University/college	10
Expecting child:	
First	8
Second	5
Third	3
Occupation:	
Working	11
Maternity leave	3
Sick leave	1
Unemployed	1

others were more open-minded but without capacity to start on their own. They hoped to start later, as they saw disadvantages in their inactivity and longed for a change in their activity level. They perceived the pregnancy mostly as a barrier to exercise but simultaneously as a motivator and a possibility for better health in the future.

Lost and lack of routines

The women all described how they had been exercising more or less earlier in life, at least during their youth while performing different types of leisure time activities and in school during sport lessons. Currently they had no routines for exercise and they expressed several reasons, including pregnancy-related problems and lack of time. These reasons were viewed as barriers that when combined were very difficult to overcome.

Starting difficulties

The further away their previous routines for exercise were, the larger the barriers had grown. They acknowledged the need for an established routine and motivation, which they lacked. The women with previous positive experience of exercise knew that they had lost a state of well-being and wanted to re-establish this in the future. The women who had not previously felt good or had fun in connection with exercise experienced an additional barrier.

And in the end I felt that I was very far from exercise and then it's also more difficult to approach it... And you have to start all over again. And that is tough! And I understand that it will be onerous in the beginning before you get going and really start to think it is fun. And I have never reached that point. (No. 9)

They found it was easy to postpone their ambitions of exercise, especially during the short period of their life when they were pregnant.

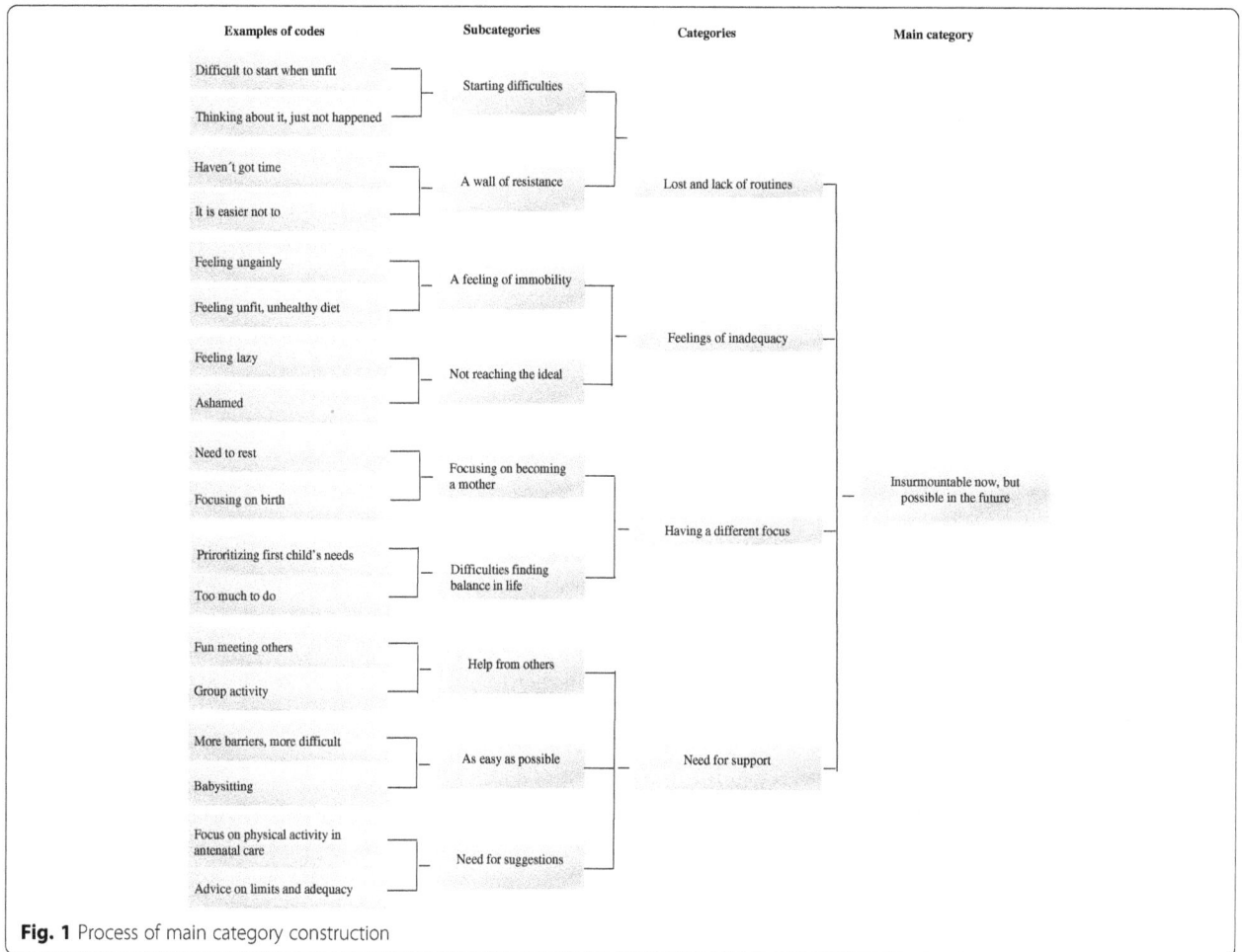

Fig. 1 Process of main category construction

And then you think that, yes, I will start next week. But now, more than half of the pregnancy has past and that week hasn't come yet. (No. 11)

They expressed a hope for a change in the future. These thoughts varied from concrete plans for how and when they would exercise, to a less precise will to start exercising later on. It could also be difficult to find the right activity which would make exercise a more attractive option. If the women had previous sport injuries, they described themselves as active persons, although in some cases it was several years since they had a continuous habit of exercise. They felt sad that they had been forced to stop exercising, but had not yet felt motivated enough to find another type of exercise.

A wall of resistance
The women described internal as well as external barriers as reasons for not exercising. Internal barriers were connected to lack of motivation, prioritizing other things or choosing the easiest alternative.

Laziness. Easy-going. It's like this, now I have worked enough for the day, now I want to go home. I don't want to get home at six or seven in the evening. I want to come home at half past four, that is reasonable. And then, to go out again when you have come home. That won't happen! Even if I have thought about doing, no, it won't happen. (No. 9)

During the interviews, the women mentioned and returned to their lack of motivation for exercise and the mechanisms that prevented them from establishing routines. They had not explored these issues in depth for themselves. They described that the problem was not that they did not know that exercise was beneficial, but that they did not do it anyway, for reasons that were not always logical or clear to the women.

I have thought that I ought to exercise, but I haven't considered it deeper than that, why you choose not to prioritize it or why you don't have time for it. It becomes some sort of defence mechanism in the head. (No. 13)

I do not know. I actually do not know. I really do not know, actually. (No. 1)

External barriers to exercising were described as the loss of routines, for example, caused by moving from one city to another, including losing friends and established activities. Linked to this was the difficulty of finding a new activity and a feeling of not knowing the existing alternatives, but still they did not seek them actively. If the woman had practised physical activity earlier but had not had a firm routine, it was common that a simple thing had permanent consequences and the routine was broken. For example, getting a cold or missing class could be reason enough for not starting again. Darkness and cold during wintertime were also mentioned as barriers to outdoor activities and a reason for not starting or continuing with, for example, walking or cycling. During pregnancy, the women experienced problems such as nausea, fatigue, and weight gain, which they considered to be major additional barriers.

Feelings of inadequacy
The women felt immobile and knew that it would be positive for them if they started to exercise, which they referred to as common knowledge. At the moment, they described a feeling of not reaching their own and society's ideal in terms of exercise.

A feeling of immobility
The women felt immobile because of lack of exercise. In addition, they experienced bodily changes due to their pregnancy and they described their condition in terms of being tired without any energy, being ungainly, heavy and stiff. This caused dissatisfaction and they missed the days when they had been more active.

And I already feel that I am not so supple as last time (during her first pregnancy). And then I feel that I have to do something before giving birth. So it won't be so tough. Because I already feel ungainly. (No. 1)

Pelvic girdle pain was expressed by two thirds of the women and this considerably added to the feeling of immobility as it restricted their general mobility as well as their self-perceived possibility to exercise.

The women looked forward to become mobile again, and for those who perceived themselves as overweight, to losing weight, which motivated them to take exercise in the future. Besides lack of exercise, these women also linked their feeling of immobility to their weight gain during pregnancy.

Not reaching the ideal
All of the women saw the advantages of exercise and described it as an ideal state. It was something they knew was beneficial, but at the moment unreachable.

Not meeting society's ideal concerning exercise was a component that contributed to a feeling of dissatisfaction.

I am a little bit ashamed of it. That I can't do something about it. And that I haven't done it in the meantime (during pregnancy). And now it's starting to feel a little bit late. (No. 15)

The women were positive to everyday activities, such as climbing stairs instead of taking the lift, to somewhat compensate for their inactivity and make them feel less discontent with their own inactivity. One woman described why she walked instead of taking the bus:

Well, I guess it's like, in my mind, you know, I can tell myself "I did do some exercise today". I wasn't just, you know, like you feel lazy and you feel "I am doing something". (No. 16)

Besides the recognition of the physical benefits of activity, the women also expressed a longing for mental satisfaction, such as becoming happier, gaining mental strength and sleeping better at night.

Having a different focus
Women described how the pregnancy had changed their focus in life and they concentrated on their pregnancy and struggled to find balance in life.

Focusing on becoming a mother.

The additional strain from pregnancy-related issues such as tiredness partly prevented the women from physical activity and made them prioritize rest during this period of life. Becoming a mother was the primary focus for the women to justify or make it acceptable for themselves to postpone their initiative to start taking regular exercise.

It feels like I'm more focused on the fact that it is will soon be due, so now I'm going to prepare mentally more than doing that (exercising). I'll have to start to exercise later instead. (No. 2)

All women had much faith in the future concerning their ambitions to exercise. They expressed hope that the parental leave would be the opportunity they needed to change their habits. Women who wished to lose weight included healthy diet in their imagined post-pregnancy concept of health. Walking with the stroller was viewed as an attractive and attainable goal.

Later on, other types of activities together with the child were a possible and positive opportunity that the women identified. The women wished to become active not only for their own sake, but also for their children's. The women explained that it was important for them to live long and healthy and to be able to play with their children.

... you have to be able to be an active parent and play with them and so on. So I believe it's better to strengthen the body and be more alert and have more strength. Just generally. If I feel well, they will too. I think so, everybody feels good if I exercise. So that's the main reason. (No. 14)

Some women mentioned that they wished to become a role model for the child regarding exercise so that early healthy lifestyle habits could be established for the children.

Difficulties finding balance in life

The women all portrayed daily life activities both as real barriers and as excuses for not exercising. Family life was highly valued and long working days were unavoidable. The pregnancy made them more tired than usual and the women felt that the days did not have enough hours. Prioritizing themselves had to be put on hold. When all compulsory daily life activities were performed, the women had little or no strength for exercise. It was easier not to be physically active and thereby gain more time for other activities.

There is a lot to do when you have a house, and stuff like that, when you come home. So then you say "I'll take it next day" and then maybe you get a cold, and some time passes, and you have to wait until you are well. And then you have a lot of other things to do because you have been ill, so it... there are excuses and that kind of thing too. (No. 5)

The women prioritized previous children before spare time of their own, but sometimes the children's needs promoted shared physical activities when playing together or for example when cycling or walking in the forest.

Need for support

Initiating exercise after or during pregnancy was perceived as easier with support from others and if the women knew about easily accessible alternatives suitable for pregnant women, such as group activities or easy exercises to perform at home.

Help from others

There were divergent opinions about the degree to which a significant other person, such as husband or friend, or a group activity was valued. Both the presence of an inspiring instructor and being accompanied by a friend could be motivating. Several of the women referred to their partner as actively trying to encourage them to start exercising.

Some women described how a group of other pregnant women would be beneficial as they would exercise on the same terms. Nevertheless, it was difficult to start on their own if the women classified themselves as untrained, as they imagined it to be uncomfortable when being both pregnant and a beginner among non-pregnant participants or pregnant participants who were used to taking exercise.

I have read that they will have some kind of yoga for pregnant women. But I feel I am totally unfit. So it feels silly to go there by myself. That's how I feel. (No. 11)

While some women solely referred to their own motivation as the crucial factor for starting to exercise, others referred to the organization of Swedish antenatal care, with just a few antenatal visits in early pregnancy. This was pointed out as a problem, if the women wished to be active but were in need of professional support.

...and that is probably another thing, not having that (antenatal visits) regular... you have a gap from about week 9 or 10 to week 25, when you are just kind of on your own and you feel OK, but you just carry on without doing it... so you don't have that reminder or kind of pressure. (No. 14)

As easy as possible

At the same time as there was a need for routines, it was felt that exercise should ideally be easily accessible as regards both time and location. A long distance to the sport facilities or limited opportunities to choose a suitable time were perceived as barriers by the women.

The smallest barrier is just to put on trainers and maybe a warm coat, and take a walk. For the more barriers you build, the more difficult are they to overcome. You have to book, rebook and you have to go there, and you have to take a shower, and you have to fix and plan. And then it falls through just from thinking about it. So it has to be, it will probably be walks and running again, for that is the smallest barrier. (No. 7)

It was suggested that exercise should be more mandatory and not in forms that could be questioned. For example, having a dog or getting a formal physical activity prescription from antenatal care would make it easier as this would be perceived as not having a choice.

This is an area that has to be prioritized more; that it is incorporated (in the antenatal programme) like a natural part as much as many other parts, so to speak... Because I think it would be, sometimes you should not have the feeling of too much of a free choice. That it's included. (No. 3)

Although the women planned to become more physically active after birth, they also recognized that their time would be limited and they would have to prioritize the newborn baby's needs before their own. It was considered difficult to have too detailed plans in advance, but activities that allowed them to bring their child along was one option identified by the women.

Need for suggestions

It was not considered necessary that the midwife should be an expert on exercise, but the women would like her to be a catalyst that presented alternatives suitable for pregnant women and could refer them to suitable activities or, for example, to a physiotherapist. Just to have knowledge about organized alternatives in the neighbourhood would have been of value for the women or to know about instructive exercise websites targeting pregnant women. Furthermore, the women called for recommendations for suitable mild forms of activities that could be performed at home and easily incorporated into daily life. It was a common experience that the subject of exercise was only taken up at the beginning of pregnancy and the women wished that exercise should also be discussed during subsequent antenatal visits. Instead it was suggested to be practised or at least followed up as pregnancy gradually influenced the women's abilities and possibilities to be active. The pregnancy generated additional questions concerning suitable forms of exercise to be performed and how these should be adapted, in case of health problems such as pelvic girdle pain.

I think that it should be more in focus and that they should discuss it more often. You know, present recommendations and focus more on it at the appointments with the midwife. So you are updated on how it goes, if there are any difficulties with it, like that. And maybe have some information about why it is good for you. (No. 4)

To practise some kind of exercise in connection with antenatal care or antenatal class and not just to discuss it was one solution mentioned.

Furthermore, as other issues seemed to be more in focus, the women did not consider introducing exercise as a topic themselves and it was therefore important that the subject was initiated by the midwife if the exercise was to be acknowledged during pregnancy for these non-exercising women.

Discussion

This study explored non-exercising pregnant women's views and experiences of exercise and found that in general the women had a positive attitude towards exercise. However they did not find it possible to practise during pregnancy – at least not without active support from antenatal care providers or significant others. Some women viewed exercise as impossible, even with support, while others were more open minded but without own capacity to start. They hoped to start later, as they saw disadvantages of their inactivity and longed for a change in their activity level. They perceived the pregnancy mostly as a barrier to exercising but at the same time as a motivator and a possibility for better health in the future.

Not overcoming barriers

The participants in this study were not comfortable with their level of exercise, but experienced more barriers than resources to mobilize themselves to engage in exercise. The barriers experienced were lack of time and physical pregnancy-related symptoms, as also shown by other researchers [22, 23]. Additionally, this group of non-exercising pregnant women had lost, and therefore lacked, routines for exercise. This generated great initial difficulties which diverges from previous research showing that experiences and already established habits could be helpful in overcoming barriers [24].

Intentions to exercise

According to the current results, the women were aware of the benefits of exercise but found it difficult to combine with their major focus on becoming a mother. Among the women who had an intention to start exercising during pregnancy, but had not managed it, some had difficulties explaining why. Other studies have shown that many women consider rest to be more important than activity and exercise during pregnancy [29, 30]. The belief that rest is beneficial during pregnancy has been shown to be supported by women's networks [30], but not shown in the current study, where partners were referred to as potential supporters concerning exercise. Family members' strong normative influence on women's exercise during pregnancy and postpartum has been recognized by Symons Downs and Hausenblas [31]. However, other and stronger forces were explained as preventing the women in the current study from exercising. An interesting result of this study was the women's intention and willingness to start exercising after the birth. ACOG [2] states that it is important to support lifelong health habits during pregnancy and exercise between pregnancies may have positive impact on fitness, mood and weight loss [32]. The latter is important as weight gain between pregnancies increases the risk of adverse pregnancy outcomes including stillbirth [33, 34]. The women described that they wanted to be role models for their children in relation to exercise. This is an important result as there is some evidence that maternal inactivity during pregnancy may contribute to child obesity risk in both active and inactive children 3–9 years old [35].

Need for support from care givers

The women's need for support from antenatal health care professionals varied concerning both extent and shape, stressing the need for individualized care. Although some women did not imagine that any support would help them to start exercising during pregnancy, most regretted the lack of *continuous* support for exercise during pregnancy that could be in accordance with their evolving physical changes due to pregnancy. The women even called for elements of mandatory exercise in antenatal care. Interventions during pregnancy, especially face-to-face counselling, have shown some success in reducing the decline of physical activity in pregnant women [36]. A qualitative study with participants having lifestyle discussions in a health centre setting has shown that a desire to make a lifestyle change combined with sensitivity in the discussion are basic conditions for success [37]. Furthermore, this is in line with the experiences of pregnant women participating in group exercise sessions [24].

Group interventions exclusively for pregnant women may be warranted as the women in the current study pointed out that it was important for them in order to dare as beginners and that the exercise programme should be adapted to their pregnancy. Hinton and Olson [18] have shown that self-efficacy is a predictor of change in physical activity. However, a systematic review evaluating the evidence for different interventions aiming at improving physical activity during pregnancy concluded that in general little is known about the efficacy of the interventions [38].

The women's individual needs of support underline the importance of health professionals following the current recommendations for counselling on exercise. ACOG [2] states that an exercise programme meeting the recommendations should be developed with the woman and adjusted when medically indicated, but the result of our study reflects a lack of such structured support. An interview study with 41 midwives counselling on physical activity, showed that this was a complex task containing both opportunities and challenges, for example difficulties in responding to divergent needs while struggling with lack of resources and fear of failure as expressed by the midwives [39]. To improve counselling, further training for midwives and resources should be introduced [39]. This is especially important for preventing social differences in health, as both previous Swedish and international research has identified social inequality in meeting the recommendations for exercise during pregnancy [5, 18, 21].

To understand why pregnant women do not start exercising, the theory of planned behaviour [40] may be of use. The theory includes the concept of perceived behavioural control which describes a person's perception of how easy or difficult it is to perform specific behaviours. Perceived behavioural control may include both practical issues, which in the current context for example can be explained as easy access to exercise, and the perception of one's own abilities. A person's level of perceived behavioural control, combined with the level of intention (motivation), may in this context potentially determine whether the pregnant woman actually starts to exercise or not. According to Ajzen [40], the level of intention is influenced by a person's attitude to the behaviour as well as perceived social pressure. Interventions targeting exercise should acknowledge the complexity in a woman's decisions concerning exercise during pregnancy.

Limitations

The sample of women in this study was diverse as regards socio-demographic characteristics such as age and level of education as well as parity. Nevertheless the study only covers three antenatal care centres in Sweden and the results should be interpreted in this context. The transferability to women in developing countries with less well-organized health systems is low or not possible. All authors participated in the analysis process by analysing first individually and then comparatively to increase the confirmability. All authors have preunderstanding as midwives and two of the authors, HKH and MB, have in addition preunderstanding from previous research on physical activity among pregnant women, but not among non-exercising women. The authors' preunderstanding was recognized and discussed in relation to the analysis.

As the midwives who informed about the study also were the ones that had to counsel the women on exercise, this could be a potential source of bias, as it cannot be excluded that this may have resulted in more focus on counselling on exercise from the midwives during the study period which may have affected the women's experiences. However since the results of the study revealed a need for further support and continuous follow-up during antenatal care, this effect is likely to have been limited.

Clinical implications

The fact that the women in this study did not have any current routines for exercise led to an increased need for support compared to women practising exercise pre-pregnancy. An easily implementable implication of this study is to present local alternative examples of exercise offered during pregnancy in the antenatal care setting, as the women in this study were in need of suggestions. Ideally exercise in groups could be incorporated as the social element and having fun with other pregnant women is an aspect that could be a strong facilitator for exercise according to the results of the current study.

The results clearly showed that the women liked to start exercising after birth. Postpartum walking with baby stroller was judged as realistic by the women and could be encouraged as a part of the woman's individual plan or as a part of the postpartum health care.

Conclusion

The results provide a deeper understanding of non-exercising pregnant women's situation and the barriers they try to overcome with respect to exercise, including their lack of routines. Health professionals should take into consideration that the pregnancy is viewed both as a barrier preventing exercise and as a motivator for a healthier lifestyle and therefore a possibility for exercise promotion. Exercise should not only be supported at the beginning of the pregnancy but must be emphasized throughout the pregnancy. As the result showed that these women were highly motivated to a lifestyle change post-pregnancy, it may be crucial to support non-exercising women postpartum.

It is essential to conduct further research developing a behaviour-change intervention targeting non-exercising pregnant women, including continuous support during and after pregnancy followed by a RCT.

Acknowledgements
The authors thank the participating women and the antenatal care units.

Funding
The research network LuCare, Lund University, https://www.med.lu.se/lucare_network
The funding bodies had no influence on study design and have no role in data acquisition, data analyses and interpretation or manuscript preparation.

Authors' contributions
The study was initiated by ME and HH who conceptualized the idea and design of the study. ME conducted the interviews and all authors contributed to the subsequent analysis and interpretation of data. ME drafted the first version of the article and HH, MB and ML all critically revised it for important intellectual content. The final manuscript was approved for publication by all authors.

Competing interests
The authors declare that they have no competing interests.

Author details
[1]Department of Health Sciences, Lund University, PO Box 157, S-22100 Lund, Sweden. [2]Department of Obstetrics, Copenhagen University Hospital, Rigshospitalet, Copenhagen, Denmark. [3]The Research Unit Women's and Children's Health, The Juliane Marie Centre, Copenhagen University Hospital, Rigshospitalet, Blegdamsvej 9, 2100 Copenhagen, Denmark. [4]The Institute of Clinical Medicine, Faculty of Health and Medical Sciences, University of Copenhagen, Blegdamsvej 3, Copenhagen, Denmark. [5]Department of Gynecology and Obstetrics, Zealand University Hospital, Sygehusvej 10, 4000 Roskilde, Denmark.

References
1. ACOG Committee Opinion No. 267. Exercise during pregnancy and the postpartum period. Int J Gynaecol Obstet. 2002;77(1):79–81.
2. ACOG Committee Opinion No. 650. Physical activity and exercise during pregnancy and the postpartum period. Obstet Gynecol. 2015;126(6):e135–42. https://doi.org/10.1097/AOG.0000000000001214.
3. Evenson KR, Barakat R, Brown WJ, Dargent-Molina P, Haruna M, Mikkelsen EM, Mottola MF, Owe KM, Rousham EK, Yeo S. Guidelines for physical activity during pregnancy: comparisons from around the world. Am J Lifestyle Med. 2014;8(2):102–21.
4. American College of Sports Medicine. ACSM's guidelines for exercise testing and prescription. 9th ed. Philadelphia: Wolters Kluwer/Lippincott Willians & Wilkins; 2014.
5. Broberg L, Ersbøll AS, Backhausen MG, Damm P, Tabor A, Hegaard HK. Compliance with national recommendations for exercise during early pregnancy in a Danish cohort. BMC Pregnancy Childbirth. 2015;27;15:317. doi: https://doi.org/10.1186/s12884-015-0756-0.
6. Gjestland K, Bø K, Owe KM, Eberhard-Gran M. Do pregnant women follow exercise guidelines? Prevalence data among 3482 women, and prediction of low-back pain, pelvic girdle pain and depression. Br J Sports Med. 2013; 47(8):515–20. https://doi.org/10.1136/bjsports-2012-091344.
7. Owe KM, Nystad W, Bø K. Association between regular exercise and excessive newborn birth weight. Obstet Gynecol. 2009;114(4):770–6. https://doi.org/10.1097/AOG.0b013e3181b6c105.
8. Juhl M, Madsen M, Andersen AM, Andersen PK, Olsen J. Distribution and predictors of exercise habits among pregnant women in the Danish National Birth Cohort. Scand J Med Sci Sports. 2012;22(1):128–38. https://doi.org/10.1111/j.1600-0838.2010.01125.x.
9. Santos PC, Abreu S, Moreira C, Lopes D, Santos R, Alves O, Silva P, Montenegro N, Mota J. Impact of compliance with different guidelines on physical activity during pregnancy and perceived barriers to leisure physical activity. J Sports Sci. 2014;32(14):1398–408. https://doi.org/10.1080/02640414.2014.893369.
10. Russo LM, Nobles C, Ertel KA, Chasan-Taber L, Whitcomb BW. Physical activity interventions in pregnancy and risk of gestational diabetes mellitus: a systematic review and meta-analysis. Obstet Gynecol. 2015;125(3):576–82. https://doi.org/10.1097/AOG.0000000000000691.
11. Aune D, Saugstad OD, Henriksen T, Tonstad S. Physical activity and the risk of preeclampsia: a systematic review and meta-analysis. Epidemiology. 2014; 25(3):331–43. https://doi.org/10.1097/EDE.0000000000000036.
12. Liddle SD, Pennick V. Interventions for preventing and treating low-back and pelvic pain during pregnancy. Cochrane Database Syst Rev. 2015;30:9-CD001139. https://doi.org/10.1002/14651858.CD001139.pub4.
13. Domenjoz I, Kayser B, Boulvain M. Effect of physical activity during pregnancy on mode of delivery. Am J Obstet Gynecol 2014;211(4):401.e1-11doi: https://doi.org/10.1016/j.ajog.2014.03.030.
14. Daley A, Foster L, Long G, Palmer C, Robinson O, Walmsley H, Ward R. The effectiveness of exercise for the prevention and treatment of antenatal depression: systematic review with meta-analysis. BJOG. 2015;122(1):57–62. https://doi.org/10.1111/1471-0528.12909.
15. Perales M, Refoyo I, Coteron J, Bacchi M, Barakat R. Exercise during pregnancy attenuates prenatal depression: a randomized controlled trial. Eval Health Prof 2014; 38(1):59–72. pii: 0163278714533566.

16. Leppänen M, Aittasalo M, Raitanen J, Kinnunen TI, Kujala UM, Luoto R. Physical activity during pregnancy: predictors of change, perceived support and barriers among women at increased risk of gestational diabetes. Matern Child Health J. 2014;18(9):2158–66. https://doi.org/10.1007/s10995-014-1464-5.

17. Hegaard HK, Damm P, Hedegaard M, Henriksen TB, Ottesen B, Dykes AK, Kjaergaard H. Sports and leisure time physical activity during pregnancy in nulliparous women. Matern Child Health J. 2011;15(6):806–13. https://doi.org/10.1007/s10995-010-0647-y.

18. Hinton PS, Olson CM. Predictors of pregnancy-associated change in physical activity in a rural white population. Matern Child Health J. 2001;5(1):7–14.

19. Diderichsen, F. Andersoen, I. Manuel, C. Ulighed i sundhed – årsager og indsatser. Copenhagen; Sundhedsstyrelsen. 2011. http://sundhedsstyrelsen.dk/publ/Publ2011/SURA/Ulighed_i_sundhed/UlighedSundhedAarsagerIndsatser.pdf Accessed 29 December 2016. In Danish.

20. SFOG. (Swedish Society of Obstetrics and Gynecology) Mödrahälsovård, Sexuell och reproduktiv Hälsa. Report nr 59. SFOG: Stockholm; 2008. In Swedish

21. Lindqvist M, Lindkvist M, Eurenius E, Persson M, Ivarsson A, Mogren I. Leisure time physical activity among pregnant women and its associations with maternal characteristics and pregnancy outcomes. Sex Reprod Healthc. 2016;9:14–20. https://doi.org/10.1016/j.srhc.2016.03.006.

22. Duncombe D, Wertheim EH, Skouteris H, Paxton SJ, Kelly L. Factors related to exercise over the course of pregnancy including women's beliefs about the safety of exercise during pregnancy. Midwifery. 2009;25(4):430–8.

23. Evenson KR, Moos MK, Carrier K, Siega-Riz AM. Perceived barriers to physical activity among pregnant women. Matern Child Health J. 2009;13(3):364–75. https://doi.org/10.1007/s10995-008-0359-8.

24. Hegaard HK, Kjaergaard H, Damm PP, Petersson K, Dykes AK. Experiences of physical activity during pregnancy in Danish nulliparous women with a physically active life before pregnancy. A qualitative study. BMC Pregnancy Childbirth. 2010;29;10:33. doi: https://doi.org/10.1186/1471-2393-10-33.

25. Juhl M, Andersen PK, Olsen J, Madsen M, Jørgensen T, Nøhr EA, Andersen AM. Physical exercise during pregnancy and the risk of preterm birth: a study within the Danish National Birth Cohort. Am J Epidemiol 2008;1;167(7):859–866. doi: https://doi.org/10.1093/aje/kwm364.

26. Burnard P. A method of analysing interview transcripts in qualitative research. Nurse Educ Today. 1991;11:461–6.

27. Burnard P, Gill P, Stewart K, Treasure E, Chadwick B. Analysing and presenting qualitative data. Br Dent J 2008;26;204(8):429–432. doi: https://doi.org/10.1038/sj.bdj.2008.292.

28. Hsieh HF, Shannon SE. Three approaches to qualitative content analysis. Qual Health Res. 2005;15(9):1277–88.

29. Clarke P, Gross H. Women's behaviour, beliefs and information sources about physical exercise in pregnancy. Midwifery. 2004;20:133–41.

30. Newham JJ, Allan C, Leahy-Warren P, Carrick-Sen D, Alderdice F. Intentions toward physical activity and resting behavior in pregnant women: using the theory of planned behavior framework in a cross-sectional study. Birth. 2016;43(1):49–57. https://doi.org/10.1111/birt.12211.

31. Symons Downs D, Hausenblas HA. Women's exercise beliefs and behaviors during their pregnancy and postpartum. J Midwifery Womens Health. 2004;49(2):138–44.

32. Evenson KR, Mottola MF, Owe KM, Rousham EK, Brown WJ. Summary of international guidelines for physical activity after pregnancy. Obstet Gynecol Surv. 2014;69(7):407–14. https://doi.org/10.1097/OGX.0000000000000077.

33. Villamor E, Cnattingius S. Interpregnancy weight change and risk of adverse pregnancy outcomes: a population-based study. Lancet 2006;30;368(9542):1164–1170.

34. Cnattingius S, Villamor E. Weight change between successive pregnancies and risks of stillbirth and infant mortality: a nationwide cohort study. Lancet 2016;6;387(10018):558–565. doi: https://doi.org/10.1016/S0140-6736(15)00990-3.

35. Mudd LM, Pivarnik JM, Pfeiffer KA, Paneth N, Chung H, Holzman C. Maternal physical activity during pregnancy, child leisure-time activity, and child weight status at 3-9 years. J Phys Act Health. 2015;12(4):506–14. https://doi.org/10.1123/jpah.2013-0173.

36. Currie S, Sinclair M, Murphy MH, Madden E, Dunwoody L, Liddle D. Reducing the decline in physical activity during pregnancy: a systematic review of behaviour change interventions. PLoS One 2013;14;8(6):e66385. doi: https://doi.org/10.1371/journal.pone.0066385.

37. Brobeck E, Odencrants S, Bergh H, Hildingh C. Patients' experiences of lifestyle discussions based on motivational interviewing: a qualitative study. BMC Nurs. 2014;13:13. https://doi.org/10.1186/1472-6955-13-13.

38. Pearce EE, Evenson KR, Downs DS, Steckler A. Strategies to promote physical activity during pregnancy: a systematic review of intervention evidence. Am J Lifestyle Med. 2013;1:7(1). https://doi.org/10.1177/1559827612446416.

39. Lindqvist M, Mogren I, Eurenius E, Edvardsson K, Persson M. "An on-going individual adjustment": a qualitative study of midwives' experiences counselling pregnant women on physical activity in Sweden. BMC Pregnancy Childbirth 2014;30;14:343. doi: https://doi.org/10.1186/1471-2393-14-343.

40. Ajzen I. The theory of planned behavior. Organ Behav Hum Decis Process. 1991;50:179–211.

16

Childbirth fear and related factors among pregnant and postpartum women in Malawi

Madalitso Khwepeya[1,2], Gabrielle T Lee[3], Su-Ru Chen[4] and Shu-Yu Kuo[4*] [iD]

Abstract

Background: Childbirth fear is a health concern in women living in high-income countries; however, little is known about childbirth fear among women living in low-income countries like Malawi. In this study, we explored childbirth fear and associated factors among pregnant and postpartum women in Malawi.

Methods: A cross-sectional study of 152 pregnant and 153 postpartum women was conducted at a district hospital in Malawi. Participants were assessed for childbirth fear using the Wijma Delivery Expectancy/Experience Questionnaire (WDEQ). Demographic and obstetric variables were collected using a structured questionnaire. The Multidimensional Scale of Perceived Social Support (MSPSS) was used to measure social support. Using a multinomial logistic regression, factors related to childbirth fears were examined, namely demographic and obstetric characteristics, and social support.

Results: The mean age of participants was 26 (standard deviation: 6.4) years. During pregnancy, 39% women reported a low level of fear, 41% reported moderate fear, and 20% reported high fear; while after birth, 49, 41, and 10% women reported low, moderate, and high fear, respectively. Pregnant women who were illiterate (odds ratio (OR): 5.0, $p < 0.01$) or unemployed (OR: 12.6, $p < 0.01$) were more likely to report moderate and high fear. Postpartum mothers who were illiterate (OR: 4.2, $p < 0.01$) or unemployed (OR: 11.8, $p < 0.01$) were more likely to have moderate and high fear. Furthermore, postpartum women who sustained perineal tears had significantly higher odds of experiencing moderate (OR: 5.3, $p < 0.01$) or high (OR: 19.9, $p < 0.01$) fear than their counterparts.

Conclusions: Childbirth fear is common in Malawi, and pregnant women are more likely to experience high levels of fear than postpartum women. This study highlighted the connection between childbirth fear with mother's education, employment, and perineal tears during delivery. Identifying and developing interventions for women with these associated characteristics is of clinical importance for the reduction of childbirth fear before and after childbirth in Malawi.

Keywords: Childbirth, Fear, Demographics, Obstetrics, Social support, Pregnancy, Postpartum period

Background

Childbirth fear is a health concern for women and their caregivers when expectant mothers are approaching birth or are in their postpartum transition [1, 2]. During pregnancy, women with childbirth fear often experience emotional distress [3, 4], and some might even request a cesarean section (CS) because of the fear [5, 6]. The CS rate has increased worldwide in recent years, and this may be associated with elective cesarean delivery on maternal request [7, 8]. After delivery, mothers with intense childbirth fear are more likely to have difficulties with maternal adjustment [9] and mother-child adaptation [10]. Previous research suggests that early identification of women at risk of childbirth fear and initiation of appropriate interventions are essential for women's emotional well-being before and after birth [11]. However, most studies were conducted in high-income countries, and little is known regarding childbirth fear in low-income countries, such as Malawi.

* Correspondence: sykuo@tmu.edu.tw
[4]School of Nursing, College of Nursing, Taipei Medical University, 250 Wuxing Street, Taipei 11031, Taiwan
Full list of author information is available at the end of the article

Childbirth fear can be described as feelings of uncertainty and anxiousness before, during, or after the delivery [12, 13]. Childbirth fear in pregnant women is assessed based on their expectations of anticipatory delivery, while childbirth fear in postpartum women is measured with women's actual childbirth experiences [12, 13]. Evidence suggests that socio-cultural factors and health care services are likely to influence the extent of childbirth fear and the consequences associated with the fear [14, 15]. In Malawi, maternal healthcare remains a major challenge due to high birth rates (41/1000 people) [16] and the lack of resources in the health care system [17–19]. Thus, mothers' childbirth fear is often not assessed and cared for before and after the delivery. Despite considerable efforts are made to improve antenatal care (pregnant mothers have to attend at least 4 visits before delivery), hospital delivery with skilled birth attendant (i.e., by physicians or midwives), and postnatal coverage (including 1 week and 6 weeks of postpartum check-up) [18, 20, 21], mothers in Malawi are likely to be afraid of childbirth due to socio-cultural beliefs (i.e., witchcraft), health care providers' attitudes (i.e., being rude), and lack of support/companion [22]. Childbirth fear continues to have a potential impact on women's wellbeing, and this needs to be addressed directly with constant assessments and adequate care.

Childbirth fear is common in both pregnant and postpartum women in developed countries. The prevalence of childbirth fear is estimated to range from 16 to 27% during pregnancy [5, 11–13], and around 22% after birth [13]. A study in Sweden by Alehagen et al. [23] found a positive association between childbirth fear during pregnancy and postpartum period. Zar et al. reported that women who were more afraid of childbirth during pregnancy were more likely to have fears during and after labor [24]. A prospective correlational design study by Fenwick et al. found that antenatal fear significantly predicted the levels of postnatal fear [25]. A review of the existing literature suggests that most of the studies on childbirth fear have either focused on pregnant or postpartum mothers, but not on both [23]. Understanding childbirth fear in both pregnant and postpartum mothers is necessary for developing comprehensive psychological maternal care programs.

Previous studies on childbirth fear suggest that the demographic, obstetric characteristics, and social support, are potential factors associated with childbirth fear among childbearing women [26–28]. Younger women are more likely to experience elevated fears than older women during childbirth [26]. Women who are not educated or not working are more likely to be fearful than their counterparts [26, 28]. First-time mothers are more prone to have childbirth fear than parous women [11, 29]. Mothers who sustain perineal tears during

delivery are at increased risk of being fearful [27]. A lack of social support is associated with childbirth fear in women [26]. To this date, no attempt has been made to understand such factors in Malawian women. Therefore, exploring these factors affecting women's childbirth fear is the first step towards establishing regular assessments, proper educational interventions, and the provision of mental health care to childbearing women in Malawi.

Given that previous research indicated that women's childbirth fear is related to their overall health and emotional well-being, it is imperative to explore such phenomena in Malawian women. To fill in gaps in the literature, we conducted a cross-sectional study to explore factors associated with childbirth fear in pregnant and postpartum women in Malawi. The specific aims of this research were to: (1) investigate the proportion of women who experience different levels of childbirth fear, and (2) examine factors such as demographic and obstetric characteristics, and social support, associated with childbirth fear in pregnant and postpartum women.

Methods

Study design

A cross-sectional study was conducted from August to September, 2015 at a district hospital in Malawi. The study site was one of the major referral heath facilities in Malawi with more than 22 health centers referring their patients for medical care. The hospital provided services to about 538,345 people and registered at least 1500 deliveries a month [30].

Study participants

Participants in this study were pregnant and postpartum women receiving prenatal and postnatal care at this district hospital. Potential participants were approached by the researchers or were referred by the nurse-midwives to participate in the study after receiving their antenatal and postpartum care. We included pregnant and postpartum women who a) were aged ≥18 years; b) understood and spoke Chichewa; c) were in their second or third trimester with a singleton pregnancy, or d) had delivered their babies less than 6 weeks previously of the postpartum period. Women who had high-risk perinatal conditions such as preeclampsia/eclampsia, hemorrhaging, or a medical or mental illness were excluded. This was confirmed by checking on patient-held health records and medical records. Considering this is the first attempt exploring childbirth fear in Malawi, both normal vaginal delivery and cesarean section women were included. Using G*Power calculator, the sample size calculation of the study was based on previous studies by Ryding et al. [31] and Johnson et al. [32]. To obtain a power of 80% at 5% significance level with an effect size of 0.4 in a two-tailed independent t-test, a sample of 200 participants with 100 in each group was required.

The study protocol was approved by the Institutional Review Board of the National Health Science Research Committee (NHSRC), Ministry of Health, Malawi. Furthermore, an approval was obtained from the study setting to conduct the study. Eligible participants provided written informed consent prior to their participation. An informed consent form was given to each participant to read and fill out. If the participants were illiterate, the researchers read out the consent form and helped the participants to fill out the questionnaires.

Measures
Translation process
The Wijma Delivery Expectancy/Experience Questionnaire (W-DEQ) A (expectancy) and B (experience) [13] and Multidimensional Scale of Perceived Social Support (MSPSS) [33, 34] were translated into Chichewa language following recommended guidelines by Wild et al. [35]. First, we obtained the permission to use the instruments from the original authors. Second, the original English versions were translated into Chichewa by a bilingual translator (forward translation). The translated versions were then checked and discussed for wording and clarity by several Malawian-speaking experts, including the researcher who had backgrounds in midwifery (reconciliation). Third, the Chichewa versions were translated back into English by three independent bilingual translators (back translation). The original and back-translated questionnaires were discussed and compared for clarity and inconsistencies to reach a consensus on the final versions. Fourth, a pilot study was conducted to assess the wording and adequacy of translated versions. The participants in the pilot study were 15 pregnant and 15 postpartum women at the antenatal check-up and postpartum ward in Malawi.

Childbirth fear
Childbirth fear was measured using the Chichewa version of the Wijma Delivery Expectancy/Experience Questionnaire (WDEQ) versions A and B [13]. Pregnant women were assessed using version A, and postpartum women were assessed using version B. The WDEQ is a 33-item self-reported questionnaire with a 6-point Likert scale ranging from 0 (not at all) to 5 (extremely), with a total score from 0 to 165. A score of ≤37 represents low fear, of 38~65 represents moderate fear, and of ≥66 represents high fear [13]. The original WDEQ reported a Cronbach's alpha of > 0.87 in nulliparous and multiparous women [13]. Our pilot study had a Cronbach's alpha of 0.78. The content validity index (CVI) was 0.93~0.95. In this study, the Cronbach's alphas of the Chichewa version of the WDEQ ranged 0.77~0.79.

Demographic and obstetric characteristics
Demographic and obstetric variables were examined using a structured questionnaire for each participant. Furthermore, these were checked in the patient-held health records with participants' permission. Demographic characteristics included age, educational level, employment status, and monthly income [26]. Obstetric characteristics included parity, mode of birth, perineal tears, and pregnancy complications [36].

Social support
Social support was assessed using the Multidimensional Scale of Perceived Social Support (MSPSS). The original questionnaire was developed by G. Zimet [34]. The MSPSS is a 12-item self-reported questionnaire with a 7-point Likert scale that ranges from 1 (very strongly disagree) to 7 (very strongly agree), with a total score ranging 12~84 [33]. The MSPSS measures the perception of social support from family, friends, and significant others, with higher scores indicating better perceived social support. The original MSPSS reported a Cronbach's alpha of 0.88 [34]. Our pilot study had a Cronbach's alpha of 0.83. The CVI was 1. In this study, the Cronbach's alphas of the Chichewa MSPSS ranged 0.81~0.84.

Statistical analysis
The Statistical Package for Social Sciences (SPSS) version 21 (SPSS, Chicago, IL, USA) was used for all analyses. Descriptive statistics summarizing participants' characteristics included the percentage, frequency, mean, and standard deviation (SD). Of bivariate analyses, t-tests were used for continuous variables (age and childbirth fear total score), and χ^2 tests (age, educational level, employment status, income, parity, preferred/mode of birth, perineal tears, past pregnancy complications, social support, and childbirth fear class) were used for categorical variables. Potential confounding variables were identified when the variables were significant at ≤0.10 and were then included for subsequent analysis. A multinomial logistic regression was used to determine factors associated with childbirth fear, and an α level of ≤0.05 was considered significant. Missing data ranged 0%~3.9% for all variables except age and are indicated with [++] in Table 1. The age variable had 9.2% missing values due to women's high illiteracy levels. Women who did not know their birth date were coded as having a missing value.

Results
Participants
Of the 307 eligible women who were invited and agreed to participate in this study, two pregnant women were excluded due to high-risk conditions of antepartum

Table 1 Characteristics of participants

Variable	Pregnant women (N = 152)		Postpartum women (N = 153)		χ^2	p
	n	(%)	n	(%)		
Age (years)[++], Mean (SD)	26.3	(6.6)	26.1	(6.3)		
< 25	73	(48.0)	75	(49.0)	0.01	0.91
≥ 25	65	(42.8)	65	(42.5)		
Education level[++]						
Illiterate	24	(15.8)	29	(19.0)	0.66	0.72
Primary school	99	(65.1)	94	(61.4)		
Secondary and higher	28	(18.4)	30	(19.6)		
Employment status[++]						
Unemployed	23	(15.1)	13	(8.5)	3.30	0.07
Employed	128	(84.2)	140	(91.5)		
Income per month						
< MK20,000	115	(75.7)	125	(81.7)	1.66	0.20
MK20,000~ 50,000	37	(24.3)	28	(18.3)		
Parity						
Nulliparous	30	(19.7)	43	(28.1)	2.93	0.09
Multiparous	122	(80.3)	110	(71.9)		
Preferred MOD[a]/Actual MOD[b++]						
Caesarean delivery	3	(2.0)	10	(6.5)	3.70	0.05
Normal vaginal birth	145	(95.4)	143	(93.5)		
Perineal tears[++]						
Yes	~	~	20	(13.1)	~	~
No			127	(83.0)		
Past pregnancy complications[++]						
Yes	33	(21.7)	44	(28.8)	2.10	0.15
No	119	(78.2)	108	(70.6)		
Social support, Mean (SD)	5.7	(0.9)	5.4	(0.9)		
Low/Moderate	35	(23.0)	47	(30.7)	2.30	0.13
High	117	(77.0)	106	(69.3)		

SD, Standard deviation; [a] Preferred Mode of Birth for pregnant women; [b] Actual Mode of Birth for postpartum women; *MK* Malawi Kwacha currency (US$1 ≈ Malawi Kwacha (MK)725); [++]Total amounts do not either add up to n = 152 (100%) for pregnant women or n = 153 (100%) for postpartum women

hemorrhaging and preterm labor. In total, 305 women participated, including 152 pregnant and 153 postpartum women. The mean age of pregnant women was 26.3 with Standard Deviation (SD) of 6.6 (Table 1). Most pregnant women were young (< 25 years; 48%), had a primary school education (65%), were employed (84%), and earned less than Malawi Kwacha (MK) 20,000/ month (76%). The majority of women were multiparous (80%) and preferred to have a normal vaginal birth (95%) rather than a CS. More than half reported no complications of past pregnancies (78%) and received high social support (77%). Our participants are representative of the population of childbearing women in Malawi. According to the Malawi Demographic Health Survey (MDHS) and other reports, the mean age of

childbearing women is 28.3 years. About 62% of women aged 15–49 have primary education, and 70% of married women are employed [21, 37].

Characteristics of the postpartum women were similar to those of pregnant women. The mean age of postpartum women was 26.1 (SD:6.3) (Table 1). The majority of the postpartum women were young (< 25 years; 49%), had a primary school education (61%), were employed (92%), and earned less than MK20,000/month (82%). More than half were multiparous (72%), had had a normal vaginal birth (94%), and had sustained no perineal tears (83%). Most women indicated no complications with past pregnancies (71%) and received high social support (69%). The χ^2 test showed that pregnant and postpartum women had similar characteristics ($p = 0.07 \sim 0.91$), except for the preferred mode of birth/actual mode of birth.

Levels of childbirth fear in pregnant and postpartum women

Pregnant women reported higher levels of fear (mean, 47) compared to postpartum women (mean, 42) (Table 2). Of the 152 pregnant women, 59 (39%) reported low levels of fear, 62 (41%) were moderately fearful, and 31 (20%) were highly fearful. Of the 153 postpartum women, 75 (49%) reported low levels of fear, 63 (41%) were moderately fearful, and 15 (10%) were highly fearful. Overall, compared to the pregnant women, the postpartum women reported a higher proportion of low fear ($\chi^2 = 7.48$, $p = 0.02$).

Factors associated with childbirth fear

Tables 3 and 4 shows the demographic and obstetric characteristics, and social support factors for the three levels of childbirth fear in pregnant and postpartum women that were related to childbirth fear in the multinomial logistic regression using 'Low fear' (WDEQ score of ≤37) as the reference group.

Results of the univariate analyses for pregnant women showed that being illiterate, not working, and receiving less social support were significantly associated with a higher level of fear, whereas age and parity were not (Table 3). After adjusting for age, parity, educational level, employment status, and social support as the variables listed in Table 3, the adjusted ORs (aORs) of all of the variables except for social support remained significant for moderate and high fear.

Results of the univariate analysis for postpartum women showed that having an emergency CS and sustaining perineal tears significantly increased the odds of having higher fear (Table 4). After adjusting for age, parity, mode of birth, and social support as listed in Table 4, being illiterate (aOR = 4.2) and having perineal tears (aOR = 5.3) were associated with moderate fear. Not working (aOR = 11.8) and sustaining perineal tears (aOR = 19.9) increased the risk of high fear.

Table 2 Childbirth fear in pregnant and postpartum women

Variable	Pregnant women (N = 152)		Postpartum women (N = 153)		Statistical value	p
	n	(%)	n	(%)		
Childbirth fear, Mean (SD)	46.9	(18.8)	42.2	(14.6)	2.48[a]	0.01
Low (≤37)	59	(38.8)	75	(49.0)	7.48[b]	0.02
Moderate (38~65)	62	(40.8)	63	(41.2)		
High (≥66)	31	(20.4)	15	(9.8)		

Note: SD Standard deviation; [a] t-test; [b] Chi-squared test

Discussion

The purpose of this study was to examine childbirth fear and related factors in pregnant and postpartum women in Malawi. Our results indicated that over 50% of women experienced moderate or high fear during the perinatal stage. In particular, pregnant women who were illiterate or unemployed were prone to have higher levels of childbirth fear. After birth, mothers who were illiterate, were unemployed, and had sustained perineal tears were at increased risk of having elevated fears. Perceived social support was not significantly associated with childbirth fear in pregnant or postpartum women. Our study extends the literature by examining factors correlated with women's childbirth fear in Malawi, a developing country with a unique culture.

Childbirth fear

Our study revealed that childbirth fear is common in Malawi. During pregnancy, about 20% of women had a relatively high level of fear (with a score on the WDEQ-A of ≥66), a distribution similar to previous studies that used the same assessment tool in Canadian (25%) [38], Australian (24%~ 27%) [25, 39], and Swedish (26%) [24] women. A recent review suggested that most studies on childbirth fear were conducted in high-income countries, and the prevalence estimate greatly varied due to different measures and definitions [40]. Results of our study indicated that childbirth fear also exists among women in a low-income country, and the level of childbirth fear was similar to those of women in high-income countries despite differences in birth rates, medical resources and practices, and cultural values [41, 42]. Childbirth as a natural event accompanied by labor pains and potentially unpredictable variables in the process might partly explain why women in different regions or cultures also share similar levels of childbirth fear [7, 43]. A study by Fenwick et al. revealed that women were concerned about the length of time experiencing pain and were more receptive to chemical forms of pain reduction [43]. However, women in a low-resource setting might not opt to receive pain medication during childbirth, as such medications are rare and expensive [44]. Offering women the option to receive pain medication and making the medication available upon request might ease women's childbirth fears. In high-resource countries, mental health care is usually an integrated part of healthcare systems. Besides medically necessary resources, care of women's emotional well-being during and after pregnancy often includes educational sessions on childbirth, opportunities for professional consultation, and meetings with various social support groups [45–47]. Addressing mental healthcare issues can be a challenging task in Malawi. Given the country's high rates of childbirth [15],

Table 3 Relationships of baseline characteristics with childbirth fear in pregnant women (N = 152)

Variable	Low fear (n = 59)		Moderate fear (n = 62)					High fear (n = 39)				
	n	(%)	n	(%)[a]	p	aOR (95% CI)[b]	p	n	(%)[a]	p	aOR (95% CI)[b]	p
Age (years)												
< 25	31	(56.4)	26	(44.8)	0.22	0.7 (0.3~ 1.6)	0.36	16	(64.0)	0.52	1.0 (0.3~ 3.1)	0.93
≥ 25	24	(43.6)	32	(55.2)		1.00		9	(36.0)		1.00	
Parity												
Nulliparous	14	(23.7)	11	(17.7)	0.42	1.3 (0.4~ 4.3)	0.62	5	(16.1)	0.40	1.0 (0.2~ 4.9)	0.96
Multiparous	45	(76.3)	51	(82.3)		1.00		26	(83.9)		1.00	
Educational level												
Illiterate	6	(10.2)	15	(24.6)	0.01	5.0 (1.2~ 20.2)	0.03	3	(9.7)	0.44	1.8 (0.2~ 17.8)	0.61
Primary school	37	(62.7)	38	(62.3)	0.14	2.2 (0.8~ 6.1)	0.13	24	(77.4)	0.12	3.0 (0.7~ 13.1)	0.16
Secondary and above	16	(27.1)	8	(13.1)		1.00		4	(12.9)		1.00	
Employment status												
No	4	(6.8)	5	(8.2)	0.77	1.5 (0.4~ 6.3)	0.57	14	(45.2)	< 0.001	12.6 (3.1~ 50.7)	< 0.001
Yes	55	(93.2)	56	(91.8)		1.00		17	(54.8)		1.00	
Social support												
Low/Moderate	8	(13.6)	14	(22.6)	0.20	1.5 (0.6~ 4.1)	0.43	13	(41.9)	< 0.01	3.0 (0.9~ 10.2)	0.09
High	51	(86.4)	48	(77.4)		1.00		18	(58.1)		1.00	

[a]The significance level of a univariate odds ratio denoted in this column if significant. [b] Adjusted odds ratio (aOR) and its 95% confidence interval (CI), obtained after statistical adjustment for all of the variables listed in this table

maternal mortality [48], and infant mortality [49], health care for women typically focuses on physical health while ignoring mental health. Our data clearly indicated that the level of childbirth fear was similar between Malawian women and women in high-resource countries, suggesting that the need for mental health care for women in Malawi is also essential to their overall well-being.

Our data indicated that relatively few postpartum women (10%) reported a high level of fear (WDEQ ≥66), compared to pregnant women. As reported by Fenwick et al. [25] and Zar et al. [12], women's fear levels over the perinatal period decreased for nulliparous and multiparous women in the high-fear group. However, Fenwick et al. [25] also pointed out that women who experienced childbirth interventions (e.g., a CS) may have an increased level of postpartum fear, and therefore, special attention and care are necessary for this population. Our study found postpartum women had low childbirth fear and this might possibly be related to the fact that the majority of our study sample were multiparous and had had a vaginal birth without additional interventions. Although our data also indicated a low proportion of fear after delivery, women's fear did not completely cease or disappear. Therefore, it is necessary to provide assessments and care on a regular basis following childbirth in order to prevent potential adverse outcomes that might have an impact on future pregnancies and childbirths [4].

Demographic factors associated with childbirth fear

In this study, we found a significant association between childbirth fear and women's educational level. Women who were illiterate were more likely to report a higher level of childbirth fear during pregnancy and in the postpartum period than their more highly educated counterparts. Previous work by Laursen et al. [26] and Salomonsson et al. [28] also found a significant association between these two factors, although the relationship between them was not clear. It is possible that uneducated women do not usually comprehend childbirth information and make informed choices. Conversely, Saisto et al. found no significant association between women's educational backgrounds and their fear of childbirth [50]. More research is needed to examine the association between women's educational level and childbirth fear. In any case, providing educational programs designed specifically for illiterate women in Malawi may help reduce their fears and promote their emotional well-being before and after childbirth.

We found that a woman's unemployment status was significantly associated with a higher level of fear during pregnancy and after childbirth. Our results concurred with previous studies in Denmark [26] and Finland [50], which also suggested that unemployed women were at higher odds of having childbirth fear. Saisto et al. [50] suggested that unemployment was a socioeconomic factor that may be linked to women's childbirth fear. On the contrary, other researchers reported that employed

Table 4 Relationships of baseline characteristics to childbirth fear in postpartum women (N = 153)

Variable	Low fear (n = 75)		Moderate fear (n = 63)					High fear (n = 15)				
	n	(%)	n	(%)[a]	p	aOR (95% CI)[b]	p	n	(%)[a]	p	aOR (95% CI)[b]	p
Age (years)												
< 25	36	(49.3)	31	(56.4)	0.43	1.0 (0.4~ 2.4)	0.99	8	(66.7)	0.27	1.8 (0.3~ 11.5)	0.52
≥ 25	37	(50.7)	24	(43.6)		1.00		4	(33.3)		1.00	
Parity												
Nulliparous	17	(22.7)	21	(33.3)	0.16	2.1 (0.8~ 5.9)	0.16	5	(33.3)	0.38	1.9 (0.3~ 14.2)	0.52
Multiparous	58	(77.3)	42	(66.7)		1.00		10	(66.7)		1.00	
Educational level												
Illiterate	9	(12.0)	17	(27.0)	0.21	4.2 (1.1~ 16.3)	0.04	3	(20.0)	0.63	0.3 (0.0~ 8.4)	0.47
Primary school	52	(69.3)	33	(52.4)	0.39	1.2 (0.4~ 3.3)	0.77	9	(60.0)	0.77	2.2 (0.3~ 17.0)	0.45
Secondary and above	14	(18.7)	13	(20.6)		1.00		3	(20.0)		1.00	
Employment status												
No	4	(5.3)	6	(9.5)	0.35	3.0 (0.6~ 14.6)	0.17	3	(20.0)	0.07	11.8 (1.3~ 108.4)	0.03
Yes	71	(94.7)	57	(90.5)		1.00		12	(80.0)		1.00	
Mode of birth												
Caesarean delivery	3	(4.0)	3	(4.8)	0.83	0.2 (0.0~ 2.4)	0.23	4	(26.7)	< 0.01	8.4 (0.8~ 86.7)	0.08
Normal vaginal birth	72	(96.0)	60	(95.2)		1.00		11	(73.3)		1.00	
Perineal tears												
Yes	5	(6.7)	9	(15.3)	0.12	5.3 (1.1~ 25.3)	0.04	6	(46.2)	< 0.01	19.9 (2.4~ 162.7)	< 0.01
No	70	(93.3)	50	(84.7)		1.00		7	(53.8)		1.00	
Social support												
Low/Moderate	23	(30.7)	17	(27.0)	0.64	0.8 (0.3~ 1.9)	0.61	7	(46.7)	0.24	1.7 (0.3~ 8.4)	0.53
High	52	(69.3)	46	(73.0)		1.00		8	(53.3)		1.00	

[a] The significance level of a univariate odds ratio denoted in this column if significant. [b] Adjusted odds ratio (aOR) and its 95% confidence interval (CI), obtained with statistical adjustment for all of the variables listed in this table

women were more likely to experience childbirth fear and seek treatment for psychological well-being [39, 51]. Toohill et al. [39] further reported that mothers who were employed were more likely to have a high level of fear, compared to mothers who were not engaged in paid work. Given the mixed results of women's employment status with childbirth fear, it is important to conduct more studies to further understand such associations in Malawian women. Our results suggest a need to incorporate mental health care into perinatal care for unemployed women in Malawi.

Obstetric factors associated with childbirth fear

The mode of birth was significantly related to childbirth fear in this study. However, the result was statistically insignificant after adjusting for other variables. Our results are similar to previous findings by Fenwick et al. [25] and Johnson et al. [32], who found no association between childbirth fear and a CS delivery. Johnson et al. in their study specified that most women were generally more frightened of childbirth (mean scores of the WDEQ of >60) across all types of delivery [32].

However, Ryding et al. did not find the same association but found that women who underwent a CS were at a greater risk of anxiety, had poorer stress-coping abilities, and had higher levels of childbirth fear [52]. Childbirth fear being associated with a CS may be attributed to negative birth experiences, and some women considered such a birth intervention to be a traumatic event [53]. Additionally, a CS is major surgery usually accompanied by poor physical and psychological outcomes [54–56]. Medical systems and cultural factors of different countries might contribute to the mixed results of childbirth fear and CS delivery [25]. In our study, most mothers clearly indicated their preference for a vaginal birth as opposed to a CS. As the CS rate is rising globally (26%) [8], the rate in Malawi is only around 5% [57], possibly due to limited access to CSs in Malawi. Although current conditions in Malawi do not allow women to have a CS by choice, this might not necessarily have an adverse impact on their childbirth fear. Instead, this creates an opportunity for women to reflect on their childbirth experiences in relation to their fears under professional guidance as recommended by other studies

[46] and not to choose a CS due to fear of childbirth. Future investigations on the association between a CS delivery and childbirth fear among perinatal women are needed.

We found that women with perineal damage (tears) after delivery tended to be at risk of childbirth fear. A study by Areskog et al. reported that women's fears were associated with physical damage to themselves [58]. Serçekuş et al. also reported a similar result in their qualitative study that women's fears may be associated with episiotomies [27]. A study conducted in Australia reported that concern about perineal tearing may lead to childbirth fear in childbearing women and the decision to have a CS as an easier option for birth [43]. In Malawi, episiotomy is not a standard practice. Therefore, the significant association between women's fear and perineal tears might be related to pains experienced during and after suturing. Furthermore, potential complications that underline sexual activities resulting from perineal tears might be of concern for some women [59]. Concerns about perineal damage by Malawian women warrant the need for healthcare professionals to attend to women's pain levels by administering anesthesia upon a woman's request, provide instructions for perineal management, inform the patient about potential complications, and facilitate checkup visits [60]. Furthermore, it is important that healthcare professionals take cautious actions to minimize the extent of perineal damage during birth in order to optimize birth and emotional outcomes.

Social support
Women in our study who received less social support during pregnancy reported higher levels of childbirth fear. However, the result was statistically insignificant after adjusting for other variables. Previous studies also reported that a woman's lack of social support was associated with childbirth fear [7, 26, 61], as having social support may act as a buffer in stressful situations [62]. However, Haines et al. refuted such a relationship and found that personal or social characteristics of women had no connection with childbirth fear, especially in rural townships with a sense of community that reduced the need for direct support [63]. This potentially explains why the results were not significant after adjusting for other confounders in our study. In Africa including Malawi, reproductive health issues such as childbirth are considered a woman's responsibility [64, 65]. Thus, women rely on each other in times of childbirth [66], hence fostering community support. Although social support was not significant after adjusting for other variables in pregnant women, identifying and providing long-lasting social support [50, 61] by families and significant others are vital during pregnancy.

Study limitations
When interpreting results of this study, some limitations need to be considered. Our study used a cross-sectional design to explore possible factors associated with childbirth fear which cannot show the cause-and-effect relationships. However, as the first study investigating childbirth fear in Malawi, our findings provide a basis for understanding childbirth fear in pregnant and postpartum women. Future studies can consider study designs that are longitudinal in nature to draw such causal inferences. The generalizability of results to high-risk women and other hospitals is limited, because our study only included women with no complications in a single hospital. We recommend further studies to incorporate high-risk women and women in various districts and central hospitals for the purpose of increasing generalizability. As most women in our study were illiterate, the researchers helped the illiterate participants to fill out the questionnaires. This could potentially underestimate their responses if they perceived less privacy.

Conclusions
Childbirth fear is common in Malawian women. Pregnant women tend to report high levels of childbirth fear, compared to postpartum women. The demographic and obstetric characteristics of the women were associated with childbirth fear during pregnancy and after childbirth. Early identification of women at risk of childbirth fear is of clinical importance in order to improve the health care for women during pregnancy and after the delivery in Malawi. Therefore, clinical attention to childbirth fear with comprehensive assessments and mental health care in Malawi is warranted.

Abbreviations
MK: Malawi Kwacha; MSPSS: Multidimensional Scale of Perceived Social Support; NHSRC: National Health Science Research Committee; WDEQ: Wijma Delivery Expectancy/Experience Questionnaire

Acknowledgements
Our appreciation goes to all the women who took part in this study and for their patience.

Funding
This study has been supported by research grants awarded by Ministry of Science and Technology (MOST 104–2314-B-038-008).

Authors' contributions

MK designed the study, prepared the data, and drafted the manuscript. GTL interpreted the data, read the entire manuscript critically, and revised the "Introduction" and "Discussion". SC participated in the design of the study and interpreted the data. SK designed the study, prepared data and statistical analysis, directed and revised the manuscript, and approved the final manuscript. All authors read and approved the final manuscript.

Authors' information

MK is a Registered Nurse Midwife at Machinga District Hospital, Malawi, and currently a doctoral student at the School of Nursing, College of Nursing, Taipei Medical University, Taipei, Taiwan. GTL is an Assistant Professor in the Faculty of Education at Western University in London, Canada. She is a licensed psychologist in Michigan, USA and a board certified behavior analyst. SC is an Associate Professor at School of Nursing, College of Nursing, Taipei Medical University, Taipei, Taiwan. SK is the Director and Associate Professor at School of Nursing, College of Nursing, Taipei Medical University, Taipei, Taiwan. SK is a registered nurse in the US and Taiwan and specializes in maternal and child health care.

Competing interests

The authors declare that they no competing interests.

Author details

[1]School of Nursing, College of Nursing, Taipei Medical University, Taipei, Taiwan. [2]Maternity Department, Machinga District Hospital, Liwonde, Malawi. [3]Applied Psychology, Faculty of Education, Western University, London, ON, Canada. [4]School of Nursing, College of Nursing, Taipei Medical University, 250 Wuxing Street, Taipei 11031, Taiwan.

References

1. Eriksson C, Westman G, Hamberg K. Content of childbirth-related fear in swedish women and men—analysis of an open-ended question. J Midwifery Womens Health. 2006;51(2):112–8.
2. Hofberg K, Ward M. Fear of pregnancy and childbirth. Postgrad Med J. 2003; 79(935):505–10.
3. Zar M, Wijma K, Wijma B. Relations between anxiety disorders and fear of childbirth during late pregnancy. Clin Psychol Psychother. 2002;9(2):122–30.
4. Hanna-Leena Melender R. Experiences of fears associated with pregnancy and childbirth: a study of 329 pregnant women. Birth. 2002;29(2):101–11.
5. Nieminen K, Stephansson O, Ryding EL. Women's fear of childbirth and preference for cesarean section–a cross-sectional study at various stages of pregnancy in Sweden. Acta Obstet Gynecol Scand. 2009;88(7):807–13.
6. Nilsson C, Lundgren I, Karlström A, Hildingsson I. Self reported fear of childbirth and its association with women's birth experience and mode of delivery: a longitudinal population-based study. Women Birth. 2012; 25(3):114–21.
7. Saisto T, Halmesmäki E. Fear of childbirth: a neglected dilemma. Acta Obstet Gynecol Scand. 2003;82(3):201–8.
8. Souza JP, Gülmezoglu A, Lumbiganon P, Laopaiboon M, Carroli G, Fawole B, et al. Caesarean section without medical indications is associated with an increased risk of adverse short-term maternal outcomes: the 2004-2008 who global survey on maternal and perinatal health. BMC Med. 2010;8(1):71.
9. Rouhe H, Salmela-Aro K, Toivanen R, Tokola M, Halmesmäki E, Ryding E-L, et al. Group psychoeducation with relaxation for severe fear of childbirth improves maternal adjustment and childbirth experience–a randomised controlled trial. J Psychosom Obstet Gynecol. 2015;36(1):1–9.
10. Salmela-Aro K, Read S, Rouhe H, Halmesmäki E, Toivanen RM, Tokola MI, et al. Promoting positive motherhood among nulliparous pregnant women with an intense fear of childbirth: Rct intervention. J Health Psychol. 2012; 17(4):520–34.
11. Salomonsson B, Alehagen S, Wijma K. Swedish midwives' views on severe fear of childbirth. Sex Reprod Healthc. 2011;2(4):153–9.
12. Wijma K. Why focus on 'fear of childbirth'? J Psychosom Obstet Gynaecol. 2003;24(3):141–3.
13. Wijma K, Wijma B, Zar M. Psychometric aspects of the w-deq; a new questionnaire for the measurement of fear of childbirth. J Psychosom Obstet Gynecol. 1998;19(2):84–97.
14. Stoll K, Fairbrother N, Thordarson DS. Childbirth fear: relation to birth and care provider preferences. J Midwifery Womens Health. 2018;63(1):58–67.
15. Morris T, McInerney K. Media representations of pregnancy and childbirth: an analysis of reality television programs in the United States. Birth. 2010; 37(2):134–40.
16. The world factbook [https://www.cia.gov/library/publications/the-world-factbook/fields/2054.html]. 22 Jan 2018.
17. Palmer D. Tackling malawi's human resources crisis. Reprod Health Matters. 2006;14(27):27–39.
18. Kongnyuy EJ, Hofman J, Mlava G, Mhango C, Van Den Broek N. Availability, utilisation and quality of basic and comprehensive emergency obstetric care services in Malawi. Matern Child Health J. 2009;13(5):687–94.
19. Leigh B, Mwale TG, Lazaro D, Lunguzi J. Emergency obstetric care: how do we stand in Malawi? Int J Gynecol Obstet. 2008;101(1):107–11.
20. Mamba KC, Muula AS, Stones W. Facility-imposed barriers to early utilization of focused antenatal care services in Mangochi district, Malawi–a mixed methods assessment. BMC Pregnancy Childbirth. 2017;17(1):444.
21. Office NS: Malawi demographic and health survey 2015–16. In.; 2017.
22. Kumbani L, Bjune G, Chirwa E, Odland JØ. Why some women fail to give birth at health facilities: a qualitative study of women's perceptions of perinatal care from rural southern Malawi. Reprod Health. 2013;10(1):9.
23. Alehagen S, Wijma B, Wijma K. Fear of childbirth before, during, and after childbirth. Acta Obstet Gynecol Scand. 2006;85(1):56–62.
24. Zar M, Wijma K, Wijma B. Pre-and postpartum fear of childbirth in nulliparous and parous women. Scand J Behav Ther. 2001;30(2):75–84.
25. Fenwick J, Gamble J, Nathan E, Bayes S, Hauck Y. Pre-and postpartum levels of childbirth fear and the relationship to birth outcomes in a cohort of australian women. J Clin Nurs. 2009;18(5):667–77.
26. Laursen M, Hedegaard M, Johansen C. Fear of childbirth: predictors and temporal changes among nulliparous women in the danish national birth cohort. BJOG Int J Obstet Gynaecol. 2008;115(3):354–60.
27. Serçekuş P, Okumuş H. Fears associated with childbirth among nulliparous women in Turkey. Midwifery. 2009;25(2):155–62.
28. Salomonsson B, Gullberg MT, Alehagen S, Wijma K. Self-efficacy beliefs and fear of childbirth in nulliparous women. J Psychosom Obstet Gynecol. 2013; 34(3):116–21.
29. Spice K, Jones SL, Hadjistavropoulos HD, Kowalyk K, Stewart SH. Prenatal fear of childbirth and anxiety sensitivity. J Psychosom Obstet Gynecol. 2009; 30(3):168–74.
30. Machinga district hospital [https://www.malawiproject.org/machinga-district-hospital/]. 26 June 2018.
31. Ryding E, Wijma B, Wijma K, Rydhström H. Fear of childbirth during pregnancy may increase the risk of emergency cesarean section. Acta Obstet Gynecol Scand. 1998;77(5):542–7.
32. Johnson R, Slade P. Does fear of childbirth during pregnancy predict emergency caesarean section? BJOG Int J Obstet Gynaecol. 2002;109(11):1213–21.
33. Zimet GD, Powell SS, Farley GK, Werkman S, Berkoff KA. Psychometric characteristics of the multidimensional scale of perceived social support. J Pers Assess. 1990;55(3–4):610–7.
34. Zimet GD, Dahlem NW, Zimet SG, Farley GK. The multidimensional scale of perceived social support. J Pers Assess. 1988;52(1):30–41.
35. Wild D, Grove A, Martin M, Eremenco S, McElroy S, Verjee-Lorenz A, et al. Principles of good practice for the translation and cultural adaptation process for patient-reported outcomes (pro) measures: report of the ispor task force for translation and cultural adaptation. Value Health. 2005; 8(2):94–104.
36. Rouhe H, Salmela-Aro K, Halmesmäki E, Saisto T. Fear of childbirth according to parity, gestational age, and obstetric history. BJOG Int J Obstet Gynaecol. 2009;116(1):67–73.
37. Malawi [https://knoema.com/atlas/Malawi/topics/Demographics/Fertility/Age-of-childbearing]. 22 June 2018.
38. Hall WA, Hauck YL, Carty EM, Hutton EK, Fenwick J, Stoll K. Childbirth fear, anxiety, fatigue, and sleep deprivation in pregnant women. J Obstet Gynecol Neonatal Nurs. 2009;38(5):567–76.

39. Toohill J, Fenwick J, Gamble J, Creedy DK. Prevalence of childbirth fear in an australian sample of pregnant women. BMC Pregnancy Childbirth. 2014;14(1):275.

40. O'Connell MA, Leahy-Warren P, Khashan AS, Kenny LC, O'Neill SM. Worldwide prevalence of tocophobia in pregnant women: systematic review and meta-analysis. Acta Obstet Gynecol Scand. 2017.

41. Stilwell B, Diallo K, Zurn P, Vujicic M, Adams O, Dal PM. Migration of health-care workers from developing countries: strategic approaches to its management. Bull World Health Organ. 2004;82(8):595–600.

42. Geubbels E. Epidemiology of maternal mortality in Malawi. Malawi Med J. 2006;18(4):208–28.

43. Fenwick J, Toohill J, Creedy D, Smith J, Gamble J. Sources, responses and moderators of childbirth fear in australian women: a qualitative investigation. Midwifery. 2015;31(1):239–46.

44. Kumbani LC, Chirwa E, Odland JØ, Bjune G. Do malawian women critically assess the quality of care? A qualitative study on women's perceptions of perinatal care at a district hospital in Malawi. Reprod Health. 2012;9(1):30.

45. Waldenström U, Hildingsson I, Ryding E-L. Antenatal fear of childbirth and its association with subsequent caesarean section and experience of childbirth. BJOG Int J Obstet Gynaecol. 2006;113(6):638–46.

46. Saisto T, Salmela-Aro K, Nurmi J-E, Könönen T, Halmesmäki E. A randomized controlled trial of intervention in fear of childbirth. Obstet Gynecol. 2001; 98(5):820–6.

47. Toohill J, Fenwick J, Gamble J, Creedy DK, Buist A, Turkstra E, et al. A randomized controlled trial of a psycho-education intervention by midwives in reducing childbirth fear in pregnant women. Birth. 2014;41(4):384–94.

48. The world factbook [https://www.cia.gov/library/publications/the-world-factbook/fields/2223.html]. 23 Jan 2018.

49. The world factbook [https://www.cia.gov/library/publications/the-world-factbook/fields/2091.html]. 30 Jan 2018.

50. Saisto T, Salmela-Aro K, Nurmi JE, Halmesmäki E. Psychosocial characteristics of women and their partners fearing vaginal childbirth. BJOG Int J Obstet Gynaecol. 2001;108(5):492–8.

51. Sydsjö G, Sydsjö A, Gunnervik C, Bladh M, Josefsson A. Obstetric outcome for women who received individualized treatment for fear of childbirth during pregnancy. Acta Obstet Gynecol Scand. 2012;91(1):44–9.

52. Ryding EL, Wijma K, Wijma B. Psychological impact of emergency cesarean section in comparison with elective cesarean section, instrumental and normal vaginal delivery. J Psychosom Obstet Gynecol. 1998;19(3):135–44.

53. Ryding EL, Wijma B, Wijma K. Posttraumatic stress reactions after emergency cesarean section. Acta Obstet Gynecol Scand. 1997;76(9):856–61.

54. Lobel M, DeLuca RS. Psychosocial sequelae of cesarean delivery: review and analysis of their causes and implications. Soc Sci Med. 2007;64(11):2272–84.

55. Chen MM, Hancock H. Women's knowledge of options for birth after caesarean section. Women Birth. 2012;25(3):e19–26.

56. Rowlands IJ, Redshaw M. Mode of birth and women's psychological and physical wellbeing in the postnatal period. BMC Pregnancy Childbirth. 2012; 12(1):138.

57. Cavallaro FL, Cresswell JA, França GV, Victora CG, Barros AJ, Ronsmans C. Trends in caesarean delivery by country and wealth quintile: cross-sectional surveys in southern asia and sub-saharan africa. Bull World Health Organ. 2013;91(12):914–22D.

58. Areskog B, Uddenberg N, Kjessler B. Fear of childbirth in late pregnancy. Obstet Gynecol Surv. 1982;37(5):313.

59. Signorello LB, Harlow BL, Chekos AK, Repke JT. Postpartum sexual functioning and its relationship to perineal trauma: a retrospective cohort study of primiparous women. Am J Obstet Gynecol. 2001;184(5):881–90.

60. Macarthur AJ, Macarthur C. Incidence, severity, and determinants of perineal pain after vaginal delivery: a prospective cohort study. Am J Obstetrics Gynecol. 2004;191(4):1199–204.

61. Toohill J, Fenwick J, Gamble J, Creedy DK, Buist A, Ryding EL. Psycho-social predictors of childbirth fear in pregnant women: an australian study. Open J Obstet Gynecol. 2014;4(09):531.

62. Turner RJ, Grindstaff CF, Phillips N. Social support and outcome in teenage pregnancy. J Health Soc Behav. 1990:43–57.

63. Haines H, Pallant JF, Karlström A, Hildingsson I. Cross-cultural comparison of levels of childbirth-related fear in an australian and swedish sample. Midwifery. 2011;27(4):560–7.

64. Kabagenyi A, Jennings L, Reid A, Nalwadda G, Ntozi J, Atuyambe L. Barriers to male involvement in contraceptive uptake and reproductive health services: a qualitative study of men and women's perceptions in two rural districts in Uganda. Reprod Health. 2014;11(1):21.

65. Kululanga LI, Sundby J, Chirwa E. Striving to promote male involvement in maternal health care in rural and urban settings in Malawi-a qualitative study. Reprod Health. 2011;8(1):36.

66. Rosato M, Mwansambo CW, Kazembe PN, Phiri T, Soko QS, Lewycka S, et al. Women's groups' perceptions of maternal health issues in rural Malawi. Lancet. 2006;368(9542):1180–8.

Foetal weight prediction models at a given gestational age in the absence of ultrasound facilities: application in Indonesia

Dewi Anggraini[1,2]* iD, Mali Abdollahian[1] and Kaye Marion[1]

Abstract

Background: Birth weight is one of the most important indicators of neonatal survival. A reliable estimate of foetal weight at different stages of pregnancy would facilitate intervention plans for medical practitioners to prevent the risk of low birth weight delivery. This study has developed reliable models to more accurately predict estimated foetal weight at a given gestation age in the absence of ultrasound facilities.

Methods: A primary health care centre was involved in collecting retrospective non-identified Indonesian data. The best subset model selection criteria, coefficient of determination, standard deviation, variance inflation factor, Mallows C_p, and diagnostic tests of residuals were deployed to select the most significant independent variables. Simple and multivariate linear regressions were used to develop the proposed models. The efficacy of models for predicting foetal weight at a given gestational age was assessed using multi-prediction accuracy measures.

Results: Four weight prediction models based on fundal height and its combinations with gestational age (between 32 and 41 weeks) and ultrasonic estimates of foetal head circumference and foetal abdominal circumference have been developed. Multiple comparison criteria show that the proposed models were more accurate than the existing models (mean prediction errors between − 0.2 and 2.4 g and median absolute percentage errors between 4.1 and 4. 2%) in predicting foetal weight at a given gestational age (between 35 and 41 weeks).

Conclusions: This research has developed models to more accurately predict estimated foetal weight at a given gestational age in the absence of ultrasound machines and trained ultra-sonographers. The efficacy of the models was assessed using retrospective data. The results show that the proposed models produced less error than the existing clinical and ultrasonic models. This research has resulted in the development of models where ultrasound facilities do not exist, to predict the estimated foetal weight at varying gestational age. This would promote the development of foetal inter growth charts, which are currently unavailable in Indonesian primary health care systems. Consistent monitoring of foetal growth would alleviate the risk of having inter growth abnormalities, such as low birth weight that is the most leading factor of neonatal mortality.

Keywords: Fundal height, Gestational age, Estimated foetal head circumference, Estimated foetal abdominal circumference, Regression analysis, Foetal weight estimation, Absence of ultrasound facilities, Primary health care centre, Prediction accuracy, Indonesia

* Correspondence: dewi.anggraini@rmit.edu.au; dewi.anggraini@ulm.ac.id
[1]School of Science (Mathematical and Geospatial Sciences), College of Science, Engineering, and Health, RMIT University, GPO BOX 2476, Melbourne, VIC 3001, Australia
[2]Study Program of Statistics, Faculty of Mathematics and Natural Sciences, University of Lambung Mangkurat (ULM), Ahmad Yani Street, Km. 36, Banjarbaru, South Kalimantan 70714, Indonesia

Background

Birth weight is a primary measurement and significant indicator to ensure the optimal growth, survival, and future well-being of new-borns. Deviation from normal delivery weights (2500–3999 g), such as low birth weight (LBW) (< 2500 g) and macrosomia (> 4000 g) could lead to some negative consequences on neonatal health [1–3]. While macrosomia may cause neonatal and maternal morbidity [4], LBW is well-documented to be one of the most contributing factors to the neonatal mortality [1]. LBW is defined as weight less than 2500 g at birth regardless of gestational age (GA) and can be caused by preterm birth or intrauterine growth restriction [5]. In this paper, LBW includes both preterm and term new-borns of appropriate for GA.

Routine and reliable estimates of foetal weight at a given GA throughout pregnancy are vital. These estimates could create evidence-based track records/analysis to assist medical practitioners to detect the signs of potential LBW during pregnancy and provide the appropriate interventions. Although a wide range of simple and advanced multivariate weight prediction models based on clinical and ultrasonic measurements has been developed, most are only based on maternal or foetal factors [6–25]. Less is known about the combinations of these characteristics to estimate foetal weight during pregnancy despite the fact that birth weight is significantly associated with characteristics of both mother and foetus [1, 26].

Several models based on combined maternal and neonatal characteristics have been developed and reviewed, these existing models were mostly developed based on the information available at delivery time [27, 28]. In most developing countries, the availability of foetal biometric measurements during pregnancy is low, particularly in rural areas due to limited access to ultrasound machines and skilled personnel [29]. Westerway et al. (2000), Loughna et al. (2009), and Papageorghiou et al. (2014) have used a large number of ultrasonic measurements to develop formulas that estimate foetal biometric characteristics at a given GA [30–32]. These formulas then could be used to fill the foetal database gaps during pregnancy when ultrasound facility is absent.

The present research develops foetal weight prediction models based on combined maternal and estimated foetal biometric characteristics to estimate foetal weight at any given GA. The proposed models can be simply implemented in low-resource primary health care centres where ultrasound machines and trained ultra-sonographers are not always available. The predicted foetal weight will assist in the development of foetal growth charts for Indonesia. No such charts currently exist for the Indonesian population.

Methods
Study design and setting

A quantitative and analytic study based on a retrospective pregnancy cohort analysis was carried out. Unidentified secondary quantitative data were collected and analysed to (1) assess the adequacy of the existing ultrasonic models in estimating foetal biometric characteristics, (2) develop new foetal weight prediction models based on both maternal and estimated foetal biometric characteristics, (3) assess the accuracy of the proposed models in predicting foetal weight between 35 and 41 weeks of GA, and (4) carry out a comparison study between the proposed and commonly used models. The study was conducted in a primary health care centre in South Kalimantan province, Indonesia. The locality was selected because it is one of the five provinces with the highest neonatal mortality in the country [33–35].

Conceptual framework

Figure 1 shows the framework used in this study, along with the selected possible predictors of foetal weight estimation.

Data source

Study data were sourced primarily from a paper-based pregnancy register of pregnant women who received antenatal care (ANC) services and gave birth in the selected primary health care centre from January 2013 to August 2015. Prior to delivery, GA, fundal height (FH), foetal head engagement/foetal station (FS), and recorded foetal weight estimation (EFW$_r$) at a given GA were measured and recorded by the assigned midwives. At delivery time, actual birth weight (ABW), neonatal head circumference (HC), and neonatal abdominal circumference (AC) were also measured and recorded.

Data management

Data was recorded in Microsoft Excel and the statistical analyses were performed using Minitab version 17 and R. The ordinary least square (OLS) and robust regression (the weighted likelihood estimation) were carried out by using *lm* function and *wle.lm* function, respectively in R [36–39].

Statistical analysis
The adequacy assessment of existing ultrasonic models to estimate foetal biometric characteristics during pregnancy

The existing ultrasonic formulas to estimate foetal HC and foetal AC which were developed based on the Australian foetal biometry data (measured between 11 and 41 weeks), the UK foetal biometry data (measured between 13 and 42 weeks), and the international foetal biometry data (measured between 14 and 42 weeks or until birth) [30–32] (provided in Additional file 1: Table S1) were applied to estimate foetal HC and foetal AC at a given GA for Indonesian foetus (n = 127). A reliability analysis using intraclass correlation coefficient (ICC) [40, 41] was performed to assess the consistency of the ultrasonic

Foetal weight prediction models at a given gestational age in the absence of ultrasound...

179

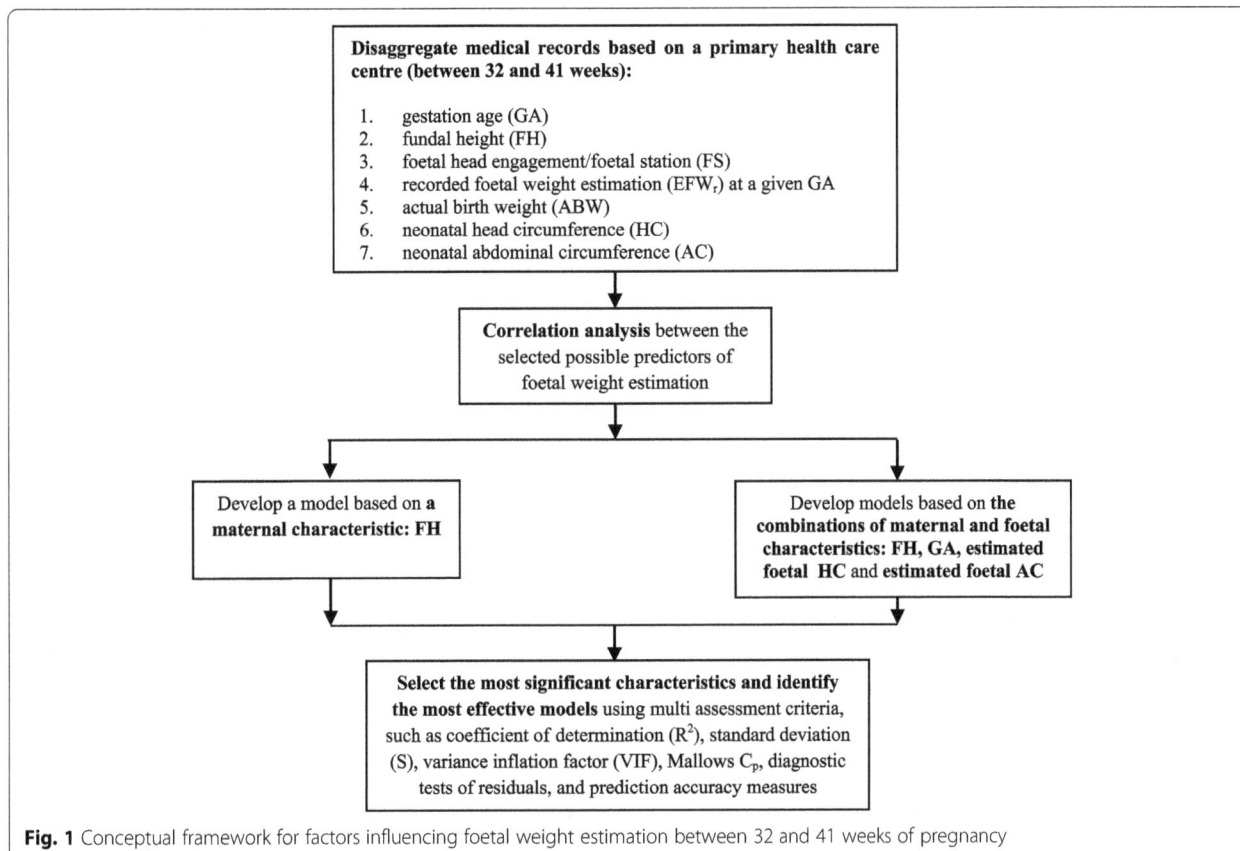

Fig. 1 Conceptual framework for factors influencing foetal weight estimation between 32 and 41 weeks of pregnancy

formulas for Indonesian population. The obtained ICC values (provided in Additional file 2: Table S2) were computed by single-rating, consistency, and two-way random effects models for the foetal biometrics with three raters (different ultrasonic formulas) across 127 subjects (pregnant women). Interclass (Pearson) correlation coefficient was also analysed to assess whether there is a significant relationship between the predicted foetal biometrics and the neonatal measurements recorded at delivery time (provided in Additional file 3: Table S3).

The development of new foetal weight prediction models based on combinations of maternal and estimated foetal biometric characteristics

Bernoulli distribution with the event probability (p) of 70% was used to randomly divide our data into two sets: model development (training) data ($n = 89$) and model efficacy assessment (testing) data ($n = 38$).

Based on the training data set, simple and multivariate linear regressions were used to develop our proposed models. The best subset selection methodology together with correlation coefficient (r), coefficient of determination (R^2), standard deviation (S), Mallows C_p, and variance inflation factor (VIF) were deployed to identify the most suitable subset of predictors. Analysis of variance (ANOVA) together with t-test statistics was used to

simultaneously and partially confirm the significance of predictors' contribution in the regression models. Diagnostic tests of residuals were used to confirm the validity of the regression models.

Since our aim is to investigate whether a combination of maternal and foetal factors could improve foetal weight prediction accuracy, we have utilised the most commonly recommended formulas of ultrasonic foetal measurement standards (based on GA) to predict the measurements of foetal biometrics in our local population. This prediction is one way to fill in the foetal database gaps during pregnancy in the absence of ultrasound. The estimates of these two most significant characteristics of foetal biometry, such as HC and AC were then combined with maternal FH to develop the prediction models. The idea of this combination was to evaluate whether it could improve the prediction accuracy of foetal weight.

Our delivery date in our data ranged from 32 to 41 weeks. The ultrasonic formulas were deployed to estimate foetal HC and foetal AC at the given GA for each individual patient and used to estimate the delivery weight. Therefore, the mean time between the last measurements of FH and GA as well as the last estimates of foetal HC and foetal AC and birth was assumed to be 0 days.

The efficacy assessment of the proposed models

The testing data set was used to validate and assess the efficacy of the proposed models. The potential bias due to growth between the last measurements and birth of the developed models for estimating foetal weight was assessed by calculating the mean prediction error [the average of the differences between the ith actual values of birth weight (ABW_i) and the ith predicted values of foetal weight based on the proposed models (EFW_{p_i})]$= \sum_{i=1}^{n} \frac{(ABW_i - EFW_{p_i})}{n}$. The mean absolute percentage prediction error or $MAPE = \sum_{i=1}^{n} \frac{|(\frac{ABW_i - EFW_{p_i}}{ABW_i} \times 100)|}{n}$ was also calculated to represent the dispersion of the errors [42]. In addition, the median absolute percentage prediction error or $MEDAPE = Median |(\frac{ABW_i - EFW_{p_i}}{ABW_i} \times 100)|$ was measured and used for assessing the efficacy of the models. The later measurement is more resistant to outlier distortion (due to the presence of extreme deviations) than the mean; therefore, deploying $MEDAPE$ would eliminate the false interpretation of forecast accuracy [43].

The efficacy of the proposed models was also assessed by the number of estimates within 10% of ABW. A two independent sample t-test was used to decide if there is a significant difference between the observed or actual values of birth weight (ABW), EFW_p, and estimated foetal weights based on the proposed models (EFW_p). Multiple comparisons were carried out between our proposed models, eleven existing clinical models, and six existing ultrasonic models to select the most effective models for estimating foetal weights at a given GA.

Results

Out of 146 women who received ANC services and gave birth in the selected primary health care centre, 127 (87%) women met the study criteria (Fig. 2). These women delivered live singletons with normal delivery weights between 32 and 41 weeks of GA. We excluded 19 (13%) women due to incomplete information on the required characteristics listed in Fig. 2, such as no records of GA, FH, and FS ($n = 3$), GA > 41 weeks ($n = 2$), been referred to hospitals due to pregnancy complications ($n = 6$), and abnormal birth weight babies ($n = 8$).

General information on the study population

Descriptive statistics on baseline characteristics of mother and new-born of the study population ($n = 127$) are presented in Table 1. Overall, the pregnant women were well-nourished (arm circumference = 25.5 cm) and had normal haemoglobin level (11.6 g/dl) and body mass index (24.4 kg/m^2). The median age, height, weight, and FH for women were 28 years (range 16–44 years), 156 cm (range 148–176 cm), 60 kg (range 44–83 kg), and 32 cm (range 27–

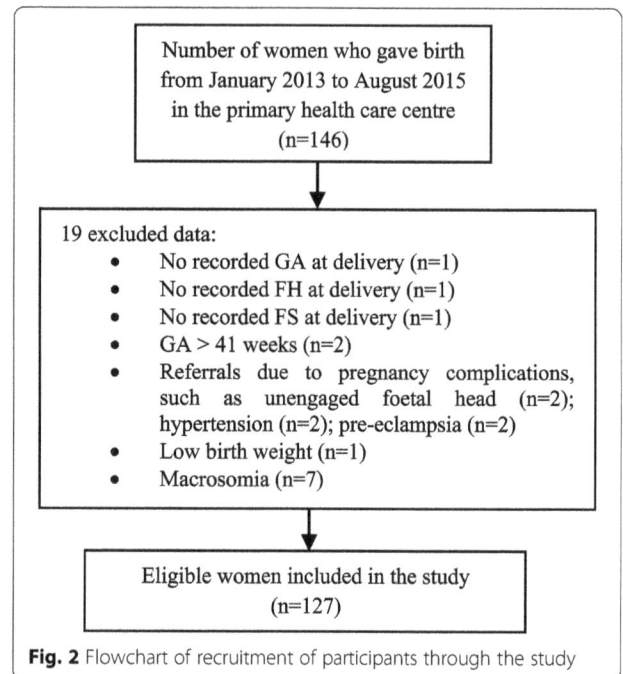

Fig. 2 Flowchart of recruitment of participants through the study

36 cm), respectively. The outcomes of pregnancy were in a normal average of GA (38 weeks), delivery weight (3252.8 g), birth length (50.2 cm), neonatal HC (33.5 cm), and neonatal AC (34.5 cm).

The reliability assessment of existing ultrasonic formulas in estimating foetal biometrics

This section presents the results of reliability analysis among three existing ultrasonic formulas [30–32] listed in Additional file 1: Table S1 in predicting foetal biometrics when ultrasound facilities are not accessible.

The intraclass and interclass correlation coefficient analyses are presented in Additional files 2 and 3: Table S2 and S3, respectively. The results presented in Additional file 2: Table S2 indicate that all three formulas have excellent reliability/consistency in predicting foetal HC and foetal AC at a given GA (the obtained ICC values are 0.957 and 0.996, respectively). Therefore, either of the existing formulas can be deployed in our study population.

Additional file 3: Table S3 shows that the estimated ultrasonic HC has a significant relationship with the neonatal HC (p-value < 0.0005) based on the existing models although the relationship was weak ($0.191 < r < 0.212$). Meanwhile, there is no significant correlation between the estimated ultrasonic AC and the neonatal AC ($0.076 < r < 0.078$, p-value > 0.05). However, since the Australian standard formulas produced slightly higher interclass correlation coefficients (between the estimates of foetal biometrics and the neonatal measurements) and more estimates falling within 10% of the neonatal measurements; therefore, the ultrasonic formulas based

Table 1 Maternal and neonatal baseline characteristics of study population ($n = 127$)

Characteristics	Missing data	Mean	Standard deviation	Median	Minimum	Maximum
Maternal age (years)	–	27.6	4.9	28	16	44
Maternal height (cm)	3	156.5	5.0	156	148	176
Maternal weight (kg)	–	59.9	7.5	60	44	83
Maternal body mass index (kg/m^2)	3	24.4	3.1	24.3	16.5	34.2
Maternal arm circumference (cm)	1	25.5	1.7	25	22	31
Maternal haemoglobin level (g/dl)	–	11.6	0.7	11.4	9	13.2
Maternal fundal height (FH) at delivery time (cm)	–	32.2	2.4	32	27	36
Gestational age (GA) at delivery time (weeks)	–	38.6	1.5	39	32	41
Actual birth weight (ABW) (g)	–	3252.8	340.8	3300	2600	4000
Neonatal birth length (cm)	–	50.2	2	50	40	56
Neonatal head circumference (HC) (cm)	–	33.5	1.3	33	29	37
Neonatal abdominal circumference (AC) (cm)	–	34.5	1.9	35	28	37

on the Australian population will be deployed to fill the foetal database gaps and assist the development of our proposed models.

Correlation analysis

Prior to developing models, correlations between the potential predictors of foetal weight estimation based on 127 data were investigated. The correlation analysis is presented in Additional file 4: Table S4.

Additional file 4: Table S4 shows that maternal FH has a significant correlation with the EFW$_r$ and the ABW (r = 0.952, p-value < 0.0005 and r = 0.795, p-value < 0.0005, respectively). Unlike FH, GA has no significant correlation with the EFW$_r$ and ABW.

Optimal models based on the best subset selection algorithm

Deploying the best subset selection algorithm, we have summarised the models developed based on the EFW$_r$ (provided in Additional file 5: Table S5). These models were based on one, two, and three independent variables. The table also lists their corresponding R^2, Mallows Cp, S, and VIF statistics.

Additional file 5: Table S5 shows that the first model incorporated only one predictor: FH. The second, third, and fourth models incorporated two predictors: FH and GA, FH and estimated foetal HC, and FH and estimated foetal AC, respectively. The last model was developed based on three predictors: FH, estimated foetal HC, and estimated foetal AC.

Overall, the developed models had equal capability in predicting foetal weight estimation (coefficient of determination between 88.3 and 88.8%). However, using Mallows Cp index and S, we concluded that Models (3) and (4) were the best fit models with the least predicting errors. Models based only on estimated foetal HC or estimated foetal AC was excluded from the analysis due to

the insignificant R^2. Model (5) was excluded due to the presence of severe multicollinearity ($VIF > 193$) (provided in Additional file 5: Table S5).

Table 2 presents the coefficients of the predictors for the chosen models together with the corresponding p-values of ANOVA, t-test statistics, and diagnostics of residuals.

Table 2 shows that for each individual model, the p-value corresponding to independent predictors is significant. Since our sample size is large, statistically significant non-normality of residuals was accepted. However, the authors have deployed robust regression to find the best fit models. Unfortunately, the best fit models proposed by robust regression had slightly larger prediction errors than those selected through the best subset models. Therefore, our further analysis is carried out using the OLS regression models presented in Table 2.

The accuracy comparison of the proposed and existing models

The two most commonly used models in Indonesia for estimating delivery weight are the Johnson-Toshach and the Risanto models. Both models estimate foetal weight based on FH. However, the Johnson-Toshach formula, which is nationally well-recognised, requires additional information on the status of the FS [44].

As listed in Table 2, the first model recommended through the best selection algorithm was Model (1) which is also developed based on FH only. Therefore, the authors carried out further comparisons between the proposed Model (1) and the widely used the Johnson-Toshach [14, 15] and the Risanto models [22, 23] as well as other existing models for estimating foetal weight based only on FH (the Niswander, the modified Niswander, the Mhaskar, the Gayatri-Afiyanti, the Buchmann-Tlale, the Santjaka-Handayani, the Mongelli-Gardosi, and the Yiheyis [16–18, 22–25, 45]). We also compared Models (2), (3), and (4) with the existing models based on ultrasonic measurements of foetal

Table 2 Predictor analysis of the proposed models

Model	Parameters	Estimated coefficients	Simultaneous p-value (ANOVA)	Partial p-value (t-test)	VIF	Residuals
(1)	β_0 (Intercept)	− 1538.3	< 0.0005[***]	2.66e-12[***]	–	Non-normal (p-value < 0.005)
	β_1 (FH)	150. 3		< 2e-16[***]	–	
(2)	β_0 (Intercept)	− 959	< 0.0005[***]	0.011[*]		Non-normal (p-value < 0.005)
	β_1 (GA)	−15.8		0.071[*]	1.01	
	β_2 (FH)	151.2		< 0.0005[***]	1.01	
(3)	β_0 (Intercept)	− 634.3	< 0.0005[***]	0.2304	–	Non-normal (p-value < 0.005)
	β_1 (FH)	151.2		< 2e-16[***]	1.01	
	β_2 (estimated HC)	−2.8		0.0682[*]	1.01	
(4)	β_0 (Intercept)	−996.8	< 0.0005[***]	0.00548[**]	–	Non-normal (p-value < 0.005)
	β_1 (FH)	151.2		< 2e-16[***]	1.01	
	β_2 (estimated AC)	−1.6		0.07066[*]	1.01	

[***]Significant at p-value < 0.0005
[**]Significant at p-value < 0.05
[*]Significant at alpha p-value < 0.1

biometrics, such as foetal HC and foetal AC (the Jordaan, the Weiner, the Hadlock 1984, and the Stirnemann [10, 42, 46, 47]). Details for the proposed and existing models are presented in Additional file 6: Table S6.

The prediction accuracy of the proposed (Models (1), (2), (3), and (4) in Table 2) and the existing models were assessed using the testing data set. The predicting errors were calculated as the mean prediction error (the average of the differences between ABW_i and EFW_{p_i}), the $MAPE$, and the $MEDAPE$. The results are presented in Table 3.

Table 3 shows that the mean prediction errors recorded for the proposed models are significantly smaller (between − 0.2 and 2.4 g) than those recorded for other existing models. Similarly, the MAPEs and MEDAPEs recorded for the proposed models are significantly smaller (between 5.0 and 5.1% and between 4.1 and 4.2%, respectively) than those recorded for other existing models. Therefore, we concluded that our four proposed models were capable to predict estimated foetal weight with less errors compare with the existing models between 35 and 41 weeks of pregnancy. The visualisation of these multiple comparisons can be seen in Fig. 3.

Furthermore, a two independent sample t-test (provided in Additional file 7: Table S7) was also used to investigate if there is a significant difference between the observed and estimated foetal weights based on the proposed models. The results show that there is no significant difference between the observed and estimated foetal weights based on the proposed models (p-value > 0.05).

Assessing the prediction accuracy based on proportion falling between 10% of actual values

Table 3 presents the prediction ability of the proposed models, 11 existing clinical models (based on FH only),

and 6 existing ultrasonic models (based on ultrasonic measurements of foetal HC and foetal AC as well as based on GA only). The table provides the total number of predictions falling within 10% of ABW.

Table 3 shows that 92% of the predicted values produced by our proposed Model (1) fall within the 10% of ABW compared with 89% for the Johnson-Toshach model and 84% of the Risanto models. However, Model (1) only uses FH to predict foetal weight, while the Johnson-Toshach model requires information on FH as well as FS. Therefore, we recommend that Model (1) be used instead of the Johnson-Toshach model.

Model (1) (based on FH only) is equally capable to estimate foetal weight as Models (2) and (4). These results imply that the inclusion of GA (which is not a biometric measurement of foetus) and estimated foetal AC do not have an impact on estimated foetal weight accuracy. Our results are in agreement with the previous study conducted by Huber (2014) [48].

Comparing the accuracy of Model (3) (based on FH and estimated foetal HC) and Model (4) (based on FH and estimated foetal AC) with the Hadlock 1984 model (based on ultrasonic measurements of foetal HC and foetal AC) [10], we concluded that both proposed Models (3) and (4) were significantly more capable in predicting foetal weight than the Hadlock model. Table 3 shows that the proportion of predicted birth weights falling within the 10% of ABW for Models (3) and (4) are more than double the proportion based on the Hadlock model.

Discussion

Our study highlights that the use of combined maternal and estimated foetal biometric characteristics can provide a reliable estimate of delivery weights

Table 3 Accuracy comparisons between the proposed and existing models

Sample size $n = 38$

(ABW - EFW$_p$)	Mean prediction error (g)	MAPE (%)	MEDAPE (%)	Error distribution	Number of estimates within 10% of ABW (%)
Our recommended models					
Model (1)	2.42	5.01	4.10	Normal (*p*-value > 0.05)	92
Model (2)	−0.20	5.10	4.16		92
Model (3)	−1.62	5.10	4.22		89
Model (4)	−0.29	5.10	4.16		92
Existing clinical models					
Johnson (1957) [15]	31.18	5.28	4.73	Normal (*p*-value > 0.05)	89
Risanto I (1995) [22]	149.56	5.95	5.37		84
Risanto II (2014) [23]	152.37	6.00	5.45		84
Niswander (1970) [16]	400.95	12.24	12.07		37
Mod Niswander (1999) [17]	457.68	13.70	14.16		29
Mhaskar (2003) cited in [65]	405.26	12.59	12.86		32
Gayatri (2006) [24]	471.05	14.02	15.15		26
Buchmann-Tlale (2009) [18, 66]	571.05	17.12	18.18		11
Santjaka (2011) [25]	− 2411.95	75.33	72.24		0
Mongelli-Gardosi (2004) [19]	1348.35	41.93	42.40		0
Yiheyis (2016) [45]	363.95	11.12	11.05		45
Existing ultrasonic models					
Jordaan (1983) [46]	− 277.09	14.64	14.43	Normal (*p*-value > 0.05)	39
Weiner II (1985) cited in [60]	486.29	15.90	12.86		32
Hadlock 1984 [10]	−96.83	12.67	12.64		45
Hadlock 1991 [67]	− 42.75	11.74	9.88		50
Stirnemann 2016 [42]	−31.46	12.20	10.88		39
Sotiriadis 2017 [68]	230.72	10.88	9.43		50

between 35 and 41 weeks of GA. This result confirms the previous study that shows a significant association between birth weight and characteristics of mother and foetus [1, 26].

Both clinical and estimates of ultrasonic predictors are used in our proposed models. Maternal FH measurement was selected as one of the clinical predictors as it is one of the most recommended and accessible predictors to estimate foetal weight and monitor foetal growth during pregnancy [3, 23, 49, 50]. Although the clinical approach using FH screening had reportedly low sensitivity for detecting intergrowth and birth weight abnormalities (ranged 16–45%) [51, 52], it is a simple and inexpensive clinical activity [29, 53], especially true in rural areas where ultrasound machines and skilled personnel are not always available. The utility of FH remains an important first level screening tool, widely used during routine ANC in both high and low income settings [29] even though it had high false-negative rates for small for GA [53].

In ultrasonic settings, foetal biometric characteristics monitored during pregnancy include HC, biparietal diameter (BPD), occipitofrontal diameter (OFD), AC, and femur length (FL). These characteristics are routinely measured by ultrasound every 5 weeks after the first initial dating scan (between 8 and 14 weeks' gestation). The standard ranges for ultrasonic measurements are (14–18), (19–23), (24–28), (29–33), (34–38), and (39–42) weeks [54] or at least once every trimester of pregnancy, i.e. between weeks 10–14 (first trimester), 20–24 (second trimester), and 30–32 (third trimester) [55].

Assessment of foetal biometric characteristics during ANC is vital to ensuring normal foetal size and safe delivery. In the absence of ultrasound facility, particularly in low-resource primary health care settings, the measurements of these characteristics are not always accessible. Therefore, a reliable prediction of these characteristics during pregnancy would be a proxy of foetal biometrics and vitally improve the quality of

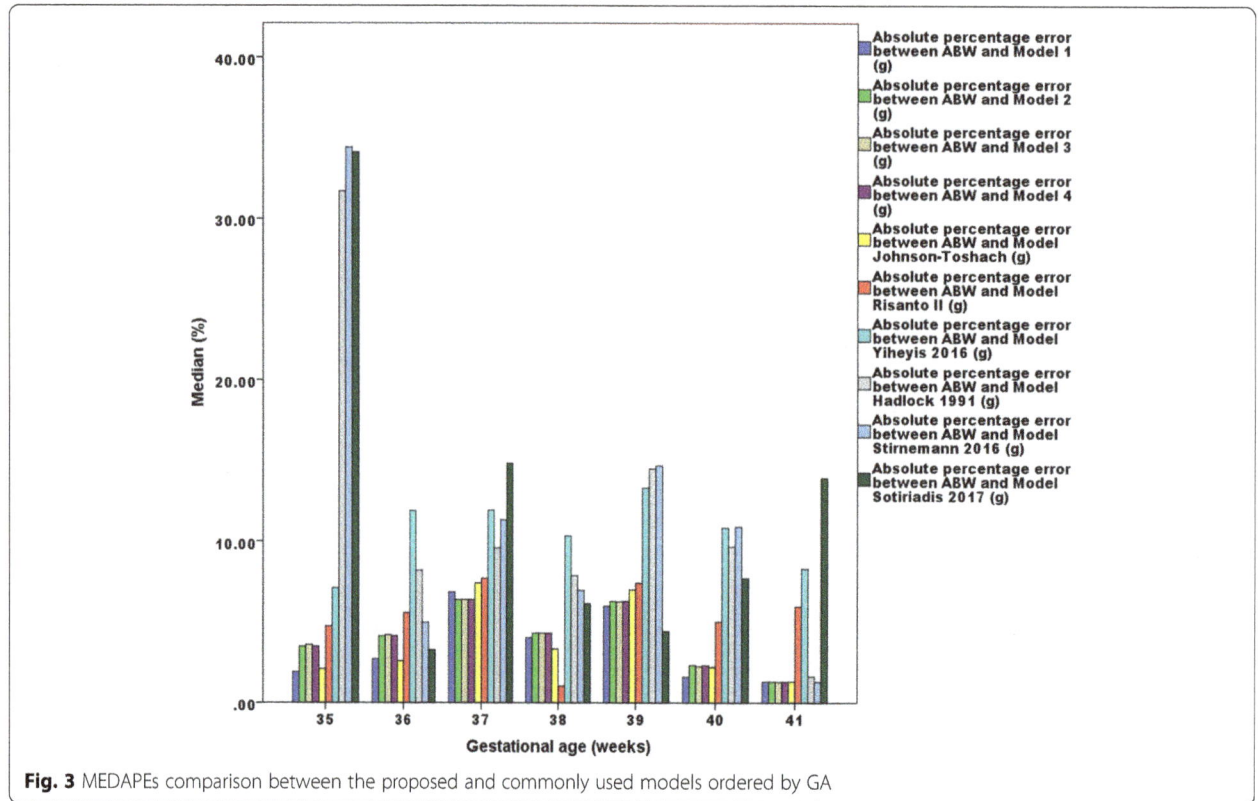

Fig. 3 MEDAPEs comparison between the proposed and commonly used models ordered by GA

ANC services in monitoring foetal inter growth assessment which currently remain low due to the database gaps [56–59].

Several ultrasonic formulas to estimate the foetal characteristics at different GA have been developed [30–32]. The foetal HC and foetal AC are widely recognised as the most influential predictors for predicting foetal weight [10, 11, 46, 60, 61]. Our results show that the best fit formulas to estimate these foetal characteristics at a given GA in our population were based on the Australian population [30].

To the best of our knowledge, in the majority of Indonesian primary health care centres where ultrasound facility is not accessible, none of the existing ultrasonic formulas were adopted to estimate foetal HC and foetal AC. Therefore, the formulas potentially can be deployed to fill in the database gaps on the inter growth process of foetus during pregnancy. Consequently, early informed intervention could be initiated to prevent abnormal growth and delivery weights.

Several techniques have been available to reduce collinearity, such as centering, multiplying variables by various constants (scaling), the use of orthogonal polynomials, and other transformations [62]. Currently, the use of automated machine learning, such as Genetic Algorithm rather than a conventional fractional polynomial approach has also been applied to

model multiple biometric variables of foetus that are highly correlated [54].

In this paper, we used the best subset selection algorithm to prevent the inclusion of highly correlated variables and select the best subset of predictors to be included in the models. It has been emphasized that a formula for estimating foetal weight should be simple and straightforward to be used by doctors and midwives and be easily understood by patients [63]. This would improve the quality of communication, information, and education as part of routine ANC service in low-resource primary health care centres.

Based on our comparison analysis, the proposed Models (1), (2), (3), and (4) produced the least mean prediction errors (between – 0.2 and – 2.4 g), the MAPEs (between 5.01 and 5.10%), and the MEDAPEs (between 4.10 and 4.22%). The mean percentage prediction error (MPE) steadily tended towards zero as the time interval between the last scan and birth decreased [42]. Our MPEs were ranged between – 0.1 and – 0.3% in those born within 0 day ($n = 38$) which are lower than the previous research [42] reported by – 0.8% in those born within 1 day ($n = 198$).

Our proposed models were unbiased for predicting weight between 35 and 41 weeks of GA. In the group born within 0 day of the last measurements, the MAPEs were ranged between 5.0 and 5.10% with 89–92% of

Foetal weight prediction models at a given gestational age in the absence of ultrasound...

185

predicted weights falling within 10% of the true birth weights which are smaller than those reported in previous study [42]. This was particularly for Model (1) which was simply developed based on FH only.

The comparison between the proposed Model (1) and the widely used Johnson-Toshach model shows that Model (1) (developed based on the Indonesian data) was more accurate in predicting the estimated foetal weight than the Johnson-Toshach model (developed based on the United States data). Furthermore, the Johnson-Toshach model requires the knowledge of FS. The results presented in Table 3 also shows that the inclusion of FS in the model has not reduced the prediction errors in foetal weight estimations yet raise a subjectivity issue unless there is a standard protocol to determine FS with less error [20]. Therefore, we recommend the proposed Model (1) be deployed in Indonesia and other countries with similar health systems and challenges for weight prediction.

Our comparison study confirms that the proposed Models (3) (based on FH and estimates of foetal HC) and (4) (based on FH and estimates of foetal AC) perform better than the ultrasonic models: the Jordaan, the Weiner II, the Hadlocks, the Stirnemann, and the Sotiriadis models. The incorporation of estimated foetal HC or estimated foetal AC has increased R^2 slightly (provided in Additional file 5: Table S5), but it did not improve the predicting accuracy (Table 3). However, access to these values will enable the practitioners to monitor foetal growth during pregnancy where advanced equipment, such as ultrasound, is not always available. Consequently, detecting foetal growth abnormality, such as small for GA, prematurity, intrauterine growth retardation, and LBW during pregnancy will be possible.

Strengths and limitations

Our retrospective study has investigated the utilisation of some commonly used foetal weight prediction models in Indonesia. Particularly, the combination between maternal and estimated foetal biometric characteristics was proposed. The aim of this combination was whether it could improve the prediction accuracy of foetal weight at any given GA in the absence of ultrasound machines and trained ultra-sonographers.

The retrospective cohort study was undertaken to provide baseline data on the selected primary health care centre. It is possible that women have used different health services than that reviewed in this study. Although this may result in underestimation in data records, it is unlikely to impact on the validity of the analyses. This study also encountered limitations associated with the accuracy of the information recorded on the manual pregnancy register or inaccurate data transfer to the electronic database. However, monitoring and controlling the process of data transfer was conducted to reduce potential error. Further study should be conducted to assess the efficacy of the proposed models using prospective data [64].

The proposed prediction models are linear regressions. However, the authors have investigated non-linear models. The non-linear models did not improve the estimation accuracy. Therefore, complex models do not guarantee significant improvement in the prediction accuracy. Furthermore, due to the fact that the objective of the study is to provide simple yet reliable foetal weight estimating models for low-resource areas, we are recommending the proposed models. We believe that the findings can be applied in other low-resource settings to improve ANC services.

Conclusion

This research has developed models to predict the estimated foetal weight at varying gestational age where ultrasound facilities do not exist. Since birth weight is one of the most important indicators of neonatal survival, a reliable estimate of foetal weight at different stages of pregnancy would facilitate the intervention plan for medical practitioners to prevent the risk of abnormal delivery weights. Further, the models will lead to the development of foetal inter growth charts, which are currently unavailable in the Indonesian primary health care systems.

Additional files

Additional file 1: Table S1. Existing ultrasonic formulas to estimate foetal HC and AC based on GA. Table S1 consists of the existing ultrasonic formulas to estimate foetal head circumference (HC) and foetal abdominal circumference (AC) which were developed based on the Australian foetal biometry data (measured between 11 and 41 weeks), the UK foetal biometry data (measured between 13 and 42 weeks), and the international foetal biometry data (measured between 14 and 42 weeks or until birth) [29–31]. (PDF 167 kb)

Additional file 2: Table S2. Intraclass correlation coefficient analysis of the existing ultrasonic formulas in predicting foetal biometrics. Table S2 shows a reliability analysis using intraclass correlation coefficient (ICC) to assess the consistency of the ultrasonic formulas for Indonesian population. The obtained ICC values were computed by single-rating, consistency, and two-way random effects models for the foetal biometrics with three raters (different ultrasonic formulas) across 127 subjects (pregnant women). (PDF 95 kb)

Additional file 3: Table S3. Interclass correlation coefficient analysis for predicting foetal biometrics. Table S3 describes interclass (Pearson) correlation coefficient to assess whether there is a significant relationship between the predicted foetal biometrics and the neonatal measurements recorded at delivery time. (PDF 108 kb)

Additional file 4: Table S4. Correlation coefficient of the potentially clinical predictors of foetal weight estimation. Table S4 presents the investigation of correlations between the potential predictors of foetal weight estimation based on 127 data. (PDF 91 kb)

Additional file 5: Table S5. Models recommended by the best subset selection algorithm together with corresponding analysis of variance information. Table S5 summarises the models developed based on the recorded estimated foetal weight (EFW$_r$) using the best subset selection algorithm. These models were based on one, two, and three independent variables. The table also lists their corresponding R^2, Mallows C$_p$, S, and VIF statistics. (PDF 171 kb)

Additional file 6: Table S6. List of the proposed and existing models based on clinical and ultrasonic variables. Table S6 lists the proposed models and the existing clinical and ultrasonic models for estimating foetal weight. (PDF 381 kb)

Additional file 7: Table S7. Two independent sample t-tests between ABW_r, EFW_r, and EFW_p. Table S7 provides a two independent sample t-test to investigate if there is a significant difference between the observed or actual values of birth weight (ABW), recorded foetal weight estimation (EFW_r), and estimated foetal weights based on the proposed model (EFW_p). (PDF 157 kb)

Abbreviations

ABW: Actual birth weight; ABW_i: The ith actual values of birth weight; AC: Abdominal circumference; ANC: Antenatal care; ANOVA: Analysis of variance; BPD: Biparietal diameter; CIE: Communication, information, and education; EFW_p: Estimated foetal weight based on the proposed model; EFW_r: Recorded foetal weight estimation; EFW_{pi}: The ith predicted values of foetal weight based on the proposed models; FH: Fundal height; FL: Femur length; FS: Foetal head engagement/foetal station; GA: Gestational age; HC: Head circumference; ICC: Intraclass correlation coefficient; LBW: Low birth weight; MAPE: Mean absolute percentage prediction error; MEDAPE: Median absolute percentage prediction error; MPE: Mean percentage prediction error; OFD: Occipitofrontal diameter; OLS: Ordinary least square; r: Correlation coefficient; R^2: Coefficient of determination; S: Standard deviation; VIF: Variance inflation factor

Acknowledgements

We are grateful to the Australian Agency for International Development (AusAID) for funding DA's PhD scholarship in Mathematical Sciences at the School of Science, RMIT University, Melbourne, Australia.
The authors would like to thank Feri Anita Wijayanti, M.Mid, Bd. for the provision of antenatal care references in the Indonesian context. We would also thank the dedicated midwives for their roles in supervising the data measuring and recording task in the primary health care centre.
The authors are greatly indebted to the Higher Degree Research (HDR) Language and Learning Advisor of RMIT University, Dr. Ken Manson, for his roles in providing language help and proofreading the article.

Funding

Not applicable. This research did not receive any specific grant from funding agencies in the public, commercial, or not-for-profit sectors. However, the Australian Agency for International Development (AusAID) has granted DA's PhD scholarship in Mathematical Sciences at the School of Science, RMIT University, Melbourne, Australia. This analysis is part of DA's thesis.

Authors' contributions

DA and MA contributed in the conception and design of the study. DA provided the literature review and information summary on relevant research articles and policies in Indonesia. DA performed data collection, pre-processing data, analysis, and interpretation. DA prepared the manuscript. MA and KM provided data analysis, advice, proofreading, and critical revision of the manuscript. All of the authors read and approved the final manuscript.

Authors' information

DA: PhD candidate in the Mathematical Sciences (Applied Statistics), School of Science (Mathematical and Geospatial Sciences), College of Science, Engineering, and Health, RMIT University, Melbourne, Australia and Junior Lecturer at Study Program of Statistics, Faculty of Mathematics and Natural Sciences, University of Lambung Mangkurat (ULM), South Kalimantan, Indonesia.
MA: Senior Lecturer of Statistical Quality Control and its applications in: manufacturing industry, air pollution control, software quality, univariate and multivariate processes, health industry, and the banking system, School of Science (Mathematical and Geospatial Sciences), College of Science, Engineering, and Health, RMIT University, Melbourne, Australia.
KM: Senior Lecturer of Applied Statistics and Mathematics, Market Research, and Numerical Analysis in aerospace engineering, clinical sciences, geomatic engineering, and oncology and carcinogenesis, College of Science, Engineering, and Health, RMIT University, Melbourne, Australia.

Competing interests

The authors declare that they have no competing interests.

References

1. Njim T, Atashili J, Mbu R, Choukem S-P. Low birth weight in a sub-urban area of Cameroon: an analysis of the clinical cut-off, incidence, predictors and complications. BMC Pregnancy Childbirth. 2015;15(1):288.
2. Gibson KS, Waters TP, Gunzler DD, Catalano PM. A retrospective cohort study of factors relating to the longitudinal change in birth weight. BMC Pregnancy Childbirth. 2015;15(1):1.
3. Parvin Z, Shafiuddin S, Uddin MA, Begum F. Symphysio fundal height (SFH) measurement as a predictor of birth weight. Faridpur Med Coll J. 2013;7(2): 54–8.
4. Lalys L, Pineau J-C, Guihard-Costa A-M. Small and large foetuses: identification and estimation of foetal weight at delivery from third-trimester ultrasound data. Early Hum Dev. 2010;86(12):753–7.
5. Sharma SR, Giri S, Timalsina U, Bhandari SS, Basyal B, Wagle K, Shrestha L. Low birth weight at term and its determinants in a tertiary hospital of Nepal: a case-control study. PLoS One. 2015;10(4):e0123962.
6. Willocks J, Donald I, Duggan T, Day N. Foetal cephalometry by ultrasound. BJOG Int J Obstet Gynaecol. 1964;71(1):11–20.
7. Robson SC, Gallivan S, Walkinshaw SA, Vaughan J, Rodeck CH. Ultrasonic estimation of fetal weight: use of targeted formulas in small for gestational age fetuses. Obstet Gynecol. 1993;82(3):359–64.
8. Spinnato JA, Allen RD, Mendenhall HW. Birth weight prediction from remote ultrasound examination. Obstet Gynecol. 1988;71(6):893–8.
9. Shepard M, Richards V, Berkowitz R, Warsof S, Hobbins J. An evaluation of two equations for predicting fetal weight by ultrasound. Am J Obstet Gynecol. 1982;142(1):47–54.
10. Hadlock F, Harrist R, Carpenter R, Deter R, Park S. Sonographic estimation of fetal weight. The value of femur length in addition to head and abdomen measurements. Radiology. 1984;150(2):535–40.
11. Hadlock FP, Harrist R, Sharman RS, Deter RL, Park SK. Estimation of fetal weight with the use of head, body, and femur measurements—a prospective study. Am J Obstet Gynecol. 1985;151(3):333–7.
12. Campbell S, Wilkin D. Ultrasonic measurement of fetal abdomen circumference in the estimation of fetal weight. BJOG Int J Obstet Gynaecol. 1975;82(9):689–97.
13. Combs CA, Jaekle RK, Rosenn B, Pope M, Miodovnik M, Siddiqi TA. Sonographic estimation of fetal weight based on a model of fetal volume. Obstet Gynecol. 1993;82(3):365–70.

14. Johnson R, Toshach C. Estimation of fetal weight using longitudinal mensuration. Am J Obstet Gynecol. 1954;68(3):891–6.

15. Johnson RW. Calculations in estimating fetal weight. Am J Obstet Gynecol. 1957;74(4):929.

16. Niswander KR, Capraro VJ, Van Coevering RJ. Estimation of birth weight by quantified external uterine measurements. Obstet Gynecol. 1970;36(2):294–8.

17. Farid SW. Child weight prediction based on the modification of the Niswander formula (Taksasi berat badan anak berdasarkan modifikasi rumus Niswander). Majalah Obstetri dan Ginekologi Indonesia. 1999;23(4):188–93.

18. Buchmann E, Tlale K. A simple clinical formula for predicting fetal weight in labour at term: derivation and validation. SAMJ. 2009;99(6):457–60.

19. Mongelli M, Gardosi J. Estimation of fetal weight by symphysis–fundus height measurement. Int J Gynecol Obstet. 2004;85(1):50–1.

20. Bothner B, Gulmezoglu A, Hofmeyr G. Symphysis fundus height measurements during labour: a prospective, descriptive study. Afr J Reprod Health. 2000;4(1):48–55.

21. Dare F, Ademowore A, Ifaturoti O, Nganwuchu A. The value of symphysio-fundal height/abdominal girth measurements in predicting fetal weight. Int J Gynecol Obstet. 1990;31(3):243–8.

22. Siswosudarmo H. Detection of low birth weight babies at term pregnancy with fundal height measurements (Deteksi bayi berat lahir rendah pada kehamilan aterm dengan pengukuran tinggi fundus). Berkala Epidemiologi Klinik Biostatika Indonesia. 1995;1(20):78–84.

23. Siswosudarmo R, Titisari I. Developing a new formula for estimating birth weight at term pregnancy. Jurnal Kesehatan Reproduksi. 2014;1(2):145–149.

24. Gayatri D, Afiyanti Y. Validation of fetal weight estimation formula (TBJ) for prediction of birth weight based on uterine fundal height of pregnant women (Validasi rumus taksiran berat janin (TBJ) untuk prediksi berat badan lahir berdasarkan tinggi fundus uterus ibu hamil). Jurnal Keperawatan Indonesia. 2006;10(1):24–9.

25. Santjaka HI, Handayani R. Study of the accuracy of fetal weight estimates based on statistics and fundal height (Studi ketepatan taksiran berat janin berdasarkan statistik dan tinggi fundus uteri). Jurnal Bidan Prada. 2011;2(01):21–34.

26. Kiserud T, Piaggio G, Carroli G, Widmer M, Carvalho J, Jensen LN, Giordano D, Cecatti JG, Aleem HA, Talegawkar SA. The World Health Organization fetal growth charts: a multinational longitudinal study of ultrasound biometric measurements and estimated fetal weight. PLoS Med. 2017;14(1):e1002220.

27. Anggraini D, Abdollahian M, Marion K. Review of low birth weight prediction models in Indonesia. Int J Adv Sci Eng Technol. 2015;3(4):105–11.

28. Abdollahian M, Ahmad S, Huda S, Nuryani S, Anggraini D. Investigating the relationship between neonatal mortality rate and mother's characteristics. In: Proceedings of the International Conference on Information and Knowledge Engineering (IKE); The Steering Committee of the World Congress in Computer Science, Computer Engineering, and Applied Computing (WorldComp); CSREA Press; 2012. p. 1.

29. Papageorghiou AT, Ohuma EO, Gravett MG, Hirst J, da Silveira MF, Lambert A, Carvalho M, Jaffer YA, Altman DG, Noble JA. International standards for symphysis-fundal height based on serial measurements from the fetal growth longitudinal study of the INTERGROWTH-21st project: prospective cohort study in eight countries. BMJ. 2016;355:i5662.

30. Westerway SC, Davison A, Cowell S. Ultrasonic fetal measurements: new Australian standards for the new millennium. Aust N Z J Obstet Gynaecol. 2000;40(3):297–302.

31. Loughna P, Chitty L, Evans T, Chudleigh T. Fetal size and dating: charts recommended for clinical obstetric practice. Ultrasound. 2009;17(3):160–6.

32. Papageorghiou AT, Ohuma EO, Altman DG, Todros T, Ismail LC, Lambert A, Jaffer YA, Bertino E, Gravett MG, Purwar M. International standards for fetal growth based on serial ultrasound measurements: the fetal growth longitudinal study of the INTERGROWTH-21 st project. Lancet. 2014;384(9946):869–79.

33. Achadi E, Jones G. Health sector review: maternal, neonatal, and child health. In: Jakarta: Ministry of National Development Planning/Bappenas, Republic of Indonesia; 2014.

34. UNICEF-Indonesia. Issues briefs: maternal and child health. In: UNICEF Indonesia; 2012. p. 1–6.

35. MoH. Indonesia health profile (Profil kesehatan Indonesia) 2012. In: Jakarta: Ministry of Health, Republic of Indonesia; 2013.

36. Bellio R, Ventura L. An introduction to robust estimation with R functions. Proceedings of 1st International Work; 2005. p. 1–57.

37. Fox J, Weisberg S. An R companion to applied regression: Sage; 2010.

38. Renaud O, Victoria-Feser M-P. A robust coefficient of determination for regression. J Statist Plann Inference. 2010;140(7):1852–62.

39. Faraway JJ. Practical regression and ANOVA using R. In: University of Bath; 2002.

40. Landers R. Computing Intraclass Correlations (ICC) as estimates of interrater reliability in SPSS. The Winnower 2: e143518. 81744; 2015. https://doi.org/10.15200/winn.143518.81744.

41. Koo TK, Li MY. A guideline of selecting and reporting intraclass correlation coefficients for reliability research. J Chiropr Med. 2016;15(2):155–63.

42. Stirnemann J, Villar J, Salomon L, Ohuma E, Ruyan P, Altman D, Nosten F, Craik R, Munim S, Cheikh Ismail L. International estimated fetal weight standards of the INTERGROWTH-21st project. Ultrasound Obstet Gynecol. 2017;49(4):478–86.

43. Levenbach H. Training EDC: The Myth of the MAPE and how to avoid it. 2015.

44. Anggraini D, Abdollahian M, Marion K. Accuracy assessment on prediction models for fetal weight based on maternal fundal height. In: Information technology: new generations. Cham: Springer; 2016. p. 859–68.

45. Yiheyis A, Alemseged F, Segni H. Johnson's formula for predicting birth weight in pregnant mothers at Jimma University Teaching Hospital, South West Ethiopia. Med J Obstet Gynecol. 2016;4(3):1087–93.

46. Jordaan HV. Estimation of fetal weight by ultrasound. J Clin Ultrasound. 1983;11(2):59–66.

47. Weiner Z, Ben-Shlomo I, Beck-Fruchter R, Goldberg Y, Shalev E. Clinical and ultrasonographic weight estimation in large for gestational age fetus. Eur J Obstet Gynecol Reprod Biol. 2002;105(1):20–4.

48. Huber C, Zdanowicz JA, Mueller M, Surbek D. Factors influencing the accuracy of fetal weight estimation with a focus on preterm birth at the limit of viability: a systematic literature review. Fetal Diagn Ther. 2014;36(1):1–8.

49. Morse K, Williams A, Gardosi J. Fetal growth screening by fundal height measurement. Best Pract Res Clin Obstet Gynaecol. 2009;23(6):809–18.

50. Titisari HI, Siswosudarmo R. Risanto's formulas is more accurate in determining estimated fetal weight based on maternal fundal height. Indones J Obstet Gynecol. 2013;1(3):149–51.

51. Sparks TN, Cheng YW, McLaughlin B, Esakoff TF, Caughey AB. Fundal height: a useful screening tool for fetal growth? J Matern Fetal Neonatal Med. 2011; 24(5):708–12.

52. Curti A, Zanello M, De Maggio I, Moro E, Simonazzi G, Rizzo N, Farina A. Multivariable evaluation of term birth weight: a comparison between ultrasound biometry and symphysis-fundal height. J Matern Fetal Neonatal Med. 2014;27(13):1328–32.

53. Pay ASD, Wiik J, Backe B, Jacobsson B, Strandell A, Klovning A. Symphysis-fundus height measurement to predict small-for-gestational-age status at birth: a systematic review. BMC Pregnancy Childbirth. 2015;15(1):22.

54. Papageorghiou AT, Kemp B, Stones W, Ohuma EO, Kennedy SH, Purwar M, Salomon LJ, Altman DG, Noble JA, Bertino E. Ultrasound-based gestational-age estimation in late pregnancy. Ultrasound Obstet Gynecol. 2016;48(6): 719–26.

55. Postoev VA, Grjibovski AM, Nieboer E, Odland JØ. Changes in detection of birth defects and perinatal mortality after introduction of prenatal ultrasound screening in the Kola Peninsula (North-West Russia): combination of two birth registries. BMC Pregnancy Childbirth. 2015;15(1):1.

56. Gardosi J. Fetal growth standards: individual and global perspectives. Lancet. 2011;377(9780):1812–4.

57. Gardosi J. Customised assessment of fetal growth potential: implications for perinatal care. Arch Dis Child Fetal Neonatal Ed. 2012. https://doi.org/10.1136/fetalneonatal-2012-301708.

58. Moxon SG, Ruysen H, Kerber KJ, Amouzou A, Fournier S, Grove J, Moran AC, Vaz LM, Blencowe H, Conroy N. Count every newborn: a measurement improvement roadmap for coverage data. BMC Pregnancy Childbirth. 2015;15(2):S8.

59. Kerber KJ, Mathai M, Lewis G, Flenady V, Erwich JJH, Segun T, Aliganyira P, Abdelmegeid A, Allanson E, Roos N. Counting every stillbirth and neonatal death through mortality audit to improve quality of care for every pregnant woman and her baby. BMC Pregnancy Childbirth. 2015;15(2):S9.

60. Abele H, Hoopmann M, Wagner N, Hahn M, Wallwiener D, Kagan KO. Accuracy of sonographic fetal weight estimation of fetuses with a birth weight of 1500g or less. Eur J Obstet Gynecol Reprod Biol. 2010;153(2):131–7.

61. Dudley N. A systematic review of the ultrasound estimation of fetal weight. Ultrasound Obstet Gynecol. 2005;25(1):80–9.

62. Kleinbaum D, Kupper L, Nizam A, Rosenberg E. Applied regression analysis and other multivariable methods: Nelson Education; 2013.

63. Salomon LJ, Bernard JP, Ville Y. Estimation of fetal weight: reference range at 20–36 weeks' gestation and comparison with actual birth-weight reference range. Ultrasound Obstet Gynecol. 2007;29(5):550–5.

64. Asiki G, Baisley K, Newton R, Marions L, Seeley J, Kamali A, Smedman L. Adverse pregnancy outcomes in rural Uganda (1996–2013): trends and associated factors from serial cross sectional surveys. BMC Pregnancy Childbirth. 2015;15(1):1.

65. Gayatri D, Afiyanti Y. Comparison of some formulas for predicting birth weight based on height measurement of fundus uteri (Perbandingan beberapa rumus untuk memprediksi berat badan lahir berdasrkan pengukuran tinggi fundus uteri). Jurnal Keperawatan Indonesia. 2004;8(1):18–22.

66. Rusdy RS, Yasmin FA, Putri LA, Oktrian O, Pusponegoro A. Comparison of Johnson-Tohsach formula with South Africa formula in determining fetal weight estimation at Puskesmas Kecamatan Pasar Rebo, East Jakarta (Perbandingan rumus Johnson-Tohsach dengan rumus South Africa dalam menentukan taksiran berat janin di Puskesmas Kecamatan Pasar Rebo, Jakarta Timur). eJurnal Kedokteran Indonesia. 2014;2(1):33–6.

67. Hadlock FP, Harrist RB, Martinez-Poyer J. In utero analysis of fetal growth: a sonographic weight standard. Radiology. 1991;181(1):129–33.

68. Sotiriadis A, Eleftheriades M, Papadopoulos V, Sarafidis K, Pervanidou P, Assimakopoulos E. Divergence of estimated fetal weight and birth weight in singleton fetuses. J Matern Fetal Neonatal Med. 2018;31(6):761–9.

18

Effects of music intervention during caesarean delivery on anxiety and stress of the mother a controlled, randomised study

Philip Hepp[1,2]* ⓘ, Carsten Hagenbeck[2], Julius Gilles[2], Oliver T. Wolf[3], Wolfram Goertz[4], Wolfgang Janni[5], Percy Balan[2], Markus Fleisch[1], Tanja Fehm[2] and Nora K. Schaal[6]

Abstract

Background: Stress and anxiety during pregnancy and childbirth have negative consequences for both mother and child. There are indications that music has a positive effect in this situation. The present study investigates the influence of music during the caesarean on anxiety and stress of the expectant mother.

Methods: The SAMBA study is a single-centre, controlled, randomized study including 304 patients. Women in the intervention group heard music via loudspeakers from one of four self-selected genres. The control group had standard treatment without music. The caesarean was performed in regional Anesthesia. At admission, at skin incision, during skin suture and two hours after completion of surgery, different subjective (State-Trait Anxiety Inventory, visual analogue scale for anxiety) and objective parameters (salivary cortisol/amylase, heart rate, blood pressure) were collected. Mixed-factorial Analysis of variances as well as independent sample t-tests were applied for data analysis.

Results: At skin suture, significantly lower anxiety levels were reported in the intervention group regarding State anxiety (31.56 vs. 34.41; $p = .004$) and visual analogue scale for anxiety (1.27 vs. 1.76; $p = .018$). Two hours after surgery, the measured visual analogue scale for anxiety score in the intervention group was still significantly lower (0.69 vs. 1.04; $p = .018$). The objective parameters showed significant differences between the groups in salivary cortisol increase from admission to skin suture (12.29 vs. 16.61 nmol/L; $p = .043$), as well as systolic blood pressure (130.11 vs. 136.19 mmHg; $p = .002$) and heart rate (88.40 vs. 92.57/min; $p = .049$) at skin incision.

Conclusions: Music during caesarean is an easy implementable and effective way of reducing stress and anxiety of the expectant mother.

Keywords: Caesarean, Anxiety, Stress, Music intervention

Background

Almost one in three women delivers by caesarean in Germany. Thus it is the most common abdominal surgery and one of the most common operations. Although the circumstances in almost all cases give cause for joy, it is also a feared event, which is associated with a significant level of stress for the patient [1, 2]. Studies have shown adverse effects of maternal stress on the foetus and on psychological development later in life [3, 4]. In addition, it is known that increased levels of stress and anxiety can negatively affect pain perception and the usage of analgesics postoperatively [5, 6] as well as the new mothers lactation [7, 8]. In view of the limited pharmacological options of intervention for pregnant women, the need for alternative, low-risk approaches to positively influence anxiety and stress arises.

In this regard, the positive effect of music on anxiety and stress is one of the oldest treatment approaches.

* Correspondence: science@dr-hepp.de
[1]Clinic for Gynecology and Obstetrics, Helios University Hospital Wuppertal, University Witten/Herdecke, Heusnerstr 40, 42283 Wuppertal, Germany
[2]Clinic for Gynecology and Obstetrics, Heinrich-Heine-University, Düsseldorf, Germany
Full list of author information is available at the end of the article

Even Asclepius attributed a healing power to music [9]. Its positive influence in various medical interventions across all disciplines has been repeatedly examined [10–13]. Supported by a recent review by Hole et al. in the Lancet, these results also drew the attention of the wider public [14].

Nevertheless, data for music during caesarean are sparse and inconclusive [15]. Two randomized studies examining the influence of music during the pre-operative waiting time could show a positive influence of music on non-validated questionnaires as well as heart rate and heart rate variability as a surrogate for stress and anxiety. In part, this effect could still be detected six hours after the caesarean [16, 17]. A Cochrane analysis [15] investigating the effect of music during the procedure could only identify one randomized study that was able to show a positive effect of music intervention on heart rate at the end of the caesarean in 64 participants [18]. Due to their study design, no further conclusions on subjective and objective perception of anxiety were possible. Another study examined the influence of music during caesarean delivery under general anesthesia on postoperative pain and could not show any effect [19].

Therefore, the aim of the present study is to systematically examine the anxiolytic and stress reducing effect of a music intervention during the caesarean on the wake patient using validated questionnaires and a comprehensive set of objective measurements (salivary cortisol/amylase, blood pressure and heart rate).

Methods

The *SAMBA* (**S**ectio **C**aesarea und die **A**uswirkung von **M**usik**B**egleittherapie auf **A**nxiolyse; English: Caesarean and the effect of music intervention on anxiety) study is a single-centre, controlled, randomized trial conducted at the University Hospital Dusseldorf, Germany. The study adheres to the CONSORT guidelines.

Ethics, consent and permissions

The study protocol was approved by the ethics committee of the Medical Department of the Heinrich-Heine-University in Dusseldorf (No.: 3625) in accordance with the declaration of Helsinki and registered in the German registry for clinical trials (DRKS00007840) and with the WHO (Universal Trial Number U1111–1173-3204). Upon reasonable request the study protocol can be obtained via email from the corresponding author. All eligible patients gave informed written consent prior to participation.

Participants

From March 2015 to August 2017, pregnant women with an indication for primary caesarean in regional anesthesia and adequate German language comprehension were recruited.

We only included patients with normal hearing abilities. Additionally, the patients were only included when no serious comorbidities (according to the physician's assessment) were present, no significantly increased surgical risk (e.g. placental disturbances) were identified preoperatively and only if no serious condition of the foetus was known. Furthermore, only patients without any generalized anxiety disorder or other serious mental alterations were included in the study.

Outcomes, measuring instruments and procedure

The impact of music during caesarean delivery on anxiety and stress measured by State-Trait Anxiety Inventory (STAI), a visual analogue scale depicting anxiety (VAS-A) as well as on salivary cortisol and alpha-amylase were pre-specified as primary outcome measures.

To measure subjective anxiety, STAI and VAS-A were used. The STAI is an introspective inventory comprising 40 self-report items pertaining to anxiety [20]. It distinguishes between two questionnaires with 20 items each, one measuring anxiety perceived in the current situation (STAI-state) and the other evaluating a general tendency towards anxiety (STAI-trait). Participants are asked to give a response to each item on a 4-point Likert scale. A total value is calculated (possible range 20–80 for each questionnaire). Higher scores reflect higher levels of anxiety. The VAS-A comprises a 10 cm line, on which the participant marks her current degree of anxiety with the left end of the line being labelled "no anxiety" and the right end being labelled "maximum anxiety". For analysis the marking is then measured in mm from the left end.

Saliva samples were collected in order to determine cortisol and alpha-amylase levels as objective measures of stress. Salivary cortisol is a marker of the activation of the hypothalamic-pituitary-adrenal axis, whereas salivary alpha-amylase is an indirect marker of the autonomic activity [21]. For the saliva samples, patients had to thoroughly insalivate a cotton swab. The saliva samples were kept frozen at − 18 degrees until analysed, following the methods described elsewhere [22]. Heart rate and blood pressure values were taken from the anaesthesia records.

After inclusion, the computer-assisted randomization took place and divided the patients into the music group vs. control group in the ratio of one to one. Women in the music group chose their preferred music genre from lounge, classical, jazz, and meditation music.

The participating women filled in the STAI-trait when they came to the routine surgical preparation appointment 7 to14 days before the caesarean. At admission on the day of the scheduled caesarean, the VAS-A, the STAI-state and the first saliva sample were taken during the routine cardiotocogram. There was no routine preoperative medication in either group. Intraoperative, the parameters blood pressure and heart rate were recorded at skin incisions and suture. During skin suture, a second saliva sample was obtained and the patient answered the STAI-state questionnaire and the VAS-A. At the end of post-operative monitoring two hours after skin suture, a third saliva sample was taken. Furthermore, the participant answered the STAI-state questionnaire and VAS-A for a third time. Additionally, questions were asked about the music experience. Figure 1 shows the study procedure with the measurement time points schematically.

Intervention

For the music group, the music intervention started when the participant entered the operating theatre. The music was played on a CD player (TEAC CR-H 500 CD receiver) using a speaker system from Cambridge Audio 300. The participant was presented with music continuously in a standardized volume determined on the device and measured at the participants' head of 55 dB (A). All music titles had a slow tempo of 60–80 bpm in common and followed the recommendations made by Nilsson [23]. The music pool contained 60 songs. 15 tracks were each assigned to one of the 4 different genres of music. The control group received no music.

Statistical analysis

The statistical software package SPSS 24 (IBM Inc., Armonk, NY) was used for all data analyses. The group affiliation was coded and therefore the analysis was performed blind. In order to check for differences in environmental parameters between groups, which could influence the results, we compared the time of the procedure (morning vs. afternoon) using a chi-square-test and the length of the surgery with an independent sample t-test.

To compare the subjective course of anxiety on the day of the caesarean, two 2×3 mixed-factorial ANOVAs with the between-subject factor *group* (music group vs control group) and the within-subject factor *measurement*

time point (admission, skin suture, 2 h post-surgery) and the dependent variables STAI-state and VAS-A were calculated. If sphericity was not met, a correction of the degrees of freedom according to Greenhouse-Geisser was carried out. For the objective variables heart rate and systolic and diastolic blood pressure, 2×2 mixed-factorial ANOVAs were used with the factors *group* and *measurements time point* (skin incision and skin suture). In addition, direct group comparisons were performed with independent-samples t-tests. Amylase values were logarithmized analogously to the generally accepted approach [24].

An a-priori power analyses for sample-size estimation was calculated using G*Power (HHU, Düsseldorf, Germany) [25]. Given an expected small to medium effect size (d = 0.35), a power of 85% and an alpha-error of .05 the required (to be analysed) sample-size is 296 (148 per group).

Results

We screened and informed 412 patients about study participation. Sixty-two patients had to be excluded from further participation because they no longer fulfilled the inclusion criteria at the time of intervention (three had delivered spontaneously, 18 had an indication for caesarean preterm, 41 had a secondary caesarean (for example because of premature rupture of membranes)). Forty-five women did not take part due to technical difficulties (reconstruction of the operation theatre). One patient discontinued the study prematurely. In total 304 participants completed the study in accordance with the protocol (Fig. 2). The patients had a mean age of 33.6 years (range: 18–47 years) and a mean gestation age of 268.5 days. The data revealed that the two groups did not differ regarding the time of the procedure (morning vs. afternoon) [$\chi^2(1, 301) = 0.75$, $p = .388$] nor on the duration of the procedure [$t(290) = 1.36$, $p = .175$].

An overview of the descriptive data of the music and control group and the main results is given in Table 1.

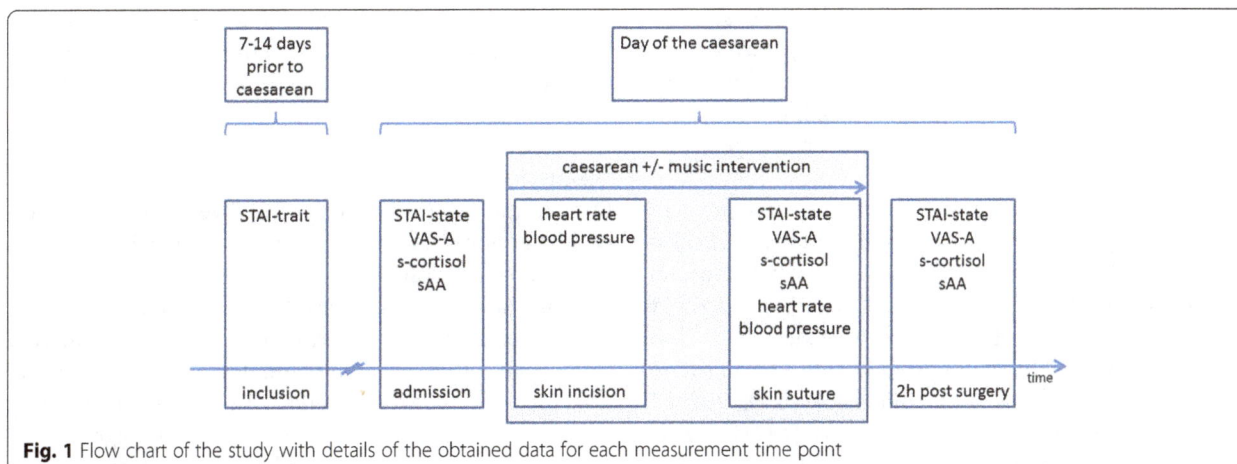

Fig. 1 Flow chart of the study with details of the obtained data for each measurement time point

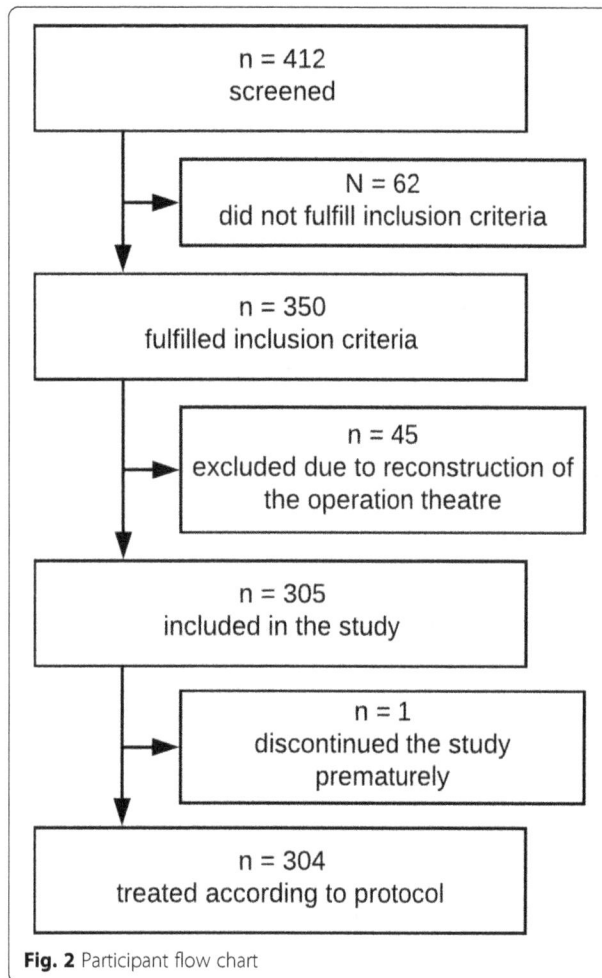

Fig. 2 Participant flow chart

Subjective parameters

For the STAI-state, significant main effects were found for the factors *measurement time point* [F (1.78, 451.28) = 454.35, $p < .001$] and *group* [F (1.254) = 4.12, $p = .043$]. The interaction was not significant [F (1.78, 451.28) = 1.47, $p = .230$]. Post-hoc comparisons showed that the two groups did not differ on admission ($p = .593$). At skin suture the music group showed significantly less anxiety compared to the control group [t (254) = 2.88, $p = .004$, mean difference = 2.72, 95% CI (0.76, 4.67), d = 0.36]. 2 h after surgery there was no significant difference ($p = .140$) (Fig. 3a).

For the VAS-A, the factors *measurement time point* [F (1.39, 301.32) = 378.50, $p < .001$] and *group* [F (1.217) = 4.51, $p = .035$] showed significant effects, whereas no interaction was present [F (1.39, 301.32) = 0.17, $p = .847$]. A post-hoc t-test showed that the level of anxiety in the two groups did not differ at admission ($p = .349$). At skin suture [t (217) = 2.39, $p = .018$, mean difference = 0.49, 95% CI (0.08, 0.89), d = 0.32] and 2 h post-surgery [t (217) = 2.38, $p = .018$, mean difference = 0.35, 95% CI (0.06, 0.64),

d = 0.32] there were significant differences in favour of the music group (Fig. 3b).

Objective parameters

Cortisol increase from admission to skin suture was significantly lower in the music group than in the control group [t (181) = 2.04, $p = .043$, mean difference = 4.32, 95% CI (0.14, 8.49), d = 0.30] (Fig. 4a). The decrease in cortisol from skin suture to 2 h post-surgery did not differ significantly between the two groups [t (193) = 1.53, $p = .121$, mean difference = 3.30, 95% CI (– 0.95, 7.55), d = 0.22]. The increase in amylase from admission to skin suture and decrease to 2 h after surgery did not differ between the two groups (p-values > .165).

For systolic blood pressure, significant main effects were found for *group* [F (1,270) = 4.73, $p = .030$] and *measurement time point* [F (1,270) = 132.58, $p < .001$] and a significant interaction revealed [F (1,270) = 8.57, $p = .004$]. At skin incision the mean systolic blood pressure was significantly lower in the music group (M = 130.11 mmHg) than in the control group (M = 136.19 mmHg) [t (270) = 3.18, $p = .002$, mean difference = 6.35, 95% CI (2.59, 10.11), d = 0.39] (Fig. 4b). There was no difference at skin suture ($p = .981$). For the diastolic blood pressure value, no significant group differences were found (p-values > .197).

Also for heart rate significant effects of the factors *group* [F (1,266) = 4.51, $p = .035$] and *measurement time point* [F (1,266) = 104.99, $p < .001$] were revealed. There was no significant interaction [F (1,266) = 0.55, $p = .457$]. Post-hoc comparisons showed that at skin incision the heart rate was significantly lower in the music group (M = 88.40) than in the control group (M = 92.57) [t (269) = 1.98 $p = .049$, mean difference = 4.13, 95% CI (0.02, 8.24), d = 0.24]. At skin suture, the groups did not differ significantly ($p = .141$) (Fig. 4c).

Acceptance of music intervention

Of the participants in the music group 95.5% stated that they would listen to music again at a possible next caesarean. Eighty-six percent were satisfied with the choice of music. In addition, 89.7% said that the music made the situation more enjoyable and 73.4% thought the music had calmed them.

Discussion

Overall, the study shows, in subjective as well as objective dimensions, an anxiety and stress reducing effect of music during caesarean.

While both groups showed high baseline values for STAI-state and VAS-A without significantly differing from each other at admission, the subjective anxiety drop in both, STAI-state and VAS-A, was significantly higher in the music group and resulted in significantly lower anxiety scores compared to the control group at

Table 1 Overview of characteristics and results

	Music group	Control group	P value
Number	154	150	
Age [years]	33.5 ± 5.4 (18–47)	33.7 ± 5.4 (21–44)	.883
Gestational Age [days]	269	268	.231
Time of procedure [morning/evening]	81/73	70/77 (3 N/A)	.388
Duration of procedure [mins]	43.0	41.6	.175
STAI-Trait	36.39 ± 8.45	37.14 ± 8.74	.474
STAI-State I	47.54 ± 10.40	48.28 ± 11.79	.593
STAI-State II	31.56 ± 6.30	34.41 ± 9.23	**.004**
STAI-State III	29.54 ± 5.91	30.91 ± 7.14	.140
VAS-A I [cm]	4.83 ± 2.61	5.18 ± 2.89	.349
VAS-A II [cm]	1.27 ± 1.20	1.76 ± 1.78	**.018**
VAS-A III [cm]	0.69 ± 0.88	1.04 ± 1.29	**.018**
C-increase I to II [nmol/L]	12.29 ± 12.15	16.61 ± 16.14	**.043**
C-decrease II to III [nmol/L]	− 13.77 ± 13.05	−17.07 ± 16.80	.128
sAA-increase [ln] I to II	1.58 ± 1.40	1.76 ± 1.24	.414
sAA-decrease II to III	−0.31 ± 1.27	−0.57 ± 1,10	.165
RR sys skin incision [mmHg]	130.11 ± 14.97	136.19 ± 16.57	**.002**
RR sys II [mmHg]	121.42 ± 12.89	121.58 ± 13.00	.981
RR dia skin incision [mmHg]	70.82 ± 9.35	72.77 ± 10.55	.106
RR dia II [mmHg]	64.65 ± 9.61	64.99 ± 9.21	.764
HR skin incision [1/min]	88.40 ± 16.23	92.57 ± 18.26	**.049**
HR II [1/min]	77.97 ± 13.91	80.51 ± 14.23	.141

N/A: data not available; I: at admission; II: at skin suture; III: 2 h post-surgery; VAS-A: Visual Analogue Scale for Anxiety; C: salivary cortisol; sAA: salivary alpha amylase; RR sys: systolic blood pressure; RR dia: diastolic blood pressure; HR: heart rate
Note: bold values indicate a significant difference between groups

skin suture. The shown positive effect of music on these subjective measures for anxiety and stress is in line with previous studies investigating the effect of music in the context of caesarean and other medical procedures [11, 13, 14, 16, 23, 26]. One of these studies showed a persisting positive effect for six hours [16]. Our data support this observation insofar that women in the music group had significantly lower scores on the VAS-A for another two hours after skin suture. This effect was not found for the STAI-state. It is likely that the STAI-state is less appropriate than the VAS-A in the obstetrical environment due to the duration of the survey?

In terms of objective parameters, the music group showed a significantly lower increase in salivary cortisol

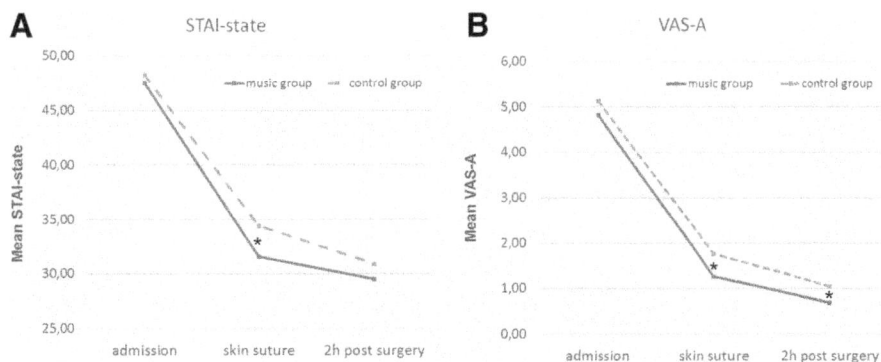

Fig. 3 The subjective course of anxiety for both groups. **a** For the STAI-state scores the music group displayed significantly lower anxiety levels at skin suture than the control group. **b** For the VAS-A scores anxiety levels of the music group are significantly below the control group at skin suture and remain lower two hours after the caesarean. * $p < .05$

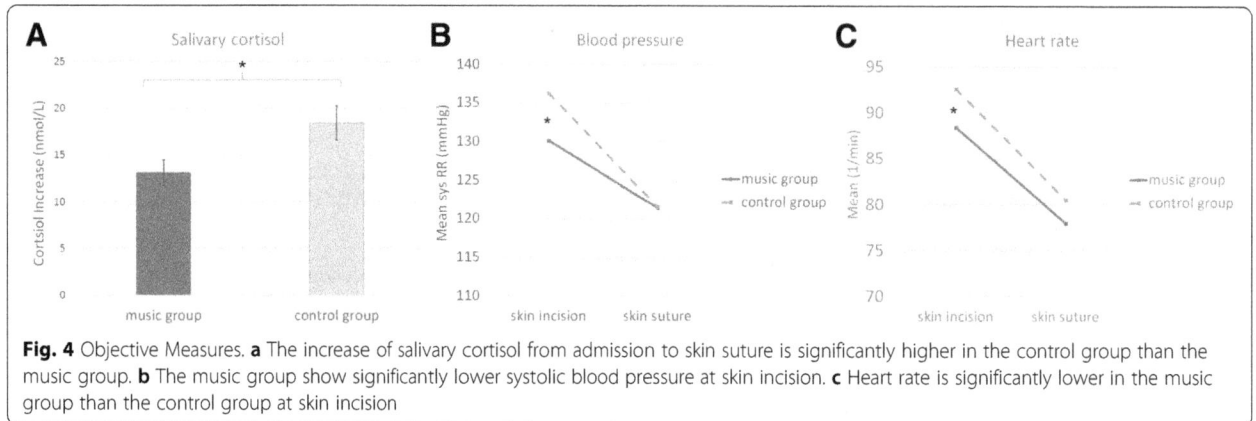

Fig. 4 Objective Measures. **a** The increase of salivary cortisol from admission to skin suture is significantly higher in the control group than the music group. **b** The music group show significantly lower systolic blood pressure at skin incision. **c** Heart rate is significantly lower in the music group than the control group at skin incision

than the control group from admission to skin suture. Saliva cortisol measures the impact of a stressor with a latency of about 30 min [27]. In this respect, the measurement at skin suture represents a large part of the objective stress sensation during the operation [2]. Therefore, the present result reflects that the music group also objectively experiences reduced stress levels during the caesarean. A lowering effect of music on cortisol could also be shown in studies in other medical fields [28].

A comparable effect could not be found for salivary amylase. Whereas cortisol represents the activity of the hypothalamic-pituitary-adrenocortical axis, salivary amylase represents the activation of the sympathetic nerve system [29]. In line with previous work on stress during surgical procedures, our study shows no measurable difference in salivary amylase between the groups [30, 31]. This might be an indication that there are unrecognized factors, which impede a reliable interpretation of the salivary amylase during surgical procedures.

A variety of studies have examined the influence of music on the cardiovascular system [32]. In addition to a direct impact on the dopaminergic mesolimbic reward centre [33], an interaction of the external musical rhythm with the internal body rhythms of heart and respiratory rate as a main carrier of the effect of music is debated [34–36]. Thereby, the value of systolic blood pressure and heart rate is well documented as objective parameters reflecting stress and anxiety [32]. In the present study, the music group showed significantly lower heart rate and systolic blood pressure levels at skin incision. This took place on average 18 min after the patient had been admitted to the operating room and the start of the music intervention. Therefore, we would argue that the calming effect of music on the expectant mother was already present at skin incision. In the case of skin suture, however, no significant difference was detectable. At this time, the new-born was usually already in the arms of the mother, so that pulse and blood pressure are certainly subject to an undetermined bias.

Besides the positive influence of music on the measured stress and anxiety of patients, the high acceptance of the intervention should also be noted. Ninety-six percent of women in the intervention group would want to hear music again during a possible repeated caesarean, regardless of any therapeutic effects. The positive response of the women regarding the music intervention alone are gratifying and should encourage the use of music in obstetrics and further research in this area.

A limitation of the study is the lack of opportunity to gain an even more comprehensive picture of the course of anxiety during caesarean through measuring more time points. For example a measurement of anxiety levels just before the women enters the operating theatre would be desirable as this time point may be the most anxious time for the women. This is partially compensated by the fact that the different measuring instruments used in this study have different latencies and thus cover a large period of time around the intervention. Additionally, in order to ensure a trial close to normal conditions of a caesarean and the needs of the woman, we decided not to use headphones, in contrast to other studies [18]. Naturally, this impeded blinding of the study staff. Using group blinded analysis and application of objective parameters such as saliva cortisol, this disadvantage was accounted for as far as possible. Another limitation which could have influenced the study results is the lack of data on the relationship and role of the nurses and other health professionals in usual interaction and information sharing with the woman during and after procedure.

We would like to emphasize that with a large sample of 304 participants and several measurement time points throughout the day of the caesarean as a strength of the study. This is the first study in this area of research that has the necessary power to detect even small effect sizes.

Conclusions

In view of the results, the present study should have implications for clinical practice. Music is a simple, inexpensive, effective and safe intervention that can be easily implemented in everyday clinical practice. Therefore, it would be desirable if the possibility to listen to music could be routinely offered to women giving birth by caesarean. However, further research should consider the impact of music on the surgical team. Although previous work showed adverse effects only for high volumes and complex interventions [37], this has not been investigated explicitly in the context of caesarean.

In conclusion, the results of the present study show that music during caesarean has an anxiety and stress soothing effect on the wake patient. Implementation in clinical routine therefore seems advisable.

Abbreviations
ANOVA: Analysis of variance; C: Salivary cortisol; CONSORT: Consolidated Standards of Reporting Trials; HR: Heart rate; Pts: Patients; RR dia: Diastolic blood pressure; RR sys: Systolic blood pressure; sAA: Salivary alpha amylase; SD: Standard deviation; STAI: State-Trait Anxiety Inventory; VAS-A: Visual analogue scale for anxiety

Acknowledgements
We'd like to thank the dedicated team of midwives of the department of gynaecology and obstetrics of the Heinrich-Heine-University Düsseldorf.

Funding
The study was funded by a research grant from the Anton-Betz-Foundation.

Authors' contributions
PH and NKS managed the project. PH, CH, WG, WJ and NKS conceived and designed the study. CH, JG, PB lead the acquisition of data. PH, JG and NKS analysed the data. PH, OTW, WG, WJ, MF, TF, NKS interpreted the data. JG, PB, and MF provided administrative, technical and logistic support. PH and NKS drafted the manuscript. All authors revised the manuscript critically for important intellectual content and approved the final version of the manuscript.

Competing interests
All authors declare that they have no competing interests.

Author details
[1]Clinic for Gynecology and Obstetrics, Helios University Hospital Wuppertal, University Witten/Herdecke, Heusnerstr 40, 42283 Wuppertal, Germany. [2]Clinic for Gynecology and Obstetrics, Heinrich-Heine-University, Düsseldorf, Germany. [3]Department of Cognitive Psychology, Institute of Cognitive Neuroscience, Faculty of Psychology, Ruhr-University Bochum, Bochum, Germany. [4]Musikerambulanz, Heinrich-Heine-University, Düsseldorf, Germany. [5]Clinic for Gynecology and Obstetrics, University Hospital Ulm, Ulm, Germany. [6]Department of Experimental Psychology, Heinrich-Heine-University, Düsseldorf, Germany.

References
1. Blüml V, Stammler-Safar M, Reitinger AK, Resch I, Naderer A, Leithner K. A qualitative approach to examine women's experience of planned cesarean. J Obstet Gynecol Neonatal Nurs. 2012;41:E82–90. https://doi.org/10.1111/j.1552-6909.2012.01398.x.
2. Hepp P, Hagenbeck C, Burghardt B, Jaeger B, Wolf OT, Fehm T, et al. Measuring the course of anxiety in women giving birth by caesarean section: a prospective study. BMC Pregnancy Childbirth. 2016;16:113. https://doi.org/10.1186/s12884-016-0906-z.
3. Mulder EJH, Robles de Medina PG, Huizink AC, den Bergh BRH V, Buitelaar JK, GHA V. Prenatal maternal stress: effects on pregnancy and the (unborn) child. Early Hum Dev. 2002;70:3–14 http://www.ncbi.nlm.nih.gov/pubmed/12441200. Accessed 15 Oct 2017.
4. O'Donnell KJ, Glover V, Barker ED, O'Connor TG. The persisting effect of maternal mood in pregnancy on childhood psychopathology. Dev Psychopathol. 2014;26:393–403. https://doi.org/10.1017/S0954579414000029.
5. Good M. Effects of relaxation and music on postoperative pain: a review. J Adv Nurs. 1996;24:905–14 http://www.ncbi.nlm.nih.gov/pubmed/8933249. Accessed 15 Oct 2017.
6. Powell R, Scott NW, Manyande A, Bruce J, Vögele C, Byrne-Davis LM, et al. Psychological preparation and postoperative outcomes for adults undergoing surgery under general anaesthesia. In: Powell R, editor. Cochrane Database of Systematic Reviews. Chichester: John Wiley & Sons, Ltd; 2016. p. CD008646. https://doi.org/10.1002/14651858.CD008646.pub2.
7. Dewey KG. Maternal and fetal stress are associated with impaired lactogenesis in humans. J Nutr. 2001;131:3012S–5S http://www.ncbi.nlm.nih.gov/pubmed/11694638. Accessed 15 Oct 2017.
8. Grajeda R, Pérez-Escamilla R. Stress during labor and delivery is associated with delayed onset of lactation among urban Guatemalan women. J Nutr. 2002;132:3055–60 http://www.ncbi.nlm.nih.gov/pubmed/12368395. Accessed 15 Oct 2017.
9. Conrad C. Music for healing: from magic to medicine. Lancet (London, England). 2010;376:1980–1 http://www.ncbi.nlm.nih.gov/pubmed/21171230. Accessed 15 Oct 2017.
10. Goertz W, Dominick K, Heussen N, Vom dahl J. Music in the cath lab: who should select it. Clin Res Cardiol. 2011;100:395–402. https://doi.org/10.1007/s00392-010-0256-1.
11. Smolen D, Topp R, Singer L. The effect of self-selected music during colonoscopy on anxiety, heart rate, and blood pressure. Appl Nurs Res. 2002;15:126–36 http://www.ncbi.nlm.nih.gov/pubmed/12173164. Accessed 14 Oct 2015.
12. Koelsch S, Fuermetz J, Sack U, Bauer K, Hohenadel M, Wiegel M, et al. Effects of music listening on cortisol levels and Propofol consumption during spinal anesthesia. Front Psychol. 2011;2:58. https://doi.org/10.3389/fpsyg.2011.00058.
13. Angioli R, De Cicco NC, Plotti F, Cafà EV, Dugo N, Damiani P, et al. Use of music to reduce anxiety during office hysteroscopy: prospective randomized trial. J Minim Invasive Gynecol. 2014;21:454–9. https://doi.org/10.1016/j.jmig.2013.07.020.
14. Hole J, Hirsch M, Ball E, Meads C. Music as an aid for postoperative recovery in adults: a systematic review and meta-analysis. Lancet. 2015;386:1659–71. https://doi.org/10.1016/S0140-6736(15)60169-6.
15. Laopaiboon M, Lumbiganon P, Martis R, Vatanasapt P, Somjaivong B. Music during caesarean section under regional anaesthesia for improving maternal and infant outcomes. Cochrane Database Syst Rev. 2009: CD006914. https://doi.org/10.1002/14651858.CD006914.pub2.
16. Li Y, Dong Y. Preoperative music intervention for patients undergoing cesarean delivery. Int J Gynaecol Obstet. 2012;119:81–3. https://doi.org/10.1016/j.ijgo.2012.05.017.
17. Kushnir J, Friedman A, Ehrenfeld M, Kushnir T. Coping with preoperative anxiety in cesarean section: physiological, cognitive, and emotional effects of listening to favorite music. Birth. 2012;39:121–7. https://doi.org/10.1111/j.1523-536X.2012.00532.x.
18. Chang S, Chen C. Effects of music therapy on women's physiologic measures, anxiety, and satisfaction during cesarean delivery. Res Nurs Health. 2005;28:453–61. https://doi.org/10.1002/nur.20102.
19. Reza N, Ali SM, Saeed K, Abul-Qasim A, Reza TH. The impact of music on postoperative pain and anxiety following cesarean section. Middle East J

Anaesthesiol. 2007;19:573–86 http://www.ncbi.nlm.nih.gov/pubmed/18044285. Accessed 15 Oct 2017.

20. Laux L, Glanzmann P, Schaffner P, Spielberger CD. Das State-Trait-Angstinventar (STAI) (Beltz-Test). Beltz Test GmbH: Göttingen; 1981.

21. Strahler J, Skoluda N, Kappert MB, Nater UM. Simultaneous measurement of salivary cortisol and alpha-amylase: application and recommendations. Neurosci Biobehav Rev. 2017;83:657–77. https://doi.org/10.1016/j.neubiorev.2017.08.015.

22. Schoofs D, Wolf OT. Are salivary gonadal steroid concentrations influenced by acute psychosocial stress? A study using the Trier social stress test (TSST). Int J Psychophysiol. 2011;80:36–43. https://doi.org/10.1016/j.ijpsycho.2011.01.008.

23. Nilsson U. The anxiety- and pain-reducing effects of music interventions: a systematic review. AORN J. 2008;87:780–807. https://doi.org/10.1016/j.aorn.2007.09.013.

24. Petrakova L, Doering BK, Vits S, Engler H, Rief W, Schedlowski M, et al. Psychosocial stress increases salivary alpha-amylase activity independently from plasma noradrenaline levels. PLoS One. 2015;10:e0134561. https://doi.org/10.1371/journal.pone.0134561.

25. Faul F, Erdfelder E, Buchner A, Lang A-G. Statistical power analyses using G*power 3.1: tests for correlation and regression analyses. Behav Res Methods. 2009;41:1149–60. https://doi.org/10.3758/BRM.41.4.1149.

26. Ikonomidou E, Rehnström A, Naesh O. Effect of music on vital signs and postoperative pain. AORN J. 2004;80:269–74, 277–8. http://www.ncbi.nlm.nih.gov/pubmed/15382598 Accessed 15 Oct 2017.

27. Khalfa S, Bella SD, Roy M, Peretz I, Lupien SJ. Effects of relaxing music on salivary cortisol level after psychological stress. Ann N Y Acad Sci. 2003;999:374–6 http://www.ncbi.nlm.nih.gov/pubmed/14681158. Accessed 15 Oct 2017.

28. Zengin S, Kabul S, Al B, Sarcan E, Doğan M, Yildirim C. Effects of music therapy on pain and anxiety in patients undergoing port catheter placement procedure. Complement Ther Med. 2013;21:689–96. https://doi.org/10.1016/j.ctim.2013.08.017.

29. van Stegeren AH, Wolf OT, Kindt M. Salivary alpha amylase and cortisol responses to different stress tasks: impact of sex. Int J Psychophysiol. 2008;69:33–40.

30. Orbach-Zinger S, Ginosar Y, Elliston J, Fadon C, Abu-Lil M, Raz A, et al. Influence of preoperative anxiety on hypotension after spinal anaesthesia in women undergoing caesarean delivery. Br J Anaesth. 2012;109:943–9. https://doi.org/10.1093/bja/aes313.

31. Sadi H, Finkelman M, Rosenberg M. Salivary cortisol, salivary alpha amylase, and the dental anxiety scale. Anesth Prog. 2013;60:46–53. https://doi.org/10.2344/0003-3006-60.2.46.

32. Koelsch S, Jäncke L. Music and the heart. Eur Heart J. 2015;36:3043–9. https://doi.org/10.1093/eurheartj/ehv430.

33. Koelsch S. Brain correlates of music-evoked emotions. Nat Rev Neurosci. 2014;15:170–80. https://doi.org/10.1038/nrn3666.

34. Bernardi L, Porta C, Casucci G, Balsamo R, Bernardi NF, Fogari R, et al. Dynamic interactions between musical, cardiovascular, and cerebral rhythms in humans. Circulation. 2009;119:3171–80 http://www.ncbi.nlm.nih.gov/pubmed/19569263. Accessed 22 Oct 2017.

35. Bernatzky G, Kreutz G. Musik und Medizin Chancen für Therapie, Prävention und Bildung. Vienna: Springer; 2015.

36. Thaut MH, McIntosh GC, Hoemberg V. Neurobiological foundations of neurologic music therapy: rhythmic entrainment and the motor system. Front Psychol. 2014;5:1185. https://doi.org/10.3389/fpsyg.2014.01185.

37. Weldon S-M, Korkiakangas T, Bezemer J, Kneebone R. Music and communication in the operating theatre. J Adv Nurs. 2015;71:2763–74. https://doi.org/10.1111/jan.12744.

19

Limits to the scope of non-invasive prenatal testing (NIPT): an analysis of the international ethical framework for prenatal screening and an interview study with Dutch professionals

A. Kater-Kuipers[1], E. M. Bunnik[1*], I. D. de Beaufort[1†] and R. J. H. Galjaard[2†]

Abstract

Background: The introduction of non-invasive prenatal testing (NIPT) for foetal aneuploidies is currently changing the field of prenatal screening in many countries. As it is non-invasive, safe and accurate, this technique allows for a broad implementation of first-trimester prenatal screening, which raises ethical issues, related, for instance, to informed choice and adverse societal consequences. This article offers an account of a leading international ethical framework for prenatal screening, examines how this framework is used by professionals working in the field of NIPT, and presents ethical guidance for the expansion of the scope of prenatal screening in practice.

Methods: A comparative analysis of authoritative documents is combined with 15 semi-structured interviews with professionals in the field of prenatal screening in the Netherlands. Data were recorded, transcribed verbatim and analysed using thematic analysis.

Results: The current ethical framework consists of four pillars: the aim of screening, the proportionality of the test, justice, and societal aspects. Respondents recognised and supported this framework in practice, but expressed some concerns. Professionals felt that pregnant women do not always make informed choices, while this is seen as central to reproductive autonomy (the aim of screening), and that pre-test counselling practices stand in need of improvement. Respondents believed that the benefits of NIPT, and of an expansion of its scope, outweigh the harms (proportionality), which are thought to be acceptable. They felt that the out-of-pocket financial contribution currently required by pregnant women constitutes a barrier to access to NIPT, which disproportionally affects those of a lower socioeconomic status (justice). Finally, professionals recognised but did not share concerns about a rising pressure to test or discrimination of disabled persons (societal aspects).

(Continued on next page)

* Correspondence: e.bunnik@erasmusmc.nl
†I. D. de Beaufort and R. J. H. Galjaard contributed equally to this work.
[1]Department of Medical Ethics and Philosophy of Medicine, Erasmus MC, University Medical Centre Rotterdam, Room 24.17, Wytemaweg 80, 3015 CN Rotterdam, The Netherlands
Full list of author information is available at the end of the article

(Continued from previous page)

Conclusions: Four types of limits to the scope of NIPT are proposed: NIPT should generate only test outcomes that are relevant to reproductive decision-making, informed choice should be (made) possible through adequate pre-test counselling, the rights of future children should be respected, and equal access should be guaranteed. Although the focus of the interview study is on the Dutch healthcare setting, insights and conclusions can be applied internationally and to other healthcare systems.

Keywords: Prenatal screening, Non-invasive prenatal testing (NIPT), Reproductive autonomy, Informed consent, Public health ethics, Ethical framework, Qualitative interview study

Background

Non-invasive prenatal testing (NIPT) is based on the analysis of cell free foetal DNA for chromosomal abnormalities [1]. Non-invasiveness refers to the way the foetal DNA sample is obtained: not from the placenta or amniotic fluid, which requires an invasive procedure, but from a blood sample of the mother. NIPT for chromosomal abnormalities was first offered in 2011, in the United States of America, Western-Europe and China [2]. In the Netherlands, prenatal screening for untreatable disorders is subjected to licensing under the Population Screening Act. NIPT has been offered to high-risk women, exclusively within the context of the TRIDENT-1 study (Trial by Dutch laboratories for Evaluation of Non-Invasive Prenatal Testing) since early 2014 [3]. When a woman received a high-risk outcome (chance ≥1:200) from the first trimester combined test (FCT) and wanted further testing, she was offered the choice between NIPT or invasive testing [3]. Low-risk pregnant women who wanted NIPT could not access NIPT in the Netherlands, and went abroad. Since April 2017, NIPT is also offered within the TRIDENT-2 study to low-risk pregnant women, who are given a choice between FCT and NIPT. The current NIPT-based prenatal test includes detection of trisomy 21 (Down syndrome), trisomy 18 (Edwards syndrome) and trisomy 13 (Patau syndrome). Compared to the FCT the sensitivity, the specificity and the positive predictive value of NIPT are remarkably high for those trisomies [3]. The positive predictive value is slightly lower in low-risk pregnant women but still higher than the positive predictive value of the FCT [1, 4, 5]. However, NIPT is not a diagnostic test. This is because of several factors. First, cell free foetal DNA circulating in maternal blood originates from the placenta, not the foetus. The presence of a chromosomal anomaly can be limited to the placenta in case of confined placental mosaicism without affecting the foetus, thus resulting in a false positive NIPT outcome. Furthermore, the presence of maternal chromosomal anomalies, including those originating from a maternal tumour, low foetal DNA fraction in maternal blood, and a vanishing twin [6, 7], may still lead to inconclusive, false positive or false negative results [8]. Yet NIPT leads to fewer unnecessary invasive follow-ups tests - through

amniocentesis and chorionic villus sampling - than the FCT. These invasive tests have a 0.1–0.2% risk, respectively, of miscarriage [3]. To minimize the need for invasive testing – and the associated risk of miscarriage – has been one of the major reasons for implementing NIPT in current screening programmes.

When genome-wide sequencing techniques are used to perform NIPT, they allow for the detection of chromosomal abnormalities other than trisomy 13, 18 and 21, and thus for an expansion of the current scope of prenatal screening [3, 9]. Several studies have indicated that additional findings could include other full trisomies, sex-chromosomal abnormalities, and sub-chromosomal aberrations, associated with rare diseases [3, 10–12]. However, the possibility to find more abnormalities has raised questions, notably the policy question whether the screening offer should be expanded to include all those abnormalities. When discussing the question whether or not to include additional conditions, experts have brought up considerations of clinical utility and concerns related to the consequences of a broader test for informed choice [13–15]. These concerns were raised 10 years ago, when genome-wide arrays were introduced in prenatal diagnosis, and are raised again with renewed urgency in the context of the introduction of NIPT [16].

Various statements and position papers about prenatal screening, issued by governmental organisations and ethical committees, have addressed ethical issues of prenatal screening [15, 17–24]. Together with scholarly studies of ethical issues in prenatal screening [25–30] these statements and position papers could be seen as an – unofficial, but broadly shared and often referred to – international ethical framework for prenatal screening. An ethical framework can be defined as a specification of general principles in a specific context, through which the scope of general principles is narrowed by spelling out why and how actions should be undertaken or avoided [31]. The aim of an ethical framework is to "provide practical guidance for public health professionals and to highlight the defining values of public health" [32].

The aim of this article is firstly to reconstruct and analyse the main tenets of the ethical framework for prenatal screening and then to compare these with the practice of prenatal screening, through interviews with professionals in the field of prenatal screening. Secondly, this article examines whether and how the ethical framework can guide an expansion of the scope of prenatal screening.

Methods

For this study we used a combination of methods, a literature study and a qualitative interview study. We conducted a comparative analysis of ethical statements about requirements for (non-invasive) prenatal testing formulated by national and international organisations or committees. Also, we conducted in-depth interviews with Dutch professionals in the field of prenatal screening. The interviews serve to illustrate how the ethical framework for prenatal screening is translated into practice, and to offer insight into professionals' moral views on recent developments in prenatal screening.

Document analysis

To identify important documents that represent an ethical framework we started with an authoritative article of the European Society of Human Genetics (ESHG) and the American Society of Human Genetics (ASHG), which offers a consensus view of responsible innovation in prenatal screening, which is also endorsed by the Human Genetics Society of Australasia and other related professional associations in Europe [15]. We built on this consensus view and postulated four pillars of an ethical framework: the aim of prenatal screening, proportionality of testing, justice, and societal aspects. Other studies and documents – notably from the World Health Organisation (WHO), UNESCO International Bioethics Committee (IBC), German Ethics Council (Ethikrat) and the Dutch Health Council (GR) – were reviewed to corroborate, adapt and complement the ethical framework. We selected these four other documents for our analysis because – in contrast to other publications we have reviewed – these documents contain discussions of issues related to all four pillars.

Interviews

For the qualitative interview study, professionals in the field of prenatal screening and follow-up diagnostic testing from six academic centres in the Netherlands were invited. In total 15 individual in-depth interviews were conducted with two midwives, seven medical specialists (three gynaecologists, four clinical geneticists specialised in prenatal diagnosis), two lab specialists working with NIPT, two test developers and two policy makers. The interviews were conducted at the respondents' work places or at Erasmus MC. A semi-structured interview guide was used. This guide included five themes: informed decision-making, proportionality, access to NIPT, societal aspects and the

scope of prenatal screening. Interviews were digitally recorded, transcribed verbatim and analysed with Atlas.ti using thematic analysis, based on the five indicated themes.

Results

The documents each point at the four pillars - the aim of screening, the proportionality of the test, justice, and societal aspects - but differ in some aspects of their interpretations. Table 1 presents an overview of interpretations of the four pillars in the five documents. Below we present the four pillars of the ethical framework for the practice of prenatal screening, complemented with results from the interviews.

Aim of prenatal screening

The first pillar of the ethical framework for prenatal screening pertains to the aim of prenatal screening for foetal abnormalities. Prenatal screening differs from other areas of public health, where the aim is reduction of morbidity and mortality associated with disorders in the population [15]. Translating this aim to prenatal screening might imply that the success of a prenatal screening programme would be defined in terms of maximisation of the termination rate of foetuses with abnormalities, which would be problematic, as abortion is often a point of controversy [15, 17, 19, 20]. Besides, prenatal screening is thought to imply discriminatory messages about the value of the lives of people living with the relevant conditions [15, 17–19]. The widely supported view therefore is that governments can only justifiably offer prenatal screening when the aim is to enable pregnant women and their partners to make autonomous reproductive choices [15, 17, 19].

Although interviewed professionals recognised informed choice as the aim of prenatal screening, some of them pointed out that prenatal screening also provides the opportunity to prepare for the birth of a disabled child and to improve the care for it. Several respondents thought that the latter should be emphasised more during pre-test counselling and that it should be made clear that prenatal screening is not exclusively aimed at offering women the opportunity to terminate an affected pregnancy.

The right not to know about the options of prenatal screening is considered very important. In the Netherlands, this has been formalised in the obligation of professionals to present women with an 'information offer' first [33], in order to stress the fact that prenatal screening for aneuploidies is not mandatory. When a pregnant woman visits the midwife or obstetrician, the professional must first ask whether the woman wants to be informed about prenatal screening at all. The woman is free to decline this information offer. Not all professionals agreed with this policy, and some argued - contra current policy - that this first question should be

Table 1 An ethical framework for prenatal screening

	ESHG/ASHG (2015)	WHO (2003)	Ethikrat (2013)	Dutch Health Council (2013)	UNESCO (2015)
Aim of prenatal screening	The aim is to enable autonomous reproductive choices, i.e. meaningful choices, related to serious health problems. The aim is achieved when women are enabled to make informed choices. Prenatal screening has a different goal than other forms of screening, because of the 'morally sensitive practice' of (selective) abortion and the stigmatisation of disabled people.	The aim is to obtain information and to promote freedom of choice and autonomy. Being able to prepare for the birth of a child with a disability is also seen as a way to exercise reproductive autonomy. Free choice requires: 1) adequate, unbiased information; 2) availability of relevant alternatives, including availability of healthcare services for disabled children or the (legal) possibility of abortion.	The aim is not specified, but prenatal screening is linked to self-determination and autonomy: "If a pregnant woman makes decisions about her pregnancy, these must be seen inter alia in the context of her right to reproductive self-determination." Reproductive decisions affect the unborn child and are thus not unlimited.	The aim is to enable and promote choice terminating or continuing the pregnancy. "Informed choice is not a condition for, but the aim of prenatal screening." The aim is not to maximise reproductive choice as such. If informed choice is not reached, the aim is not achieved.	The aim is "not health gain but to decide (…) whether to carry a pregnancy to term." Furthermore, "it allows those involved to prepare for the birth of a sick or disabled child." There is controversy about the limits of reproductive autonomy in the light of a child's right to an un-manipulated genetic make-up. Prevention, focused on "reducing care costs for people with congenital conditions or disabilities, cannot be the goal of such screening. That would imply a discriminatory practice that sends the message that these people are unwelcome in society."
Proportionality	Proportionality is defined as a balancing of benefits and harms. Benefits of NIPT include reassurance, assistance in making informed reproductive decisions, and less invasive testing. Harms of prenatal screening generally include false reassurance, stress and anxiety, and risk of miscarriage in follow-up diagnostic testing. Balancing of benefits and harms includes consideration of quality aspects of the test and adequate counselling.	Proportionality is not discussed. Benefits and burdens are included in a cost-benefit analysis. Benefits are the chance to prepare for the birth of a child that will need medical treatment or a relief of maternal anxiety. Burdens include selective abortion of a wanted pregnancy.	Proportionality is not discussed, although it is stated that quality assurance is a precondition to meeting the aim of prenatal screening. Balancing benefits and harms is difficult: "The effect of a differentiated prenatal diagnosis is ambivalent. It may relieve the pregnant woman of fears, but on the other hand there is the danger that the (…) associated burden of deciding make[s] the couple affected (…) and may even overstrain them." It is seen as a great risk that women may be insufficiently aware of the consequences of testing and subsequent decisions they will have to make.	Proportionality is a central requirement for prenatal screening. Screening is only justified when the value or utility of the offer is established and the benefits outweigh the disadvantages. Benefits of NIPT include reassurance, informed reproductive decisions and less invasive testing. 'Disadvantages' of screening include false reassurance, test-related stress and anxiety and risk of miscarriage.	Proportionality and proven usefulness are preconditions for a justified prenatal screening offer. The advantages should outweigh the disadvantages. Benefits are having freedom to choose and fewer invasive tests. Disadvantages are "routinization and institutionalization of choice of not giving birth to an ill or disabled child." If a test becomes self-evident women might feel pressured to test or stigmatised when they will not test.
Justice	Justice refers to the distribution of costs: "As health budgets are	Justice refers to the "equitable distribution of genetics services,	Justice refers to equal access to prenatal screening and to the	Justice refers to an appropriate use of healthcare resources.	Justice refers to the organisation of healthcare systems,

Table 1 An ethical framework for prenatal screening *(Continued)*

	ESHG/ASHG (2015)	WHO (2003)	Ethikrat (2013)	Dutch Health Council (2013)	UNESCO (2015)
	inevitably limited (...), opportunity costs will have to be taken into account as well." The requirement of just distribution of healthcare costs will demarcate the scope of prenatal screening.	including prenatal diagnosis, is owed first to those with the greatest medical need, regardless of ability to pay, or any other considerations." Relief of maternal anxiety has lower priority than medical indications for prenatal screening, in the just distribution of healthcare resources.	danger of "discrimination and stigmatization of people with particular genetic characteristics."	Prenatal screening can be used appropriately by couples wishing to prepare for the birth of an affected child, which is considered a justified aim of screening. Justice is also mentioned in the context of equal access to an expanded scope of prenatal screening: screening for abnormalities other than trisomy 21, 18 and 13 should not only be available for high-risk women (through invasive follow-up testing).	so that innovations are shared with society as a whole, without becoming a new source of inequality and discrimination. Justice also pertains to education: people should be actively enabled to exercise their freedom and autonomy. Finally, it refers to proper distribution of costs and investments in various fields within the healthcare system (e.g. care for people with disabilities).
Social aspects	As a public health programme, prenatal screening might have "consequences for other individuals and groups (including those living with the relevant conditions)". To avoid discriminatory messages, the aim of screening (reproductive autonomy) should be stressed. NIPT might be seen as a routine procedure, which might lead to routinisation of prenatal screening, affecting the informed choices of pregnant women.	Prenatal screening may have negative effects for people with disabilities, but does not lead to the birth of fewer people with disabilities, as long as chromosomal and single gene disorders account for only a minority of disabilities present at birth. Healthcare for people with disabilities will and should not be reduced, also to prevent 'economic eugenics' which would hinder voluntary decision-making. Although "cultures or medical settings may be implicitly coercive," these problems are seen as part of the general sociocultural context and not attributed to prenatal screening specifically.	Prenatal screening generates genetic information and could have social consequences including stigmatisation and discrimination. There is a (shared) duty to create a society without discrimination, which will be a result of interactions between people and does not depend on the presence or absence of one test. Routine offer of prenatal screening might have negative consequences for reproductive freedom and put pressure on women to test: the idea that pregnant women should take their parental responsibility and opt for testing should be avoided.	Prenatal screening programmes may have social impact but are not necessarily discriminatory, because they aim at reproductive choice and not at prevention. However, concerns related to the social impact of screening on people with a disability are realistic. Therefore ongoing ethical monitoring of screening practices is necessary. Also, the state should guarantee good-quality care for people with a disability. A simple and safe test could possibly lead to routinisation, including pressure to test. This might affect reproductive autonomy.	Prenatal screening is often not a therapeutic intervention but likely to lead to abortion and it might lead to discrimination and stigmatisation. "The adding up of a lot of individual choices to the 'acceptability' of aborting certain kinds of embryos (...) brings forward a societal phenomenon, which resembles a kind of eugenics in the search for a 'perfect child'." Non-discrimination should be emphasised and guaranteed. Prenatal screening as a 'routine measure' might negatively affect society's perception of disability and societal solidarity with disabled people and the women who give birth to them.

skipped, *"because many people actually do not know what it [prenatal screening] entails. How could you say 'yes' or 'no' to this question when you do not exactly know what this test is for?"* (I3 medical specialist)

In order to reach the aim of prenatal screening, it is of paramount importance that pregnant women or couples can make informed choices for or against a screening offer [15, 17–20]. Informed choice is often defined as "a choice that is based on relevant knowledge, consistent with the decision maker's values and behaviourally implemented" [34, 35]. This means that women should understand the purpose of the test and its potential risks and implications [36], because they may be confronted with "a large number of further decisions which [they] might have wished to avoid if [they] had been aware of the consequences before screening" [18]. To help women make informed choices pre-test counselling is offered. During pre-test counselling women are presented with information about the purpose, nature, scope and validity [18] and complete information about diseases, including e.g. "name(s) and general characteristics of the major disorder(s)," possible treatments, possible unexpected or unclear findings of the test and kinds of test-outcome [20]. Furthermore, pre-test counselling for first-trimester prenatal screening should be conducted at a designated moment, clearly separated from information provision about other aspects of antenatal care, such as lifestyle, health aspects (e.g. screening for HIV) and birth planning [15].

Many professionals noticed that when women talked about their reasons for choosing prenatal screening, they often mentioned wanting to be reassured about the health of their child. Professionals thought that women sometimes do not realise in advance what kinds of outcomes they might face and difficult choices they might have to make: women *"have to realise that if [they] opt for NIPT and a congenital disorder is found, [they] kind of jump on a train on which [they] might not want to be. [... I] hear people say that they are in a rollercoaster."* (I8, medical specialist).

Some professionals thought that especially in the case of NIPT this might be a problem. The previous screening programme in the Netherlands was step-wise: the first step was a FCT, which provided only a risk estimate for aneuploidies. Then women had to think carefully about invasive follow-up testing, taking into account the risk of miscarriage. Women could choose whether or not to undergo invasive testing to obtain a diagnostic result. Professionals thought that this step-wise process gradually prepared women for the obtaining of an abnormal test result. They thought that, with NIPT, by contrast, women will opt for an easy test and – in one single step – may be confronted with an almost 'diagnostic outcome' at once. NIPT *"gives the idea of a decisive outcome."* (I10, midwife) As said, this idea is not accurate, as diagnostic follow-up testing is required also with NIPT. The odds that the result turns out false positive, however, are much lower.

In order to protect women from the negative consequences of uninformed choices, professionals emphasised that counselling plays a crucial role. Counselling serves to explain women's options and to correct misunderstandings

of tests and disabilities, but should also explore the norms and values and the attitudes of women towards having a child with a disability. During counselling women should be encouraged to think about their views about testing, about having a child with a disability and termination of pregnancy: *"Yes, I think, that with a few standard questions [the counsellor] will [be able to] achieve a lot. Just to trigger [women], let's say [to think about the consequences of NIPT]. That does not necessarily take a lot of time. [... As a counsellor, you could ask women:] What does Down syndrome mean to you?"* (I3, medical specialist).

Respondents took the view that the current quality of counselling in the Netherlands is moderate, and needs improvement: professionals should pay more attention to and spend more time on pre-test counselling. Dedicated counselling sessions will help women understand that the aim of prenatal screening for chromosomal abnormalities is different from the aims of antenatal care (i.e. maintaining and/or improving the health of the pregnant woman and the foetus). Some respondents, who were medical specialists, feared that professionals underestimate the importance of (non-directive) counselling for NIPT and should be aware that the ease of the test, requiring only a maternal blood sample, and its high reliability may lead to less informed choices. One study suggested that professionals might indeed attach less importance to informed consent for a non-invasive test compared to an invasive test [37].

To conclude, in order to reach the aim of prenatal screening - reproductive autonomy - informed choice is of crucial importance. Counselling should be non-directive and of high quality, and include deliberation on personal values of women, in order to achieve informed choice and promote this aim.

Proportionality

In the identified ethical framework, the pillar of proportionality of screening programmes entails balancing benefits and harms, following the original screening criteria for population screening formulated by Wilson and Jungner, complemented with additional criteria from the WHO [15, 19, 38]. To assess benefits and harms, the quality of the test and the test offer, including the laboratory procedures, counselling and education of professionals should be evaluated [15]. According to the ESHG/ASHG and the Dutch Health Council, the benefits and harms or costs depend on the way NIPT will be offered, as a first-tier screening test or second-tier screening test, after FCT [15, 17]. When NIPT would replace FCT as a first-tier test, it might have the benefit of fewer false positive results for trisomy 21, 18, and 13, but on the other hand might also lead to a loss of other findings that can be identified on ultrasound as part of FCT. Experts must decide whether the benefits of a better test performance of NIPT regarding the three trisomies will outweigh this loss of diagnostic yield when the first-trimester ultrasound is removed from the screening programme.

For pregnant women or couples, prenatal screening for foetal abnormalities has the benefit of offering reproductive choices regarding an affected pregnancy, including termination of pregnancy or being able to prepare for the birth of an affected child, relief from anxiety in case of a negative test result and the reduction of invasive follow-up tests [15, 17–20]. Harms for pregnant women are related to false reassurance, burden of decision making and anxiety in case of false-positive outcomes and incidental findings, which can be of unclear clinical significance and might cause needless worries [15]. Respondents held that these harms are inevitable but acceptable. Yet the possibility of incidental findings needs to be explained during pre-test counselling. It has been suggested that making the choice to terminate a desired pregnancy after receiving an abnormal test result may be harmful, as well [20].

According to professionals, women might be faced with unwanted choices they have to make, because they may not have been fully aware of the consequences of prenatal screening beforehand, as some medical specialists indicated in the interviews: *"But sometimes I see people saying: 'I never would have wanted this choice. This is a horrible choice you're giving me. I don't want it. This is a wanted pregnancy. If I had not known that this child has Down syndrome I would go for [continuation of this pregnancy], I am sure. But now I have a choice and I am going to hesitate'."* (I7, medical specialist).

Justice

The third pillar of the ethical framework is justice. The principle of justice in prenatal screening relates to equal access to prenatal screening for all pregnant women, to policy questions concerning reimbursement of prenatal screening, and to equal distribution of healthcare resources [15, 17–20]. Equal access to prenatal screening means that differences in personal resources may not cause disparities in access to prenatal screening programmes: women's choices not to participate in screening should not be based upon a lack of financial resources [15, 17–20]. That would imply that prenatal screening should be offered especially to women with limited financial resources, either free of charge or against a small fee. On the other hand, it could be argued that a (small) payment might serve the aim of reproductive autonomy as it may "increases awareness that there is truly a choice to be made" [15].

Professionals recognised this dilemma concerning the reimbursement of prenatal screening. Respondents mentioned the impact of payment on the uptake of prenatal screening. A midwife suggested that the fee that is currently asked for FCT in the Netherlands (165 euros) has much impact and might explain the large difference in the uptake of FCT as compared to the 20-week ultrasound, which is offered free of charge: *"I am curious, when [NIPT] will be reimbursed and [as a counsellor] you explain to people the possibility of having a NIPT, whether they would say: 'If it is reimbursed and it gives information about the health of my child, of course I want [to use NIPT].' They do the same for the 20-week scan. I really wonder whether the difference [in uptake for the FCT and the 20-week ultrasound] is that big because people say: 'I [do want to] give birth to a child with Down syndrome but not to a child with spina bifida'. I do not believe that [differences in attitudes explain the] difference between 30% [the uptake of the FCT] and 95% [the uptake of the 20-week ultrasound]."* (I10, midwife)

Some professionals suggested that a financial contribution by women might serve as a helpful barrier, making women aware of the importance of the choice. It could prevent women from opting for a test 'just because it is possible and does not cost any money', and thus protect them against ill-considered testing. On the other hand, respondents mentioned two objections to payment as a barrier for test uptake. Firstly, professionals thought that some women refrain from screening because of lack of money: *"There are a lot of people for whom [165 euros] is a lot of money that can buy a lot of baby clothes."* (I13, medical specialist) They thought that lack of money is not a good reason to decline screening. Professionals think that when screening is offered, it should be reimbursed to guarantee unhindered access. Secondly, asking a contribution is in contradiction with equality in healthcare: *"Yes, it is a barrier, but for whom are you creating a barrier? For a specific group of people who cannot pay for it."* (I3, medical specialist)

Experts should understand that while requiring a personal financial contribution may serve a purpose (i.e. improving informed choice), it may also, and more importantly, create disparities in access to prenatal screening, which is undesirable and contrary to one of the moral pillars of prenatal screening: justice.

Societal aspects

Self-determination is not only a matter of individual freedom, but also has a societal dimension, and it may be threatened by for example group pressure or societal views about testing [18, 19]. One of the concerns related to group pressure is that it might lead to less-autonomous choices among pregnant women. This would be problematic, it is argued, because the aim of prenatal screening, reproductive autonomy, will not be reached when women fail to make informed choices [15, 17–20].

Furthermore, it is thought that the offer of prenatal screening for chromosomal abnormalities might also imply a discriminatory message to individuals and groups living with specific diseases [15, 17–20]. This objection is known as the 'disability rights critique' of prenatal screening and holds that discriminatory messages are inseparable from prenatal screening [15, 17]. This critique may apply both to the sheer societal availability of prenatal screening programmes and to individual women's choices. In response, it is underlined that the aim of prenatal screening is not preventing the birth of disabled people, but promoting reproductive autonomy [17]. Also, studies have shown that women's reasons for the selective termination of their pregnancies include prevention of a life of severe suffering and not being able to create the best conditions to care for a child with a disability [17, 39–43], which does not support this critique. However, with the introduction of NIPT, the uptake of first-trimester screening might increase and the number of persons with disabilities might decrease. This is not in itself problematic, but it might become problematic if a low prevalence of disabilities will negatively affect the position of persons with disabilities, and render the option to continue an affected pregnancy less attractive. Therefore the practice of prenatal screening should be evaluated continuously in comparison to its aim [17]. Moreover, a negative perception of people with a disability can be redressed with public information and education [19]. The WHO concludes that just non-discriminatory societal settings are important for making a free choice: "It is important to prevent discrimination and to provide improved support services for individuals and families with genetic conditions. The absence of adequate services for people with hereditary disabilities undermines the principle of free choice for couples at risk of having children with such disabilities" [20].

Professionals did not think that the uptake of prenatal screening would increase dramatically, although they suggested that an easier test is less likely to be declined and might become self-evident. They observed however that the need to participate in prenatal screening is not as self-evident to many pregnant women as the need for other tests in pregnancy. Besides, *"there will always be people who do not want to know [about health risks of their foetus], who just want a care-free pregnancy, and [who feel that] every child is welcome."* (I13 medical specialist) Moreover, professionals think that women will not choose to terminate pregnancies more often because women who participate in prenatal screening generally have desired pregnancies, and do not wish to undergo termination of pregnancy for trivial reasons [18]. Also, according to respondents, specific cultural aspects in the Netherlands might in part explain the low uptake of NIPT, as compared to other countries. In the Dutch prenatal screening programme, midwives play important roles in pre-test counselling, rather than medical specialists [44]. Among midwives, there is a tendency to avoid medical interference in the pregnancy. Also, in society, a rather positive public image of Down syndrome prevails. Professionals held the opinion that the fear that fewer people with Down syndrome will be born when NIPT is introduced, is not justified. Respondents thought that people with a disability are accepted in the Netherlands and that there is good care available for handicapped people. However, they agreed that care and support should be guaranteed to counteract possible negative consequences of prenatal screening, including discrimination.

In sum, societal aspects and concerns such as an increase in test uptake and a decrease in people born with disabilities are recognized, but disputed in the literature as well as among professionals. However, it is acknowledged that arrangements should be made (i.e. ensuring quality of care for the disabled) to counteract possible negative consequences.

Discussion

The four pillars of the ethical framework can be used to evaluate the potential expansion of the scope of NIPT. Below, four limits are proposed to the responsible expansion of the scope of NIPT in the future. These limits provide ethical guidance for professionals and policy-makers who are working in the field of NIPT and will be shaping its development and further implementation in the future.

Limits set by the aim of prenatal screening

In the five documents it is explicitly stated that although the aim of prenatal screening is not to maximise reproductive choice indefinitely, there is room for expansion of the screening offer [15, 17, 20]. In the interviews several professionals indicated that a broader test will contribute to the aim of prenatal screening because an expanded NIPT allows for detecting more disorders than trisomy 21, 18 and 13: *"People do not want a test for Down syndrome, but a test for a healthy child."* (I15)

However, an expanded scope might affect informed choice as a precondition of reproductive autonomy. When NIPT includes a high number of diseases, it will be difficult in pre-test counselling to discuss all possible test outcomes in detail, "including the full range of variability in the manifestations" of these diseases [15]. Testing for more abnormalities might thus "paradoxically undermine rather than serve or enhance reproductive autonomy." [15] A clinical professional feared that *"people have no idea what the results [of NIPT] can be and what these could mean to them. I am sure about this, because for Down syndrome it is already the case [that people do not understand what the outcome means to them]."* (I7, medical specialist)

This raises the question how to best inform pregnant women prior to the test. It has been suggested in documents and by some of our respondents that information about the possible outcomes of prenatal screening should be presented as categories of disorders: the scope of NIPT can be narrow or broad, with results pertaining to severe or non-severe disorders and early- or late-onset disorders. When the scope of NIPT expands to such an extent that it becomes impossible to describe in detail all possible test outcomes during pre-test counselling, the counsellor "should describe the general characteristics of the categories of disorders tested for (e.g., mental disability or neurological impairment). Women will receive intensive counselling after a foetal diagnosis." [20] This model of informed choice is sometimes referred to as 'generic consent', which is thought to be a solution for complex counselling and has already been discussed in the context of genetic screening. Generic consent aims to prevent 'information overload' and to avoid the provision of information that is "pointless or counterproductive" [45]. The question arises whether generic consent offers enough information to enable people to make a truly informed choices [46, 47]. The ESHG/ASHG and the Dutch Health Council have their reservations about generic consent [15, 17], because "the feasibility of this model has not yet been empirically tested in the prenatal context" and it remains unclear how *informed* generic consent would be [15]. The extent to which generic consent can be informed consent should be studied in line with previous studies on informed choice in the context of prenatal screening. These studies showed highly variable percentages of women having made informed choices: 89%, 77,9%, 51% and 44% [35, 48–50]. Some of that variation might be explained by variation in the nature and the quality of pre-test counselling practices, which will likely affect the 'informedness' of women's choices to a great extent, also in the context of an expanded NIPT. In practice, it is not clear whether a sufficient number of professionals will be available to counsel large numbers of pregnant women and their partners, and whether they will have enough time to explain the details of the test and facilitate informed decision-making. In some countries, measures have been put in place to counter this problem, including the use of decision aids and the additional training of midwives in NIPT counselling [51]. Another solution might be a change in the *focus* of counselling, from technical-medical aspects to women's values or goals related to screening. As respondents suggested, too, counselling is more than providing information; women should be triggered to think about why they would want prenatal screening and what they would do in case of an abnormal test result, to make them more aware of their attitude towards undergoing prenatal

screening. Attitude is defined as the general feeling of 'favourableness' or 'unfavourableness' for testing [34]. Triggering women to think about testing might lead to a process of deliberation and evaluation of pros and cons, which, according to several authors, should be part and parcel of an informed choice [49]. Professionals could play a role in this deliberation and help women to formulate their values, for instance in accordance with the interpretive model of the physician-patient relationship, as described by Emanuel and Emanuel [52]. This model entails that the healthcare professional helps to elicit the norms and values of a patient.

We would suggest that in this process, the necessary technical information about the test could support or influence the attitude, but is not sufficient or even essential to the quality of decision-making. Shifting the focus of counselling from 'conveying knowledge about screening' to 'exploring women's attitude towards screening' might improve women's and their partners' decision-making processes, even in the context of an expanded scope of screening and, in combination with decision aids, takes away the time pressure to explain all clinical and technical details of NIPT.

Professionals differed in their opinions about whether women should be given a say in decisions regarding the scope of the screening offer. Some professionals suggested that a list of options should be offered from which women could choose, whereas others believed that experts should determine which (categories of) disorders should be included in the test. The main reason for preferring a predetermined offer was that women might not have the information – or the capacity to understand the information – required to make a decision about the adequate scope of NIPT. Another study of opinions of professionals showed that a majority of respondents preferred a predetermined offer or a fixed list of disorders to be tested [53].

A second category of problems arises with the dual aim of prenatal screening within antenatal care systems [15]. Some routinely offered prenatal screening tests are used to improve pregnancy outcomes or the health condition of the mother or the baby, such as the blood test for rhesus status in RhD-negative women. The rhesus test is currently offered as a separate test but could – for reasons of efficiency – be combined in one test with NIPT for autosomal aneuploidies. An objection to a combination of this test with screening for aneuploidies is the possible confusion in women about what test they should accept or decline, and for what reasons. Prenatal screening for aneuploidies is aimed at reproductive autonomy and requires non-directive counselling [15]. The term 'non-directiveness' refers to the absence of coercion or the withholding of advice, in order to respect the autonomy of a patient [54]. According to Ten Have, as cited in Oduncu, non-directiveness means that the expert who provides information about genetic conditions "should not, in any respect, try to influence the decision made by the persons who are counselled or screened. (...) his aim is merely to provide information and to help the patients or clients to work through possible options." [54] For prevention-aimed screening in antenatal care (e.g. screening for hypertension or rhesus status), it may not be objectionable for health professionals to recommend or insist on participation, because this type of screening promotes the health of the mother and the foetus, but for autonomy-aimed screening, directive counselling is not appropriate [15, 55]. In sum, one (expanded) NIPT that combines two aims and two - opposed - modes of counselling is not desirable.

NIPT is meant to offer reproductive options, but not to screen foetuses for all kinds of medical problems. For instance, children are usually not allowed to undergo predictive testing for (untreatable) late-onset diseases because this might affect their right to an open future and their right not to know unwanted predictive information [15, 17–20]. The principle to defer testing until adulthood applies to unborn children as well. Prenatal screening is not meant as a medical screening of future children: its scope should thus be limited to those conditions for which expecting parents may consider terminating the pregnancy. To protect the unborn child's right not to know, 'conditional access' models have been proposed for women who want information about late-onset diseases: testing for late-onset diseases, including some sex chromosomal aneuploidies, will only be offered if women "expressed the clear intention to choose abortion if a predisposition for a late-onset diseases is found." [56] However, as termination of a pregnancy is, and should continue to be, the result of a voluntary decision, women who change their minds about an earlier expressed intention cannot be forced to terminate an affected pregnancy. Therefore, it cannot be excluded that children may be born in the knowledge of carrying a mutation for a late-onset disease. Further research should focus on the consequences of living with this information for both parents and children and on its effects on their relationship [18, 19].

NIPT may contribute to the aim of prenatal screening: the promotion of reproductive autonomy. On the basis of the first pillar of the ethical framework for prenatal screening, however, limits can be set to the morally responsible expansion of the scope of NIPT: NIPT should generate only test outcomes that are relevant to reproductive decision-making, and informed choice should be (made) possible through adequate pre-test counselling.

Limits set by proportionality

The expansion of the scope of NIPT also raises questions concerning proportionality. According to the Dutch Health Council, proportionality is an important requirement of

prenatal screening, and benefits of each 'test' (for each condition) to be included in the screening offer should outweigh the harms [17]. Professionals noted that it may be beneficial to include more disorders in a test because that means that more reproductive choices can be made: *"There are children who are born with a severe disorder. Then we do an exome analysis to see what the cause is. Then we find, say, in 40% of the cases, a new mutation, in a crucial gene, which the parents do not have. In the future it may be possible to detect that [mutation] in maternal blood."* (I15, lab specialist) Several professionals gave the example of the 22q11 deletion, which is associated with a severe phenotype. Studies on the attitudes of pregnant women towards an expanded scope of prenatal screening showed that women thought that it may be valuable especially to include severe disorders with no or short life expectancy in a screening test [57, 58]. Women also wanted to learn about sex chromosomal aneuploidies [59, 60] and about specific other aneuploidies, but were hesitant about learning about conditions with unknown or variable phenotypic expression. They were uncertain about what the benefit would be of knowing about such conditions [59].

Proportionality concerns might limit the expansion of the scope, on at least three points. Firstly, when genome-wide analyses are used in NIPT, it might be difficult to assess the clinical validity of many among the huge number of abnormalities that can be detected. Offering a test for disorders without knowing the validity might lead to false positives and false negatives, cause harm to pregnant women, and challenge the proportionality of including the disorders [17]. Professionals mentioned that outcomes should be actionable for pregnant women. When tests are not reliable (i.e. clinically valid), they provide few actionable options. Moreover, uncertain test outcomes might lead to unnecessary anxiety or insecurity in pregnant women, which is objectionable: *"I think that, when you introduce uncertainty in the pregnancy, it will become difficult. If you [can say that you] are sure that the child is disabled, then this is understandable for people, and they will be able to prepare [for the birth of a disabled child] or to decide that they do not want this. But if you say, 'we actually do not know what it means exactly; (...) it can turn out better than expected, but the child can also turn out severely disabled.' Well, what should you do, as parents?"* (I3, medical specialist) Several other professionals stated that in practice this should not pose a big problem, as only a small number of abnormalities that are currently being detected in labs are of unknown or little-known clinical validity. These will need to be discussed between expecting parents and clinical geneticists specialised in prenatal diagnosis.

A second point that several respondents stressed is that NIPT has shortcomings: NIPT is not a diagnostic test, and it still requires invasive follow-up. An expanded scope might lead to an increasing number of positive test results for a wide range of disorders, which will include false positive results that need confirmation by (unnecessary) invasive diagnostic testing. This is problematic, because a reduction of invasive tests as compared to FCT is seen as one of the important benefits of NIPT [15, 18, 19].

A third point that might limit the scope of NIPT is the burden of the decision to terminate a pregnancy. Some disorders may not be sufficiently severe to justify their inclusion in the NIPT; they may not meet the first screening criterion of Wilson and Jungner: "The condition sought should be an important health problem." [61] However, professionals mentioned that it is hard to define what 'serious' or 'non-serious' diseases are. In the documents it is stated, for instance, that severity should not be determined at all: "It would be dangerous to create medical, legal, or social definitions of 'serious', because these could infringe on couples' lives in several ways." [20] Expecting parents are the ones who should indicate whether they consider a disorder to be serious or not, in their life situation [20]. Although it will be difficult in practice to draw the lines, the seriousness of disorders can serve as an (arguable) limit to the expanding scope of NIPT.

From the pillar of proportionality a few additional limits can be derived for the expansion of the scope of NIPT: in order for tests to be included in an expanded scope of NIPT, they should be clinically valid. Especially the positive predictive value should be high, as confirmatory testing through invasive procedures will still be required and is associated with risks, costs and burdens. NIPT should not be offered for trivial conditions.

Limits set by justice aspects

When using the ethical framework to evaluate an expansion of the scope NIPT, the pillar of justice is less prominent than the other three pillars. However, there are three issues that arise from the pillar of justice. Firstly, when NIPT is offered as an expanded test, it should be available equally for every pregnant woman [17]. Equal access to healthcare is considered to be a fundamental right that should preclude the exclusion of specific groups from healthcare services [62]. Women should not face restrictions to having reproductive options. Ideally, all women should have access to the same information about their foetus, and the scope of first-trimester prenatal screening should be equal for all women. When expanded NIPT is made available only to women who have an increased risk of trisomy 21, 18 or 13 as a second-tier test after FTC, for instance, low-risk pregnant women will not have access to information about the foetus other than the three more common trisomies detected through FCT, whereas high-risk women will [17]. For this reason, justice would

require making NIPT available as a first-tier test to all women (or restricting the scope of NIPT as a second-tier test). Also, it is important to note that diagnostic follow-up testing should be made available to women who have undergone NIPT, in line with the criterion of Wilson and Jungner that in screening programmes, diagnostic follow-up testing should be available to those found to be at risk [38]. This is of special importance in countries in which access to follow-up testing is not self-evident.

A second aspect, according to the International Bioethics Committee, is that education is a matter of justice: "Persons with a lower education level and lower health literacy are denied the information which is required to exercise their freedom and autonomy." [19] Some women may not be able to understand all relevant information pertaining to the screening offer, which is necessary to make an informed choice. The expansion of NIPT will only exacerbate this inequality [19], it is feared, as the test becomes more elaborate and more complex, and decision-making places higher demands on women's health literacy.

A third concern is that an expanded NIPT could challenge a justifiable distribution of healthcare resources. As resources are scarce and should be distributed equally, efforts must be taken to demarcate the scope of prenatal screening tests to prevent unnecessary follow-up of clinically insignificant findings. Besides, when prenatal screening is offered within the context of a public health programme and is upheld by taxpayers, there should be transparency with regard to the utility of the test [15]. This also underlines the importance of ensuring the proportionality of a test.

When considering the costs of prenatal screening it should be noted that a widespread implementation and uptake of prenatal screening programmes is likely to lead to the birth of fewer affected children, which reduces the costs associated with their healthcare and support. Although this should not be an aim of prenatal screening, these long-term costs savings are undeniably part of a cost-effectiveness analysis of new screening tests [15].

From the pillar of justice another limitation can be derived: expanded NIPT should be available for all pregnant women, which may increase the costs of the programme. This limitation may change over time as the technology improves and becomes cheaper.

Limits set by societal aspects

In discussions on the expansion of the scope of NIPT, concerns are reiterated that have already been raised in the context of earlier prenatal screening programmes, such as discrimination and stigmatisation of people with chronic diseases. New societal aspects, unique to expanded NIPT, are raised as well. Professionals noted in the interviews, for instance, that a benefit of an expanded scope could be a removal of the focus of prenatal testing on Down syndrome. Down syndrome is the most common of the three trisomies and in the Netherlands first-trimester screening for chromosomal abnormalities is often referred to as a 'test for Down syndrome'. By expanding the scope of prenatal screening this focus could shift, which might reduce concerns related to discriminatory messages conveyed by the screening programme. This benefit of the expansion is also acknowledged by parents of children with Down syndrome, who experience the focus on Down as stigmatising for their children [63]. On the other hand, the Dutch Health Council mentioned that expanded NIPT is not free from the allegation of stigmatisation either, as, for instance, a list of selected disorders can be thought of as 'subjective' and vulnerable to stigmatisation of specific groups, too [17]. According to some professionals, an expanded scope might reduce the acceptance of children with a disability: "*With 22q11 deletion, [children] can be mentally retarded, etc. When people hear a story like that, they tend to terminate [the pregnancy]. I find it very hard. Everybody wants a healthy child; I understand that. So it is good to have these options. On the other hand, I am afraid that, when more [screening] becomes possible, what space is there for children with a disability? I find it terrible that there may be no respect or no care [for these children].*" (I10, midwife).

Adverse societal consequences of an expanded scope are also mentioned by pregnant women and parents of children with Down syndrome, who fear a loss of diversity in society and a 'slippery slope', implying that people might want to start testing for increasingly trivial abnormalities [57, 63]. However, respondents questioned whether these consequences of an expanded scope will occur and denied that society will eventually be without children with a disorder or disability. Although it is difficult to predict the societal consequences (if any) of NIPT or how these would limit the expansion of its scope, it is clear that negative consequences for people with disabilities should be mitigated, and the practice of prenatal screening should be monitored continuously, not only with a focus on the risks and benefits for individuals, but also for its wider societal implications.

Conclusion

An expansion of the scope of NIPT fits the aim of prenatal screening, as it contributes to more reproductive options for pregnant women and couples. However, drawing on the broadly shared ethical framework for prenatal screening as well as on the findings of our qualitative study of professionals' opinions and experiences of the translation of the pillars of this framework in practice, we conclude that expansion of the scope of NIPT is not unlimited. Four moral limits can be set to demarcate a responsible expansion of the scope of NIPT. Firstly, informed choice as a central precondition for prenatal screening should limit its

scope: when NIPT is expanded to include more chromosomal or sub-microscopic abnormalities, and relevant pre-test information about the test becomes more elaborate and more complex, counsellors will need to improve pre-test counselling to uphold its quality. This requires new models for counselling, with a special focus on generic information about possible test outcomes and on expecting parents' attitudes and values in relation to prenatal screening. Secondly, any expansion of NIPT should be proportionate: the test should be clinically valid and useful to women. Findings that generate mainly anxiety and for which no courses of action are available, do not meet the criterion of proportionality. Thirdly, respect for the right of the future child to an open future excludes testing for late-onset disorders when women or couples know beforehand that they will not terminate the pregnancy based on the results. Finally, healthcare resources should be justly distributed: when possible, NIPT should be made available to all pregnant women either free of charge or for a small sum. At the same time, any expansion of the scope of NIPT should be based upon a favourable assessment of the benefits of including additional 'tests' for additional disorders in proportion to the costs and burdens. Both in the literature and in our interview study of professionals' opinions, we observed differences in the sense of urgency or importance that is attributed to each of the four limitations. We contend that the criterion of reproductive autonomy as the aim of prenatal screening as well as that of proportionality – or a positive balance between the benefits and burdens for pregnant women and their future children – should together be guiding in decisions whether particular disorders should be tested or communicated to women or couples. This means that for example, depending on the test performance, disorders that are comparable to trisomies 13, 18 and 21 in terms of severity could be included in the NIPT. Over the next decade, those working in the field of NIPT may strive to maximise the potential benefits of NIPT and include more abnormalities in the screening test, keeping these moral limits to a justified scope of NIPT in mind.

Abbreviations

ASHG: American Society of Human Genetics; ESHG: European Society of Human Genetics; FCT: First trimester combined test; IBC: UNESCO International Bioethics Committee; NIPT: Non-Invasive Prenatal Test; TRIDENT-1: Trial by Dutch laboratories for Evaluation of Non-Invasive Prenatal Testing; WHO: World Health Organisation

Acknowledgements

The authors wish to thank the professionals who participated in the study.

Funding
This study is a result of a research project 'To report or not to report? The ethics of broadening the scope of (non-) invasive prenatal testing ((N)IPT)', which was funded by through Erasmus MC Grants (Mrace). The funding body had no role in the design of the study, in the collection, analysis, interpretation of data, or in writing or reviewing the manuscript.

Authors' contributions
All authors contributed to the design of the study and the interpretation of data. AKK collected and analysed the data. AKK and EMB drafted the manuscript. IDB and RJHG critically revised the manuscript for important intellectual content. All authors have read and approved the final manuscript.

Competing interests
The authors declare that they have no competing interests.

Author details
[1]Department of Medical Ethics and Philosophy of Medicine, Erasmus MC, University Medical Centre Rotterdam, Room 24.17, Wytemaweg 80, 3015 CN Rotterdam, The Netherlands. [2]Department of Clinical Genetics, Erasmus MC, University Medical Centre Rotterdam, Wytemaweg 80, 3015 CN Rotterdam, The Netherlands.

References
1. Norton ME, Jacobsson B, Swamy GK, Laurent LC, Ranzini AC, Brar H, et al. Cell-free DNA analysis for noninvasive examination of trisomy. N Engl J Med. 2015;372(17):1589–97.
2. Chandrasekharan S, Minear MA, Hung A, Allyse M. Noninvasive prenatal testing goes global. Sci Transl Med. 2014;6(231):231fs15.
3. Oepkes D, Page-Christiaens GC, Bax CJ, Bekker MN, Bilardo CM, Boon EMJ, et al. Trial by Dutch laboratories for evaluation of non-invasive prenatal testing. Part I—clinical impact. Prenat Diagn. 2016;36(12):1083–90.
4. Bianchi DW, Parker RL, Wentworth J, Madankumar R, Saffer C, Das AF, et al. DNA sequencing versus standard prenatal aneuploidy screening. N Engl J Med. 2014;370(9):799–808.
5. Meck JM, Kramer Dugan E, Matyakhina L, Aviram A, Trunca C, Pineda-Alvarez D, et al. Noninvasive prenatal screening for aneuploidy: positive predictive values based on cytogenetic findings. Am J Obstet Gynecol. 2015;213(2):214.e1–5.
6. Van Opstal D, Srebniak MI. Cytogenetic confirmation of a positive NIPT result: evidence-based choice between chorionic villus sampling and amniocentesis depending on chromosome aberration. Expert Rev Mol Diagn. 2016;16(5):513–20.
7. Bianchi DW, Wilkins-Haug L. Integration of noninvasive DNA testing for aneuploidy into prenatal care: what has happened since the rubber met the road? Clin Chem. 2014;60(1):78–87.
8. Van Opstal D, Srebniak MI, Polak J, de Vries F, Govaerts LCP, Joosten M, et al. False negative NIPT results: risk figures for chromosomes 13, 18 and 21 based on chorionic villi results in 5967 cases and literature review. PLoS One. 2016;11(1):e0146794.
9. Benn P. Expanding non-invasive prenatal testing beyond chromosomes 21, 18, 13, X and Y. Clin Genet. 2016;90(6):477–85.
10. Helgeson J, Wardrop J, Boomer T, Almasri E, Paxton WB, Saldivar JS, et al. Clinical outcome of subchromosomal events detected by whole-genome noninvasive prenatal testing. Prenat Diagn. 2015;35(10):999–1004.
11. Lau TK, Cheung SW, Lo PSS, Pursley AN, Chan MK, Jiang F, et al. Non-invasive prenatal testing for fetal chromosomal abnormalities by low-coverage whole-genome sequencing of maternal plasma DNA: review of 1982 consecutive cases in a single center. Ultrasound Obstet Gynecol. 2014;43(3):254–64.
12. Wapner RJ, Babiarz JE, Levy B, Stosic M, Zimmermann B, Sigurjonsson S, et al. Expanding the scope of noninvasive prenatal testing: detection of fetal microdeletion syndromes. Am J Obstet Gynecol. 2015;212(3):332.e1–9.
13. Brady P, Brison N, Van Den Bogaert K, de Ravel T, Peeters H, Van Esch H et al. Clinical implementation of NIPT–technical and biological challenges. Clin Genet. 2015;89(5):523–30.
14. Lo KK, Karampetsou E, Boustred C, McKay F, Mason S, Hill M, et al. Limited clinical utility of non-invasive prenatal testing for subchromosomal abnormalities. Am J Hum Genet. 2016;98(1):34–44.
15. Dondorp W, De Wert G, Bombard Y, Bianchi DW, Bergmann C, Borry P, et al. Non-invasive prenatal testing for aneuploidy and beyond: challenges of responsible innovation in prenatal screening. Eur J Hum Genet. 2015;23(11):1438–50.
16. Shuster E. Microarray genetic screening: a prenatal roadblock for life? Lancet. 2007;369(9560):526–9.
17. Gezondheidsraad. NIPT: dynamiek en ethiek van prenatale screening. Den Haag: Gezondheidsraad; 2013.
18. Deutscher Ethikrat. The future of genetic diagnosis from research to clinical practice; opinion. Berlin: Deutscher Ethikrat; 2013.
19. UNESCO. Report of the IBC on updating its reflection on the human genome and human rights. Paris: United Nations Educational Scientific and Cultural Organization; 2015.
20. Wertz DC, Fletcher JC, Berg K. Review of ethical issues in medical ethics: report of consultants to WHO. Geneva: World Health Organization; 2003.
21. Swedish National Council on Medical Ethics. Prenatal diagnosis: the ethics. 2006. Socialdepartemetet. http://www.smer.se/wp-content/uploads/2012/04/Prenatal-diagnosis-the-Ethics.pdf. Accessed 23 Aug 2017.
22. Nuffield Council on Bioethics. Critical care decisions in fetal and neonatal medicine: ethical issues: a guide to the report; 2007.
23. Skirton H, Goldsmith L, Jackson L, Lewis C, Chitty L. Offering prenatal diagnostic tests: European guidelines for clinical practice [corrected]. Eur J Hum Genet. 2014;22(5):580–6.
24. Superior Health Council of Belgium. Implementation of non-invasive prenatal genetic screening for trisomy 21 (Down Syndrome) in the practice of health care in Belgium. 2014. https://www.health.belgium.be/en/advise-8912-nipt#anchor-20611. Accessed 15 Oct 2018.
25. Minear MA, Alessi S, Allyse M, Michie M, Chandrasekharan S. Noninvasive prenatal genetic testing: current and emerging ethical, legal, and social issues. Annu Rev Genomics Hum Genet. 2015;16:369–98.
26. Allyse M, Minear MA, Berson E, Sridhar S, Rote M, Hung A, et al. Non-invasive prenatal testing: a review of international implementation and challenges. Int J Womens Health. 2015;7:113–26.
27. de Jong A. Prenatal screening à la carte?: ethical reflection on the scope of testing for foetal anomalies. Maastricht: Maastricht University; 2013.
28. Gates EA. Ethical considerations in prenatal diagnosis. West J Med. 1993; 159(3):391–5.
29. Vanstone M, King C, de Vrijer B, Nisker J. Non-invasive prenatal testing: ethics and policy considerations. J Obstet Gynaecol Can. 2014;36(6):515–26.
30. Gekas J, Langlois S, Ravitsky V, Audibert F, van den Berg DG, Haidar H, et al. Non-invasive prenatal testing for fetal chromosome abnormalities: review of clinical and ethical issues. Appl Clin Genet. 2016;9:15–26.
31. Beauchamp TL. Methods and principles in biomedical ethics. J Med Ethics. 2003;29(5):269–74.
32. Kass NE. An ethics framework for public health. Am J Public Health. 2001; 91(11):1776–82.
33. Gezondheidsraad. Juridische aspecten van prenatale screening: achtergronddocument bij prenatale screening. Den Haag: Gezondheidsraad; 2016.

34. Marteau TM, Dormandy E, Michie S. A measure of informed choice. Health Expect. 2001;4(2):99–108.

35. Lewis C, Hill M, Skirton H, Chitty LS. Development and validation of a measure of informed choice for women undergoing non-invasive prenatal testing for aneuploidy. Eur J Hum Genet. 2016;24(6):809–16.

36. Biesecker BB, Schwartz MD, Marteau TM. Enhancing informed choice to undergo health screening: a systematic review. Am J Health Behav. 2013;37(3):351–9.

37. van den Heuvel A, Chitty L, Dormandy E, Newson A, Deans Z, Attwood S, et al. Will the introduction of non-invasive prenatal diagnostic testing erode informed choices? An experimental study of health care professionals. Patient Educ Couns. 2010;78(1):24–8.

38. Andermann A, Blancquaert I, Beauchamp S, Déry V. Revisiting Wilson and Jungner in the genomic age: a review of screening criteria over the past 40 years. Bull World Health Organ. 2008;86(4):317–9.

39. van den Berg M, Timmermans DR, Kleinveld JH, Garcia E, van Vugt JM, van der Wal G. Accepting or declining the offer of prenatal screening for congenital defects: test uptake and women's reasons. Prenat Diagn. 2005;25(1):84–90.

40. García E, Timmermans DRM, van Leeuwen E. The impact of ethical beliefs on decisions about prenatal screening tests: searching for justification. Soc Sci Med. 2008;66(3):753–64.

41. Crombag NM, Bensing JM, Iedema-Kuiper R, Schielen PCJI, Visser GH. Determinants affecting pregnant women's utilization of prenatal screening for Down syndrome: a review of the literature. J Matern Fetal Neonatal Med. 2013;26(17):1676–81.

42. Crombag NMTH, van Schendel RV, Schielen PCJI, Bensing JM, Henneman L. Present to future: what the reasons for declining first-trimester combined testing tell us about accepting or declining cell-free DNA testing. Prenat Diagn. 2016;36(6):587–90.

43. Ternby E, Axelsson O, Annerén G, Lindgren P, Ingvoldstad C. Why do pregnant women accept or decline prenatal diagnosis for Down syndrome? J Community Genet. 2016;7(3):237–42.

44. Vassy C, Rosman S, Rousseau B. From policy making to service use. Down's syndrome antenatal screening in England, France and the Netherlands. Soc Sci Med. 2014;106:67–74.

45. Elias S, Annas GJ. Generic consent for genetic screening. N Engl J Med. 1994;330(22):1611–3.

46. de Wert GMWR. Met het oog op de toekomst: voortplantingstechnologie, erfelijkheidsonderzoek en ethiek. Rotterdam: Erasmus University; 1999.

47. de Jong A, Dondorp WJ, de Die-Smulders CEM, Frints SGM, de Wert GMWR. Non-invasive prenatal testing: ethical issues explored. Eur J Hum Genet. 2009;18(3):272–7.

48. van Schendel RV, Page-Christiaens GC, Beulen L, Bilardo CM, de Boer MA, Coumans ABC, et al. Trial by Dutch laboratories for evaluation of non-invasive prenatal testing. Part II—women's perspectives. Prenat Diagn. 2016;36(12):1091–8.

49. van den Berg M, Timmermans DRM, ten Kate LP, van Vugt JMG, van der Wal G. Informed decision making in the context of prenatal screening. Patient Educ Couns. 2006;63(1–2):110–7.

50. Gourounti K, Sandall J. Do pregnant women in Greece make informed choices about antenatal screening for Down's syndrome? A questionnaire survey. Midwifery. 2008;24(2):153–62.

51. Oxenford K, Daley R, Lewis C, Hill M, Chitty LS. Development and evaluation of training resources to prepare health professionals for counselling pregnant women about non-invasive prenatal testing for Down syndrome: a mixed methods study. BMC Pregnancy Childbirth. 2017;17(1):132.

52. Emanuel EJ, Emanuel LL. Four models of the physician-patient relationship. JAMA. 1992;267(16):2221–6.

53. Tamminga S, van Schendel RV, Rommers W, Bilardo CM, Pajkrt E, Dondorp WJ, et al. Changing to NIPT as a first-tier screening test and future perspectives: opinions of health professionals. Prenat Diagn. 2015;35(13):1316–23.

54. Oduncu FS. The role of non-directiveness in genetic counseling. Med Health Care Philos. 2002;5(1):53–63.

55. Bianchi DW. From prenatal genomic diagnosis to fetal personalized medicine: progress and challenges. Nat Med. 2012;18(7):1041–51.

56. de Jong A, Dondorp WJ, Frints SGM, de Die-Smulders CEM, de Wert GMWR. Advances in prenatal screening: the ethical dimension. Nat Rev Genet. 2011;12(9):657–63.

57. van Schendel RV, Kleinveld JH, Dondorp WJ, Pajkrt E, Timmermans DRM, Holtkamp KCA, et al. Attitudes of pregnant women and male partners towards non-invasive prenatal testing and widening the scope of prenatal screening. Eur J Hum Genet. 2014;22(12):1345–50.

58. van der Steen SL, Diderich KE, Riedijk SR, Verhagen-Visser J, Govaerts LC, Joosten M, et al. Pregnant couples at increased risk for common aneuploidies choose maximal information from invasive genetic testing. Clin Genet. 2015;88(1):25–31.

59. Agatisa PK, Mercer MB, Leek AC, Smith MB, Philipson E, Farrell RM. A first look at women's perspectives on noninvasive prenatal testing to detect sex chromosome aneuploidies and microdeletion syndromes. Prenat Diagn. 2015;35(7):692–8.

60. Lau TK, Chan MK, Salome Lo PS, Chan HYC, Chan WK, Koo TY, et al. Non-invasive prenatal screening of fetal sex chromosomal abnormalities: perspective of pregnant women. J Matern Fetal Neonatal Med. 2012;25(12):2616–9.

61. Wilson JMG, Jungner G. Principles and practice of screening for disease. Geneva: World Health Organization; 1968.

62. Office of the United Nations High Commissioner for Human Rights. The Right to Health. Geneva: Office of the United Nations High Commissioner for Human Rights; 2008.

63. van Schendel RV, Kater-Kuipers A, van Vliet-Lachotzki EH, Dondorp WJ, Cornel MC, Henneman L. What do parents of children with Down syndrome think about non-invasive prenatal testing (NIPT)? J Genet Couns. 2017;26(3):522–31.

20

Predictors of uterine rupture in a large sample of women in Senegal and Mali: cross-sectional analysis of QUARITE trial data

Rebecca Delafield[1]* , Catherine M. Pirkle[2] and Alexandre Dumont[3]

Abstract

Background: The purpose of this study was to investigate predictors of uterine rupture in a large sample of sub-Saharan African women. Uterine rupture is rare in high-income countries, but it is more common in low-income settings where health systems are often under-resourced. However, understanding of risk factors contributing to uterine rupture in such settings is limited due to small sample sizes and research rarely considers system and individual-level factors concomitantly.

Methods: Cross-sectional data analysis from the pre-intervention period (Oct. 1, 2007- Oct. 1, 2008) of the QUARITE trial, a large-scale maternal mortality study. This research examines uterine rupture among 84,924 women who delivered in one of 46 referral hospitals in Mali and Senegal. A mixed-effects logistic regression model identified individual and geographical risk factors associated with uterine rupture, accounting for clustering by hospital.

Results: Five hundred sixty-nine incidences of uterine rupture (0.67% of sample) were recorded. Predictors of uterine rupture: grand multiparity defined as ≥ 5 live births (aOR = 7.57, 95%CI; 5.19–11.03), prior cesarean (aOR = 2.02, 95%CI; 1.61–2.54), resides outside hospital region (aOR = 1.90, 95%CI: 1.28–2.81), no prenatal care visits (aOR = 1.80, 95%CI; 1.44–2.25), and birth weight of ≥ 3600 g (aOR = 1.61, 95%CI; 1.30–1.98). Women who were referred and who had an obstructed labor had much higher odds of uterine rupture compared to those who experienced neither (aOR: 46.25, 95%CI; 32.90–65.02).

Conclusions: The results of this large study confirm that the referral system, particularly for women with obstructed labor and increasing parity, is a main determinant of uterine rupture in this context. Improving labor and delivery management at each level of the health system and communication between health care facilities should be a priority to reduce uterine rupture.

Keywords: Uterine rupture, Sub-Saharan Africa, Delivery of health care, Dystocia, Referral and consultation

Background

Uterine rupture (UR) is a severe complication in pregnancy that involves tearing of the uterine wall during the course of pregnancy or delivery. UR is associated with a substantially increased risk of maternal and perinatal mortality and morbidity when compared to an uncomplicated delivery [1–3]. While the occurrence of UR is relatively rare, it is more frequent in low-income compared to high-income countries [3–5].

Morbidities resulting from UR include hysterectomy, massive hemorrhage, shock, post-hemorrhagic anemia, vesicovaginal fistula, infection or sepsis, and increased risk of rupture in subsequent pregnancies [3, 5, 6]. In high-income settings, the greatest risk factor is a scarred uterus, typically from a previous cesarean delivery. In contrast, while this association is also observed in low-income settings, risk for UR in these contexts

---

* Correspondence: delafiel@hawaii.edu
[1]Department of Native Hawaiian Health, John A. Burns School of Medicine, University of Hawai'i at Mānoa, 677 Ala Moana Blvd., Suite 1015, Honolulu, HI 96813-5401, USA
Full list of author information is available at the end of the article

appears largely related to factors such as parity, obstructed labor, induction of labor, use of prostaglandins, and/or breech presentation [2, 3, 7].

Research in sub-Saharan Africa highlights other risk factors for UR including lack of prenatal care, limited access to emergency obstetrical care, delays and/or poor management of care [8–12]. Yet these studies are small, frequently focus on one institution and often fail to adjust for potential confounding variables such as parity or previous cesarean delivery when characterizing health system risk factors for UR [8–11]. Published case reports of UR events provide valuable insights, but may not be applicable to the majority of cases that clinicians and health centers encounter [13–17].

Because of the severe consequences of UR, prevention is paramount. Yet, the rarity of UR makes it difficult to study. Therefore, research investigating the factors contributing to UR using large datasets with quality data collection and abstraction of data from medical records is needed. Such information can benefit clinicians, health systems, and communities that experience morbidity and mortality due to UR by identifying potential points of intervention. The purpose of this study is to investigate predictors of UR in a large sample of sub-Saharan African women.

Methods

This is a cross-sectional analysis of pre-intervention data from the QUARITE (quality of care, risk management and technology in obstetrics) trial, a cluster-randomized multicenter intervention study conducted in Mali and Senegal [18]. The QUARITE trial is registered on the Current Controlled Trials website under the number ISRCTN46950658. Data collection on all births in the study period took place at 46 public referral hospitals (district, regional, and national/teaching hospitals). For more details on the trial protocol and principal results see Dumont et al., 2009 and Dumont et al., 2013 [18, 19]. The sample includes all women ($N = 84,924$) that delivered at any of the 46 referral hospitals during the pre-intervention period (Oct. 1, 2007 – Oct. 1, 2008) of the trial. The data collection system was based on the World Health Organization (WHO) global health survey of maternal and perinatal health, which included collection of institution level and individual-level data [19, 20]. Data on the women, their pregnancy, labor and delivery were extracted from hospital and medical records into a standard one-page data collection form. Given that data were collected on all women at each participating site, the QUARITE investigators kept the data collection instrument relatively short in order to minimize the burden of the trial on health professionals working at the study sites. Trained midwives collected the data from medical records at each site. National coordinators

supervised them and data quality was monitored by random audits [18]. Complete data on UR, our principal measure of interest, were available for 84,802 women, or 99.9% of the total number of women who delivered. Records with missing values for UR ($n = 122$) were excluded from the analysis.

The outcome of interest is UR, diagnosed by a health professional. The definition used for the study was, "occurrence of clinical symptoms (pain, fetal distress, acute loss of contractions, hemorrhage) or intrauterine fetal death that lead to laparotomy, at which the diagnosis of uterine rupture was confirmed; or laparotomy for UR after vaginal birth" ([21] p6). UR has been defined similarly in previous studies [4]. UR was captured as a dichotomous variable (yes/no) in this dataset, no anatomic details of the rupture (e.g., total rupture versus dehiscence) were considered for this outcome. The literature identifies multiple risk factors for UR that fall into four categories: maternal characteristics, obstetric, institutional, and geographical factors [3, 8–12]. Maternal characteristics include a woman's age at delivery (categorized into < 20, 20–35, > 35 years), and parity for the current delivery (categorized by quartiles into ≤ 1 birth, 2 births, 3–4 births, 5 or more births). The following obstetric factors were included as dichotomous variables: induction of labor, prior cesarean delivery, comorbidity, obstructed labor (defined as slow or arrest of dilation despite ruptured membranes and oxytocin augmentation, non-engagement of presentation at full cervical dilation, or failed vacuum or forceps at full cervical dilation with engaged head), pre-eclampsia/eclampsia, hemorrhage, and $\geq$ 90th centile of birth weight ($\geq$ 3600 g) in our sample. Comorbidity was defined as having one or more co-occurring diseases or conditions such as HIV/AIDS, malaria, heart or kidney disease, chronic respiratory condition, gestational diabetes, etc., recorded on the study data collection form. For additional details please see supplementary file (Additional file 1). Mode of delivery was also collected and classified as either spontaneous vaginal delivery, cesarean delivery, and instrumental (forceps or vacuum), breech, or other. Other refers to specific obstetric maneuvers or surgical procedures (e.g., craniotomy) to achieve delivery for obstetric complications, such as fetal malformation with intrauterine fetal death, or transverse presentation or twin retention, etc. These cases may require specific obstetric maneuvers or surgical procedures (e.g., craniotomy) to achieve delivery. The number of prenatal visits (coded as none, 1–4, > 4) was also included in this analysis. The categorization of prenatal care is based on WHO guidelines for prenatal care prior to the November 2016 change, which doubled the minimum recommended prenatal care consultations to eight [22].

Institutional aspects are resources that may or may not be available at each site and included a blood bank, an adult intensive care unit, an anesthesiologist (or staff member trained in anesthesia) on call 24 h a day, and an obstetrician-gynecologist on staff (available for deliveries), each coded as dichotomous variables. Note that the institutional characteristics are not direct risk factors for UR, but serve as proxies for the level of resources available at the hospital for the care of patients. Human resources such as obstetricians-gynecologists and specialized care resources (e.g., blood bank) are associated with higher-level care facilities, but care levels are not strictly dictated by the hospital type. For example, regional hospitals can be either care level one or level two (higher-level) facilities. Higher-level facilities are presumed to provide better quality of care to patients, especially those with more complicated obstetrical conditions [19]. Geographical factors were examined to understand better the influence of geographic/spatial context and accessibility to the referral centers on UR. Previous research has indicated that disparities in mortality between rural and urban settings and delays in care are associated with transport to hospitals [23–25]. Geographical factors in this study include the country where the delivery took place (Senegal or Mali) and the type: a hospital within the capital, a regional hospital outside the capital, or a district hospital. A third geographical factor is the woman's place of residence in relation to the hospital where she delivered, categorized as: within the same town as the hospital, outside the town but within the region where the hospital is located, or outside of the region where the hospital is located. Referral from another health center, such as a community health center, which provides primary health care, (versus self-referred) is also included in this category. Ambulances will typically provide transportation for women referred from one health center to a higher-level referral hospital (a district, regional, or national/teaching hospital) [24]. An interaction term was created to combine obstructed labor (yes/no) and referred to a referral hospital (yes/no) in the final model due to the strong association between obstructed labor and referral.

Data were analyzed using STATA version 14.0 (STATA Corporation, College Texas USA). A Chi-squared test compared those who experienced UR and those who did not by each covariate individually. A P value of < 0.05 was considered statistically significant. A multiple step process tested the independent associations of each variable with UR. In cluster-randomized control trials it is assumed that the similarity or "clustering" of characteristics at any given institution will have some influence on the outcomes of each individual interacting with that specific institution. To account for the clustering of variables by institution, a mixed-effects logistic regression model assuming a random intercept was used in the analysis. A backwards elimination process was conducted to arrive at the most parsimonious model for presenting adjusted odds ratios and confidence intervals for predictors of UR. The first step was to run the full model that included each of the variables from all categories. Based on a cut-off point of a $P < 0.20$, the variable with the highest P value over 0.20 was excluded from the model and the model was run again. This step was repeated until all variables were below the cut-off point. Deletions occurred in the following order to get to the final model: adult intensive care unit, anesthesiologist on call, comorbidity, and blood bank. Excluded variables were then re-entered individually to assess the stability of the model. No meaningful changes were observed. Because of their conceptual importance, age and country were retained in the final model, even though their P values exceeded the cut-off.

Results

Among the 84,802 women in our sample for which we had full data, 569 (0.67%) experienced UR. The mean age of women in the study was 26 (range:10–56 years). The mean parity was three with a maximum of 18 births. Among the 569 women who experienced UR, 69 (12%) died. Nearly all of these deaths (62/69) were due to UR or the consequences of UR (i.e., hemorrhage). Other causes of death among those with UR included; eclampsia, infection and unspecified. Table 1 presents the frequency and percent of UR according to maternal and obstetric factors. Most of the factors identified by the literature as likely to be associated with UR were statistically significant ($P < 0.05$) in this sample, based on the bivariate analyses. The exceptions include induction and preeclampsia/eclampsia. While hemorrhage was associated with UR in this analysis, there was no information recorded on whether the hemorrhage occurred prior to the rupture and it is likely that the hemorrhage was a result of the rupture.

Table 2 presents the frequency and percent of UR according to geographical and institutional characteristics. At an institutional level, UR was less frequent when an anesthesiologist or obstetrician were available and more frequent in facilities with a blood bank or an ICU. All the geographical characteristics were significantly associated with UR in the bivariate analysis.

Table 3 presents the results of the multivariate analyses. The interaction term of obstructed labor and referral showed a strong and clear relationship between obstruction, referral, and the likelihood of UR. Of those referred, 41.25% were diagnosed with obstructed labor (not shown). The odds of UR clearly increased as parity increased and were highest for women that had a parity of five or more births

Table 1 Maternal characteristics and obstetric factors for sample and by uterine rupture

		Total sample N = 84,924 (100%)		No uterine rupture N = 84,233 (99.19%)		Experienced uterine rupture [a, b] N = 569 (0.67%)		
		n	%	n	%	n	%	p value
Maternal characteristics								
Age	< 20	16,526	19.46	16,458	99.59	45	0.27	< 0.001
	20–35	58,998	69.47	58,515	99.18	408	0.69	
	> 35	8551	10.07	8427	98.55	106	1.24	
Parity [c]	≤ 1 birth	29,502	34.74	29,418	99.72	55	0.16	< 0.001
	2 births	16,264	19.15	16,178	99.47	72	0.44	
	3 or 4 births	20,133	23.71	19,966	99.17	147	0.73	
	≥ 5 births	18,977	22.35	18,647	98.26	294	1.55	
Obstetric factors								
Mode of delivery	Vaginal	64,993	76.53	64,942	99.92	42	0.06	< 0.001
	Cesarean	16,218	19.1	15,736	97.03	477	2.94	
	Instrumental	1775	2.09	1767	99.55	8	0.45	
	Breech	1544	1.82	1539	99.68	4	0.26	
	Other	91	0.11	59	64.84	32	35.16	
Delivery induced	Yes	2484	2.92	2464	99.19	19	0.77	0.545
	No	82,162	96.75	81,598	99.31	546	0.66	
No. prenatal visits	None	8756	10.31	8592	98.13	135	1.55	< 0.001
	1 to 4	65,024	76.57	64,600	99.35	381	0.59	
	> 4	10,470	12.33	10,421	99.53	44	0.42	
Prior cesarean	Yes	5894	6.94	5771	97.91	121	2.05	< 0.001
	No	78,926	92.94	78,395	99.33	447	0.57	
Comorbidity	Yes	20,384	24.00	20,141	98.81	184	0.90	< 0.001
	No	64,502	75.95	64,086	99.36	385	0.60	
Obstructed labor	Yes	13,822	16.28	13,382	96.82	438	3.17	< 0.001
	No	70,978	83.58	70,841	99.81	130	0.18	
Pre/eclampsia	Yes	2967	3.52	2967	99.20	19	0.64	0.812
	No	81,228	96.31	81,228	99.32	550	0.67	
Hemorrhage	Yes	5220	6.15	4827	92.47	382	7.32	< 0.001
	No	79,594	93.72	79,398	99.75	186	0.23	
≥ 90% centile of birth weights	Yes	9919	11.68	9777	98.57	140	1.41	< 0.001
	No	74,529	87.76	74,097	99.42	420	0.56	

[a]Data on Uterine Rupture (yes/no) is missing for 122 women or 0.14% of the sample
[b]Missing values (of those that experienced uterine rupture): Age($n = 10$), Parity ($n = 1$), No. prenatal visits ($n = 9$), Prior cesarean delivery ($n = 1$), Mode of delivery ($n = 6$), Delivery induced ($n = 4$), Breech presentation ($n = 6$), Obstructed labor ($n = 1$), Pre/eclampsia ($n = 5$), ≥ 90th centile birth weight [3600 g] ($n = 9$), Hemorrhage ($n = 1$)
[c]Parity was categorized as ≤ 1 because there were eight deaths of women prior to delivery among the total sample. Among women who experienced UR, there were no nulliparous women

compared to women with lower parity even after adjusting for previous cesarean delivery. It should be noted that there were no URs among nulliparous women, so data in the lowest parity category represent women with a parity of one for the current pregnancy. Maternal age was not significant in this model either as a categorical variable or as a continuous variable (not shown).

Discussion

UR in this large sample was significantly influenced by multiple factors which corroborate maternal and obstetrical risk factors identified in smaller studies [9–12]. An important contribution of this study is the pronounced relationship between obstructed labor and referral to a referral hospital. This finding, in conjunction with the independent association between UR and birth weight ≥ 3600 g raises

Table 2 Geographical & institutional characteristics for sample and by uterine rupture

		Total sample N = 84,924 (100%)		No uterine rupture N = 84,233 (99.19%)		Experienced uterine rupture [a, b] N = 569 (0.67%)		
		n	%	n	%	n	%	p value
Geographical characteristics								
Country	Senegal	45,687	53.80	45,338	99.24	278	0.61	0.018
	Mali	39,237	46.20	38,895	99.13	291	0.74	
Hospital type	Capital	37,247	43.86	37,117	99.65	121	0.32	< 0.001
	Regional	29,211	34.40	28,835	98.71	293	1.01	
	District	18,466	21.74	18,281	99.00	155	0.84	
Location of residence	In town of hospital	72,339	85.18	71,867	99.35	433	0.60	< 0.001
	Outside town, same region	9550	11.25	9451	98.96	76	0.80	
	Outside of region	2751	3.24	2683	97.53	56	2.04	
Referral	Yes	21,028	24.76	20,526	97.61	424	2.02	< 0.001
	No	63,871	75.21	63,689	99.72	144	0.23	
Institutional characteristics								
Blood bank	Yes	43,695	51.45	43,181	98.82	410	0.94	< 0.001
	No	41,229	48.55	41,052	99.57	159	0.39	
Adult intensive care	Yes	31,468	37.05	31,123	98.90	268	0.85	< 0.001
	No	53,456	62.95	53,110	99.35	301	0.56	
24-h a day anesthesiologist	Yes	45,742	53.86	45,417	99.29	275	0.60	< 0.001
	No	39,182	46.14	38,816	99.07	294	0.75	
Obstetrician	Yes	73,744	86.84	73,190	99.25	457	0.62	< 0.001
	No	11,180	13.16	11,043	99.77	112	1.00	

[a] Data on Uterine Rupture (yes/no) is missing for 122 women or 0.14% of the sample
[b] Missing values (of those that experienced uterine rupture): Location of residence (n = 4), Referral (n = 1)

concerns about quality of care. Specifically, concerns about the timing and accuracy of the diagnosis and management of obstructed labor, as well as concern about referral systems and timely transportation to referral hospitals. Calls for improving quality of care for maternal and child health are not new but should be heeded to prevent the high levels of maternal morbidity and mortality in sub-Saharan Africa and elsewhere [26]. Interventions that address these system issues, particularly improvement in the management of labor and referral processes for women with obstructed labor, have the potential to improve the effectiveness of emergency obstetric interventions at the level of a referral hospital.

The higher odds of UR at regional compared to district hospitals (with fewer resources to manage obstetric emergencies) is likely due to selection processes with high-risk cases being referred to regional facilities. While regional referral hospitals have resources to perform interventions that may prevent UR (e.g., cesarean delivery), our work suggests that the usefulness of certain institutional level interventions could be constrained by other factors. Delay in care is a significant contributor to maternal mortality and morbidity [3, 23–25]. This analysis cannot provide details on specific sources of delay, but

results suggest that delay in seeking care, delay in decision to refer for obstructed labor (which may indicate poor labor and delivery management) or delay in transportation to a referral hospital likely impact this outcome. With regard to transportation, previous studies have noted poor roads as well as long distances and lack of available transport as obstacles to care [24, 25].

Previous work in Western Mali examined in-hospital maternal mortality by time traveled for women who underwent a cesarean section and those who did not. The authors observed that among women who traveled 4 h or more, case-fatality was dramatically higher among women who underwent a cesarean delivery compared to those who did not [24]. The authors noted that these women likely arrived at the hospital beyond the point at which the cesarean delivery was an effective intervention. Instrumental delivery (forceps or vacuum) is another intervention that could prevent UR [27]. Research conducted at a busy referral hospital in Uganda found a decrease in UR with increased use of vacuum extraction [27]. Instrumental delivery was used in only 2% of deliveries in our study. It is possible that interventions to increase appropriate use of vacuum extraction may help to reduce the incidence of uterine rupture in this context,

Table 3 Mixed-effects logistic regression analysis of predictors for uterine rupture[a]

		n	%[b]	aOR	SE	95%CI	p value
Geographical characteristics							
Country	Senegal	278	48.86	Ref			
	Mali	291	51.14	1.33	0.24	0.94–1.89	0.112
Hospital Type	Capital	121	21.27	Ref			
	Regional	293	51.49	1.59	0.32	1.08–2.34	0.018
	District	155	27.24	1.22	0.24	0.82–1.80	0.327
Location of residence	In town of hospital	433	76.10	Ref			
	Out of town, same region	76	13.36	1.06	0.19	0.75–1.50	0.736
	Outside of region	56	9.84	1.90	0.38	1.28–2.81	0.001
Maternal characteristics							
Age	< 20	45	7.91	1.06	0.21	0.71–1.56	0.789
	20–35	408	71.70	Ref			
	> 35	106	18.63	1.09	0.13	0.85–1.38	0.498
Parity[c]	1 birth	55	9.67	Ref			
	2 births	72	12.65	2.74	0.56	1.84–4.07	< 0.001
	3 or 4 births	147	25.83	4.89	0.96	3.33–7.19	< 0.001
	≥ 5 births	294	51.67	7.57	1.45	5.19–11.03	< 0.001
Obstetric factors							
No. Prenatal Visits	None	135	23.73	1.80	0.21	1.44–2.25	< 0.001
	1 to 4	381	66.96	Ref			
	≥ 4	44	7.73	0.98	0.17	0.70–1.36	0.891
Prior Cesarean	Yes	121	21.27	2.02	0.23	1.61–2.54	< 0.001
	No	447	78.56	Ref			
Obstructed labor + Referral	Not obstructed or referred	43	7.56	Ref			
	Not obstructed, Referred	87	15.29	7.61	1.50	5.17–11.19	< 0.001
	Obstructed, Not referred	101	17.75	23.65	4.57	16.20–34.53	< 0.001
	Obstructed + Referred	336	59.05	46.25	8.04	32.90–65.02	< 0.001
≥ 90th centile birth weight	Yes	140	0.25	1.61	0.17	1.30–1.98	< 0.001
	No	420	0.75	Ref			

[a]Missing values: Age (n = 10), Parity (n = 1), No. Prenatal Visits (n = 9), Referral (n = 1), Prior cesarean delivery (n = 1), Obstructed labor (n = 1), ≥ 90th centile birth weight [3600 g] (n = 9), Location of residence (n = 4)
[b]Percentage of uterine rupture cases
[c]Among cases of uterine rupture all women in the lowest parity category were parity = 1 representing the current pregnancy

similar to what was found in the intervention study in Uganda [27]. Based on our work and other studies in sub-Saharan Africa, it appears that even when resources for obstetric emergencies are available at referral hospitals, often interventions are provided too late for many women with obstructed labor, leading to UR [24, 27].

The association of UR with birth weight ≥ 3600 g suggests problems with cephalopelvic disproportion (a risk factor for obstructed labor). Neither breech presentation nor induction, risk factors identified in previous work, were significantly associated with UR in our study [3]. Because breech and induction are potential contributors to obstructed labor, an independent association may have been masked by the strong association between obstructed labor and UR.

Another important finding is the clear pattern of increased odds of UR with increasing parity after controlling for covariates. Other authors have found an increase in UR with higher parity [3, 7, 9]. For example, a study examining risk of complete UR in Norway found women (without a previous cesarean delivery) with a parity of three or more had 2.4 greater odds of complete UR compared to women with less than three births [7]. Results on the influence of grand multiparity compared to lower parity (2–4 births) on UR from studies in low-income countries are mixed [3]. This may be due to smaller sample sizes and lack of statistical control for covariates. Our study adds to the literature by capturing the increase in risk for UR at more discrete levels of parity and controlling for covariates such as previous cesarean delivery. The higher odds of UR as the number of deliveries increases may be due to weakening of the uterus or factors not captured in this study [3]. Based on these findings, interventions to address unmet contraceptive needs in multiparous women and/or programs that support multiparous women with parity greater than three to deliver at a hospital may help to reduce UR in these communities.

Lack of prenatal care was associated with increased odds of UR. As others have noted, the absence of prenatal care suggests women at greater risk for UR are not engaging with the health system, which may impact their decisions about when to seek care at the point of childbirth [3, 25]. Improved access/utilization of the health care system during the prenatal and pre/interconception period could help reduce UR in this sample. More research at the community and institution levels could add to our understanding about how obstructed labor is identified and addressed, how referrals and transportation to referral centers are managed, and how decisions to refer or to seek services from the health care system are made.

This study has several strengths. The enrolled institutions represent 94% of all referral hospitals in Mali and Senegal; therefore, this work may be generalizable to other countries in the region with similar health care systems. The data collection and abstraction were audited for completeness as part of the QUARITE protocol, which minimized problems due to missing data and concerns about the data quality. The large sample size allowed evaluation of associations between variables while controlling for multiple covariates, which may not be feasible in other studies.

Limitations should also be noted. Because the primary focus of the QUARITE trial was maternal mortality, certain variables potentially pertinent to UR were absent (e.g. interconception intervals, quantification of the number of previous cesarean deliveries, exposure to trauma, or scarring of the uterus due to reasons other than prior cesarean delivery). Also, while this study is likely to be representative of factors that impact deliveries in the referral hospitals, a significant proportion of births in Mali and Senegal take place at home (43.4% and 27% respectively); therefore, our results may not be generalizable beyond the scope of referral hospitals [28, 29].

Conclusions

The results of this large study confirm the strong influence of the referral system as a major determinant of UR, particularly for women with obstructed labor in Senegal and Mali. This work also provides evidence of a dose-response relationship between parity and the odds of experiencing UR in this context. Improving labor and

delivery management at each level of the health system and communication between health care facilities should be a priority to reduce UR. Furthermore, efforts to improve interventions upstream from delivery such as addressing unmet needs in family planning and increasing access and engagement in prenatal care could help decrease the risk of UR for women in such settings.

Abbreviations
aOR: Adjusted odds ratio; CI: Confidence interval; QUARITE: Quality of care, risk management and technology in obstetrics; SE: Standard error; UR: Uterine rupture

Acknowledgements
We wish to thank CIHR for funding of the QUARITE trial and NIMHD and NIH for the funding of our secondary data analysis. We thank Sarah Hipp for her assistance with formatting and copy editing.

Funding
Full funding for QUARITE was provided by the Canadian Institutes of Health Research (CIHR) under grant number 200602MCT-1587547-RFA-CFC-100169. CIHR awards grants through an external peer review process that examines scientific quality and merit. CIHR played no role in conducting the research or writing the paper. This secondary data analysis of pre-intervention period data and was supported in part by the National Institute on Minority Health and Health Disparities (U54MD007584), National Institutes of Health (NIH). The content is solely the responsibility of the authors and does not necessarily represent the official views of the NIMHD or NIH.

Authors' contributions
The QUARITE trial was conceived and designed by AD and others. This secondary analysis of the pre-intervention data was conceived and designed by RD and CP. The data from the QUARITE trial was provided by the Principal Investigator of that study and co-author AD. RD conducted the analysis of the data with substantial mentorship and detailed guidance from CP and AD on approach and interpretation. RD drafted the manuscript. CP and AD critically reviewed the manuscript multiple times and provided edits to the text, suggestions for revisions to analysis and discussion points. All authors approved of the final version before submission.

Competing interests
The authors declare that they have no competing interests.

Author details
[1]Department of Native Hawaiian Health, John A. Burns School of Medicine, University of Hawai'i at Mānoa, 677 Ala Moana Blvd., Suite 1015, Honolulu, HI 96813-5401, USA. [2]Office of Public Health Studies, University of Hawai'i at

Mānoa, 1960 East-West Road, BioMed T102, Honolulu, HI 96822-2319, USA.
³Research Institute for Development, Université Paris Descartes, Sorbonne Paris Cité, Research Unit 196 (CEPED), Paris, France.

References

1. Mirza FG, Gaddipati S. Obstetric emergencies. Semin Perinatol. 2009;33(2): 97–103.

2. Hofmeyr GJ, Say L, Gülmezoglu AM. WHO systematic review of maternal mortality and morbidity: the prevalence of uterine rupture. BJOG. 2005;112: 1221–8.

3. Berhe Y, Wall LL. Uterine rupture in resource-poor countries. Obstet Gyneco Surv. 2014;69(11):695–701.

4. Zwart JJ, Richters JM, Ory F, de Vries JIP, Bloemenkamp KWM, van Roosmalen J. Uterine rupture in the Netherlands: a nationwide population-based cohort study. BJOG. 2009;116(8):1069–80.

5. Motomura K, Ganchimeg T, Nagata C, Ota E, Vogel JP, Betran AP, et al. Incidence and outcomes of uterine rupture among women with prior caesarean section: WHO multicountry survey on maternal and newborn health. Sci Rep. 2017;7:44093.

6. Kwee A, Bots ML, Visser GHA, Bruinse HW. Uterine rupture and its complications in the Netherlands: a prospective study. Eur J Obstet Gynecol Reprod Biol. 2006;12(1):257–61.

7. Al-Zirqi I, Daltveit AK, Forsén L, Stray-Pedersen B, Vangen S. Risk factors for complete uterine rupture. Am J Obstet Gynecol 2017;216(2):165.e1–165.e8.

8. Igwegbe AO, Eleje GU, Udegbunam OI. Risk factors and perinatal outcome of uterine rupture in a low-resource setting. Niger Med J. 2013;54(6):415–9.

9. Kadowa I. Ruptured uterus in rural Uganda: prevalence, predisposing factors and outcomes. Singap Med J. 2010;51(1):35–8.

10. Fofie CO, Baffoe P. A two-year review of uterine rupture in a regional hospital. Ghana Med J. 2010;44(3):98–102.

11. Eze JN, Ibekwe PC. Uterine rupture at a secondary hospital in Afikpo. Southeast Nigeria Singapore Med J. 2010;51(6):506–11.

12. Astatikie G, Limenih MA, Kebede M. Maternal and fetal outcomes of uterine rupture and factors associated with maternal death secondary to uterine rupture. BMC Pregnancy Childbirth. 2017;17(1):117.

13. Getahun BS, Yeshi MM, Roberts DJ. Case 34-2012. N Engl J Med. 2012; 367(19):1839–45.

14. Nelson JP. Posterior uterine rupture secondary to use of herbs leading to peritonitis and maternal death in a primigravida following vaginal delivery of a live baby in western Uganda: a case report. Pan Afr Med J. 2016;23:81.

15. Fouelifack FY, Fouogue JT, Messi JO, Kamga DT, Fouedjio JH, Sando Z. Spontaneous second-trimester ruptured pregnancy of rudimentary horn: a case report in Yaounde. Cameroon Pan Afr Med J. 2014;18:86.

16. Nkwabong E, Kouam L, Takang W. Spontaneous uterine rupture during pregnancy: case report and review of literature. Afr J Reprod Health. 2007; 11(2):107–12.

17. Egbe TO, Halle-Ekane GE, Tchente CN, Nyemb JE, Belley-Priso E. Management of uterine rupture: a case report and review of the literature. BMC Res Notes. 2016;9(1):492.

18. Dumont A, Fournier P, Fraser W, Haddad S, Traore M, Diop I, et al. QUARITE (quality of care, risk management and technology in obstetrics): a cluster-randomized trial of a multifaceted intervention to improve emergency obstetric care in Senegal and Mali. Trials. 2009;10:85.

19. Dumont A, Fournier P, Abrahamowicz M, Traoré M, Haddad S, Fraser WD, et al. Quality of care, risk management, and technology in obstetrics to reduce hospital-based maternal mortality in Senegal and Mali (QUARITE): a cluster-randomised trial. Lancet. 2013;382(9887):146–57.

20. Shah A, Faundes A, Machoki M, Bataglia V, Amokrane F, Donner A, et al. Methodological considerations in implementing the WHO global survey for monitoring maternal and perinatal health. Bull World Health Organ. 2008; 86(2):126–31.

21. Ndour C, Dossou Gbété S, Bru N, Abrahamowicz M, Fauconnier A, Traoré M, et al. Predicting in-hospital maternal mortality in Senegal and Mali. PLoS One. 2013;8(5):e64157.

22. World Health Organization. WHO recommendations on antenatal care for a positive pregnancy experience. 2016. http://apps.who.int/iris/bitstream/10665/250800/1/WHO-RHR-16.12-eng.pdf. Accessed 26 Apr 2017.

23. Thaddeus S, Maine D. Too far to walk: maternal mortality in context. Soc Sci Med. 1994;38:1091–110.

24. Pirkle CM, Fournier P, Tourigny C, Sangaré K, Haddad S. Emergency obstetrical complications in a rural African setting (Kayes, Mali): the link between travel time and in-hospital maternal mortality. Matern Child Health J. 2011;15(7):1081–7.

25. Gabrysch S, Campbell OMR. Still too far to walk: literature review of the determinants of delivery service use. BMC Pregnancy Childbirth. 2009;11(9):34.

26. Lawn JE, Blencowe H, Kinney MV, Bianchi F, Graham WJ. Evidence to inform the future for maternal and newborn health. Best Pract Res Clin Obstet Gynaecol. 2016;36:169–83.

27. Nolens B, Lule J, Namiiro F, van Roosmalen J, Byamugisha J. Audit of a program to increase the use of vacuum extraction in Mulago hospital. Uganda BMC Pregnancy Childbirth. 2016;2(16):258.

28. Planning and Statistics Unit (CPS / SSDSPF), National Institute of Statistics (INSTAT / MEFB), INFO-STAT and ICF International. Demographic and Health Survey Mali 2012–2013: Synthesis Report. Rockville, Maryland, USA: CPS, INSTAT, INFO-STAT and ICF International, 2014. https://dhsprogram.com/what-we-do/survey/survey-display-405.cfm. Accessed 1 July 2018.

29. Agence Nationale de la Statistique et de la Démographie (ANSD) [Sénégal], and ICF International. Senegal Demographic and Health and Multiple Indicator Cluster Survey (EDS-MICS) 2010–2011. Rockville, Maryland, USA: ANSD and ICF International, 2012. https://dhsprogram.com/publications/publication-fr258-dhs-final-reports.cfm. Accessed 1 July 2018.

21

The Indigenous Birthing in an Urban Setting study: the IBUS study

A prospective birth cohort study comparing different models of care for women having Aboriginal and Torres Strait Islander babies at two major maternity hospitals in urban South East Queensland, Australia

Sophie Hickey[1], Yvette Roe[1], Yu Gao[1,2], Carmel Nelson[3], Adrian Carson[3], Jody Currie[4], Maree Reynolds[5], Kay Wilson[5], Sue Kruske[3], Renee Blackman[4], Megan Passey[6], Anton Clifford[1], Sally Tracy[6], Roianne West[7], Daniel Williamson[8], Machellee Kosiak[9], Shannon Watego[5], Joan Webster[10] and Sue Kildea[1,2*] ⓘ

Abstract

Background: With persisting maternal and infant health disparities, new models of maternity care are needed to meet the needs of Aboriginal and Torres Strait Islander people in Australia. To date, there is limited evidence of successful and sustainable programs. Birthing on Country is a term used to describe an emerging evidence-based and community-led model of maternity care for Indigenous families; its impact requires evaluation.

Methods: Mixed-methods prospective birth cohort study comparing different models of care for women having Aboriginal and Torres Strait Islander babies at two major maternity hospitals in urban South East Queensland (2015–2019). Includes women's surveys (approximately 20 weeks gestation, 36 weeks gestation, two and six months postnatal) and infant assessments (six months postnatal), clinical outcomes and cost comparison, and qualitative interviews with women and staff.

Discussion: This study aims to evaluate the feasibility, acceptability, sustainability, clinical and cost-effectiveness of a Birthing on Country model of care for Aboriginal and Torres Strait Islander families in an urban setting. If successful, findings will inform implementation of the model with similar communities.

Keywords: Indigenous, Maternity, Midwifery, Health services research, Aboriginal and Torres Strait Islander, Health disparities, Birthing on Country, Prospective birth cohort, Preterm birth, Child mortality

* Correspondence: sue.kildea@mater.uq.edu.au
[1]Midwifery Research Unit, Mater Research Institute-University of Queensland, Brisbane, QLD, Australia
[2]School of Nursing, Midwifery and Social Work, University of Queensland, Brisbane, Australia
Full list of author information is available at the end of the article

Background

Maternal and infant health disparities have persisted between Aboriginal and Torres Strait Islander people and non-Indigenous Australians, with Aboriginal and Torres Strait Islander women having disproportionately higher rates of: maternal mortality (~ 3 times higher) [1]; preterm births (14% vs. 8%); low birth weight infants (liveborn: 12% vs. 6%); and perinatal deaths (12 vs. 9/1000) [2, 3]. Preterm birth is a leading cause of perinatal mortality, serious neonatal morbidity, and moderate to severe childhood disability [4]. It contributes to more than two-thirds of perinatal mortality (fetal loss and neonatal death) [5] and is associated with diabetes, cardiovascular and renal disease in adulthood [6]. Queensland [7] and Western Australian [8] research suggests the majority of perinatal deaths are associated with preterm birth and low birth weight, which in turn are linked to modifiable risk factors: maternal psychosocial stress [9], infections in pregnancy [10], smoking in pregnancy [11], limited maternal education and young maternal age [12]. An Australian Indigenous study found preterm births and perinatal deaths decrease as the number of antenatal consultations increases [13]. Targeting the antenatal period with interventions that are culturally safe and high quality are essential to addressing these health disparities [14–16].

Birthing on Country

The Australian National Maternity Services Plan [17] identified three priority areas for improving services for Aboriginal and Torres Strait Islander women: 1) developing and expanding culturally competent maternity care; 2) developing and supporting an Aboriginal and Torres Strait Islander maternity workforce; and 3) developing dedicated programs for 'Birthing on Country' (best practice maternal and infant services for Aboriginal and Torres Strait Islander women).

An international literature review on Birthing on Country [14] was commissioned by the Australian government who defined Birthing on Country as:

> 'Maternity services designed and delivered for Indigenous women that encompass some or all of the following elements: are community based and governed; allow for incorporation of traditional practice; involve a connection with land and country; incorporate a holistic definition of health; value Indigenous and non-Indigenous ways of knowing and learning; risk assessment and service delivery; are culturally competent; and developed by, or with, Indigenous people' (p. 5).

The review assisted in identifying the characteristics of successful services [14] and at a national Birthing on Country workshop [18] participants described Birthing on Country as:

> 'a metaphor for the best start in life for Aboriginal and Torres Strait Islander babies and their families, an appropriate transition to motherhood and parenting for women, and an integrated, holistic and culturally appropriate model of care for all' (p. 25).

Aboriginal participants described Birthing on Country as 'the most powerful thing' stating it was 'about cultural choice' and 'being able to have babies safely on country' (p. 33):

> 'not only bio-physical outcomes ... it's much, much broader than just the labour and delivery ... (it) deals with socio-cultural and spiritual risk that is not dealt with in the current systems' (p.24).

Workshop recommendations called for widespread system reform and the development of exemplar models of Birthing on Country in urban, rural and remote areas [18]. Guiding Principles for Developing a Birthing on Country Service Model and Evaluation Framework were subsequently developed and endorsed by the Australian Health Ministers Advisory Council based on the literature and a national workshop [19]. The key components of successful programs that should be integrated in Birthing on Country service models are shown in Table 1. To date, implementation and evaluation of such models has been limited.

Caseload midwifery models

Continuity of care and carer has been identified as an important characteristic of culturally safe care for Aboriginal and Torres Strait Islander women [20]. Caseload midwifery (or midwifery group practice, MGP) is one such model that delivers continuity of midwifery carer throughout pregnancy, labour, birth and the early postnatal period [21]. MGP has been found to significantly improve outcomes for women and babies including reductions in preterm birth and increased satisfaction, breastfeeding, and cost savings [22, 23]. Only 10% of Australian women currently have access to caseload midwifery models, with only a disproportionately small number of Aboriginal and Torres Strait Islander women receiving this model of service delivery [24, 25]. Few services exclusively target Aboriginal and Torres Strait Islanderwomen and many women do not receive continuity of care across the maternity episode; therefore, there is a paucity of research in the area [26].

The research gap

The main methodological limitations of published interventional studies aimed at improving care and services

Table 1 Key components of successful, culturally competent Birthing on Country Service Models, reproduced with permission [19]

Birthing on Country
    Maternity services designed by & delivered for Aboriginal & Torres Strait Islander women & families

Governance
    Indigenous control, community development approach, shared vision cultural guidance & oversight

Philosophy & Overarching Principles
    Respect for & incorporation of Indigenous knowledge & traditional practice; respect for family & mens' involvement; partnership approach;
    women's business; continuity of carer; connection with country/land; capacity building approach - particularly with training & education;
    holistic definition of health; choice; evidenced-based clinical practice; social model of health & wellbeing

Skill Acquisition, Training & Education	*Service Characteristics*	*Monitoring & Evaluation*
Partnership approach/ two-way learning; appropriately trained & supported; competency based; delivered on-site; career pathway from maternity workers to midwifery; health literacy for women & families	Culturally competent service & staff; community based; specific location; designated ongoing funding; welcoming flexible service focusing on relationships & trust; outreach, transport, child friendly & group sessions; social, cultural, biomedical & community risk assessment criteria; clinical & cultural governance, interdisciplinary perinatal committee; effective IT; integrated services	Designated funding for monitoring & evaluation; continuous quality assurance; audit activities & recall register

Results
    Community healing as evidenced by: reduced family separation at critical times, restoration of skills & pride; capacity building in the community;
    supporting community & family relationships; reduced family violence; increased communication & liaison with other health professionals & service
    providers; comprehensive, holistic, tailored care; improved maternal & infant health outcomes.

for Aboriginal and Torres Strait Islander mothers and babies are small sample sizes, short-term evaluations and a lack of an appropriate comparison group [14–16]. Although several studies show promising results, most lack appropriate methodology and/or statistical power. Birthing on Country is a complex intervention that has not yet been rigorously evaluated in an urban Australian setting. The current study will contribute to addressing this knowledge gap by employing a methodologically rigorous study design and participatory research methods to evaluate an urban Birthing on Country continuity of care model for Aboriginal and Torres Strait Islander families in Australia.

Methods/Design

Aims

This research project aims to evaluate the feasibility, acceptability, sustainability, clinical and cost-effectiveness, of maternity care for Aboriginal and Torres Strait Islander families in South East Queensland. Specifically, this study aims to:

1. Restructure services to incorporate the key characteristics of a Birthing on Country Service Model of maternity services for Indigenous women in an urban setting, including an enhanced midwifery group practice
2. Conduct an evaluation of the restructure using a prospective cohort study
3. Utilise participatory action research methods to 'fine tune' the restructure of services
4. Determine if women receiving this new model have improved maternal and infant health outcomes

when compared to women receiving other models of care and baseline data
5. Determine the acceptability and sustainability of this new model of care
6. Evaluate the economic impact of this model
7. Explore the pregnancy and early parenting (six months postnatal) experiences of 20 women using an ethnographic approach accessing different models of care.

Study setting

South East Queensland comprises one of the largest and fastest growing Aboriginal and Torres Strait Islander populations of Australia [27]. The Birthing in Our Community service, launched in 2013, is a new model of care informed by the Birthing on Country literature and Guiding Principles. This model of care is available to women having Aboriginal and Torres Strait Islander babies at the Mater Mothers' Hospital (MMH), one of the largest tertiary maternity hospitals in Australia. Birthing in Our Community is conducted in partnership with two local Aboriginal Community Controlled Health Organisations: the Institute for Urban Indigenous Health (IUIH) and the Aboriginal and Torres Strait Islander Community Health Service Brisbane Limited (ATSICHS). The partnership is underpinned by a Memorandum of Understanding and Statement of Commitment to share resources to redesign maternal and infant health services. Service characteristics were based on the literature review [14] and the workshop report [18] as well as tailoring to the local context following recommendations from a World Café attended by 60 local stakeholders [28]; which resulted in the partnership. The overarching aim of the Birthing in Our

Community partnership is to close the gap in Aboriginal and Torres Strait Islander maternal and infant health outcomes, particularly preterm birth, through the translation of evidence-based strategies into the Birthing in Our Community program.

In developing the evaluation of the Birthing in Our Community program we aimed to compare outcomes for mothers and infants with a similar cohort of women receiving standard care. After reviewing the statistics from across South East Queensland, the most appropriate comparison cohort was women attending the Royal Brisbane and Women's Hospital (RBWH) where senior managers and researchers agreed to collaborate on a joint project and funding submission. However, as the funding was being awarded, the RBWH also changed their model of care (2013) for Aboriginal and Torres Strait Islander women through the Ngarrama Indigenous Maternity Service and it is no longer standard care. The Ngarrama Service is a government-funded midwifery continuity of care service for women having an Aboriginal and/or Torres Strait Islander baby/ies and planning to birth at the RBWH (located fewer than six kilometres north of the MMH). Thus we have agreed to evaluate both new services, Birthing in Our Community and the Ngarrama Service, and will compare them to each other, and to women receiving standard care and to baseline data from both hospitals. (Note: not all women having Aboriginal and Torres Strait Islander babies at both MMH and RBWH access the Indigenous-specific models of care hence the concurrent comparison with standard care). Table 2 outlines the components of the different models of care available to women having Aboriginal and Torres Strait Islander babies at the MMH and RBWH. For the first time, researchers will test the effectiveness of caseload midwifery in an urban setting where 100% of the midwives' caseload are women having Aboriginal and Torres Strait Islander babies receiving care across the maternity continuum (antenatal, birth, until 6 weeks postnatal).

Study design

This study underwent peer review by the funding body, the National Health and Medical Research Council. This study will consist of a prospective cohort study comparing:

1. *Maternal and infant health outcomes*: women booked to receive maternity care through MMH or RBWH, by model of care and Aboriginal and Torres Strait Islander status of baby and/or mother (see Table 3). Routinely collected clinical outcomes for mothers and infants will provide data on the effectiveness of the programs since they commenced in late 2013 and be compared across

groups for the duration of the study (ending in 2019), and to baseline data for both hospitals (2009–2013). Infant assessments will be undertaken at two and 6 months postnatally for Groups 1 and 4.

2. *Service acceptability, effectiveness and cost-effectiveness*: Maternal surveys will be undertaken as early as possible antenatally (~ 20 weeks and 36 weeks antenatally, two and six months postnatally). An ethnographic component will also explore the pregnancy and early parenting (to six months postnatal) experiences of ~ 20 women from each Birthing in Our Community and the Ngarrama Service using a longitudinal, ethnographic approach: 'Tell My Story' substudy. Cost-effectiveness analysis will be conducted from the broader 'societal' perspective which will include not only the cost to the hospital (Routine data) but the cost to the women (Women's surveys) and partner organisations (Routine data).

3. *Service sustainability and feasibility*: Staff perspectives and experiences will be compared across the services to determine the sustainability and feasibility from a workforce perspective.

Birthing in Our Community is a complex intervention with multifaceted components; identifying its 'active ingredients' is vital to evaluating effectiveness and replicating the intervention in other settings [29]. As with the Ngarrama Service, an appropriate monitoring and evaluation framework [29, 30] is needed that enables all stakeholders to understand not only what components are integral to success or failure but why these components are so important and influential. A Program Logic Model will be used for the monitoring and process evaluation to assess if the services are being implemented as planned [28]. Program logic is essentially a conceptual 'road map' that presents the thinking/theory behind the expected outcomes of research activities.

A mixed-methods research design has therefore been selected as the most appropriate to achieve these goals, with equal weight given to both qualitative and quantitative approaches. Incorporating participatory action research [31] (PAR), as recommended for Indigenous research [32], will allow the research team to be responsive to evaluation findings throughout the duration of the study. In line with a PAR approach, the IBUS research team will meet regularly to discuss relevant issues and collaboratively plan research-related activities, with regular reflections on previous steps, progress to date, and future expectations/aspirations [31]. Regular Steering Committee meetings provide a mechanism (Birthing in Our Community only) enabling timely feedback and regular reporting to key stakeholders.

Table 2 Models of care available to Aboriginal and Torres Strait Islander families at study sites

Birthing in Our Community (Group 1)	Standard Care (Groups 2, 5)	Ngarrama Maternity Service (Group 4)
Indigenous governance (operating through a Steering Committee) functioning in accordance with Terms of Reference and underpinned by a MOU A community-based Midwifery Group Practice (MGP), which provides continuity of care to enrolled women throughout pregnancy, birth and up to six weeks postnatally Care is provided according to hospital guidelines and protocols in the home and at community venues where regular cultural and education days are held 24/7 access to caseload midwife who works in MGP of 4FTE on annualised salary with each woman allocated a primary midwife. Midwife support during birthing is likely to be by a known midwife. Location for birth is the Birth Suite (no homebirth or Birth Centre services provided)[a] Indigenous Maternal Infant Health/ Family Support Workers and Indigenous student midwives work with the caseload midwives to provide culturally tailored care Referral to and integration with Indigenous community support agencies as required; All women are offered a formal handover to child health services with other referrals as required (e.g. paediatric, allied health) Clinical and cultural supervision for staff.	Antenatal care may be received from community based general practitioner, hospital based midwives or doctors who rotate throughout the service on rosters. Midwife support during birthing is likely to be by a midwife the woman has never met. Postnatal care or phone call from a rostered community midwife might take place if the woman meets the criteria for early discharge—before 48h for vaginal birth and 72h for caesarean section usually for up to less than two weeks No 24/7 access to MGP midwife but can call hospital birthing suite in emergency Location for birth same as other groups for the hospitals	A hospital-based Midwifery Group Practice (MGP) with a community clinic one day a week, which provides continuity of care to enrolled women throughout pregnancy, birth and up to six weeks postnatally. Care is provided according to hospital guidelines and protocols, regardless of setting (women's homes, community venues or hospital) 24/7 access to MGP midwives who work in a small team and are on annualised salary with each woman allocated a primary midwife. Midwife support during birthing is likely to be by a known midwife. Location for birth may be in the Birth Suite or the co-located Birth Centre (eligibility criteria apply); Access to Cultural Capability Officers of the regional (Metro North) Aboriginal and Torres Strait Islander Health Unit who provide additional cultural guidance and support.

Indigenous Liaison Officers are based in the hospitals to strengthen culturally responsive care and support
Access to medical staff, allied health professionals, social workers, child safety officers and other professionals (e.g. diabetic educator) as required
Discharge letter to referral doctor and referrals to community support agencies as required

[a]Despite community recommendations for an Indigenous Birthing Centre, funding has not yet been secured

Study participants
Inclusion/exclusion criteria

Women's surveys, Tell My Story and Infant Assessments Women are eligible to participate if they:

- Are having an Aboriginal and/or Torres Strait Islander baby;
- Receive their maternity care through the Birthing in Our Community program and are planning to birth at the MMH (Group 1); receive their maternity care through the Ngarrama Indigenous Maternity Service and are planning to birth at the RBWH (Group 4); receive standard maternity care and birth at the MMH or RBWH (Groups 2 & 5); and
- Consent to participate.

Table 3 Timeline of groups by model of care and research data available

Year	2009	2010	2011	2012	2013	2014	2015	2016	2017	2018	2019
Groups by model of care						Group 1: Birthing in Our Community, MMH (Indigenous)					
	Group 2: Standard care, MMH (Indigenous)										
	Group 3: Standard care, MMH (Non-Indigenous)										
						Group 4: Ngarrama Indigenous Maternity Service, RBWH (Indigenous)					
	Group 5: Standard care, RBWH (Indigenous)										
	Group 6: Standard care, RBWH (Non-Indigenous)										
Research data (Groups)	*Baseline*					*Study period*					
	Routine Data (2, 3, 5, 6)					Routine Data (1–6)					
						Women's Surveys (1, 2, 4, 5)					
						Tell My Story (1, 4)					
						Infant Assessments (1, 2, 4, 5)					
						Staff Interviews (1, 4)					

Women are not eligible to participate if they:

- Have been transferred into the RBWH or the MMH from out of area for high-level specialist services or received no antenatal care.

Infants are eligible if:

- They are Aboriginal and/or Torres Strait Islander and their mothers received care through either of these hospitals and were recruited to the study.

Routinely collected clinical and costing data (Groups 1–6) Women and infants will be excluded if they have been transferred into the RBWH or the MMH from out of area for high-level specialist services or received no antenatal care.

Staff surveys, interviews, and focus groups (Groups 1–6) Staff are eligible to participate in the staff surveys, interviews and focus groups if they have been involved in the planning and/or provision of maternity care services for Aboriginal and Torres Strait Islander families in South East Queensland during the study period; and consent to participate.

Power and sample size

This study has been powered to detect changes in clinical outcomes and the number of women accessing care per annum in each program [33]. During the 3.5-year recruitment period, we will aim to access routinely collected data for approximately 420 women at MMH, and 350 from RBWH (based on an estimated 20% attrition rate). The change in outcomes has been estimated based on changes seen in the Townsville Mums and Bubs program that reported a reduction in preterm birth [34] (Table 4).

The sample size for the ethnographic component of the study ('Tell My Story') will involve a smaller group of women from each cohort. The project aims to recruit up to 25 women from each cohort, which factors in a 20% attrition rate (25*.8 = 20).

Participant recruitment and informed consent

Written informed consent to participate in the study will be obtained from all participants. The privacy, wellbeing

and safety of all participants is a paramount consideration, and will be ensured by strict adherence to eligibility criteria, ensuring the relevant Participant Information and Consent Form has been read and understood, and reminding participants of their right to withdraw from the study at any time, without penalty. Study data collection will not commence until the requisite site-specific Human Research Ethics Committee and Research Governance approvals have been secured.

Women's surveys and Infant Assessments (Groups 1, 2, 4, 5)
Written information about the study will be provided to all women at both sites when they book into the hospital. Recruiting staff (midwives, health workers, and liaison officers) will fill out an 'Expression of Interest' referral form with women interested and willing for IBUS research staff to contact her to tell her more about the study. Women will then be contacted by IBUS research staff who will explain the study in more detail and invite them to participate. Women who agree to participate will be given, mailed or emailed the Participant Information and Consent Form, with verbal information provided by the research staff. Written informed consent to participate will be obtained by member/s of the research team who will meet women at their next antenatal visit or to ring them to discuss the study in more detail.

In line with the NHMRC *Values and Ethics Guidelines for Ethical conduct in Aboriginal and Torres Strait Islander Health Research* [32], women will be reminded that they may defer making a decision until they have had time to discuss the information with any "interested parties … formally constituted bodies … collectives or community elders" (p.14). Provision will also be made for answering any outstanding questions. Consent to participate will be obtained by member/s of the research team who will offer to meet them at their next antenatal visit or to ring them to discuss the study in more detail.

Although this study is not specifically targeting young women, we are guided by the National Statement in that they will not be excluded on the basis of age alone [35]. The study will also be guided by usual practice employed for clinical procedures whereby the best interests of the young woman, and her capacity to consent, will be assessed on an individual basis. Hence, young women "who are mature enough to understand and consent,

Table 4 Power calculations with $n = 350$ in each arm + 20% for attrition

Outcome	From %	To %	No./ cohort	Power
Proportion of women who attend ≥ 5 antenatal visits	81.0	90.0	261	0.924
Proportion of women who were smoking after 20 weeks	42.0	31.0	318	0.858
Preterm birth < 37 weeks pregnancy	16.0	9.0	350	0.801
Exclusive Breast feeding at discharge (2007–09 Mater data)	78.0	88.0	240	0.942

and are not vulnerable through immaturity in ways that warrant additional consent from a parent or guardian" (p. 65) will be invited to consent in their own right [35]. Where there is any concern that immaturity renders a young woman vulnerable, she will not be invited to participate.

Routinely collected data (Groups 1–6)

We are seeking a waiver of consent to access routinely collected data for the all cohorts of women in order to satisfactorily answer the outcome measures. This will include both clinical and costing data. For women who participate in the IBUS surveys, consent will be sought to link IBUS survey data to routinely collected data. Initially the data will be collected in an identifiable form so we can be assured that data from different sources can be merged with each participant given one unique identifier. Once this is completed all identifiable data (e.g. name, address) will be removed and kept only in the participant log, which will be used to contact participants at different time points.

Tell My Story (Groups 1 & 4)

A smaller group of women will be invited to participate in the Tell My Story qualitative component. Women in the IBUS study who are interested in participating in further qualitative antenatal and postnatal follow-up will be approached by the IBUS research team.

Staff interviews and focus groups (Groups 1 & 4)

All staff members involved in planning or providing specialized maternity care to women having Aboriginal and/or Torres Strait Islander babies at MMH or RBWH will be eligible to participate in these individual and focus groups interviews. Staff will be invited to participate by the IBUS research team. A researcher will explain the staff interview process to the staff either face-to-face or on the phone using the Participant Information and Consent Form for Staff which will be emailed in advance. Staff who provide written consent to participate will be interviewed either annually or when exiting a role. Interviews will be conducted one-on-one or in small focus groups. Interview participants will be reimbursed for parking costs and given a small gift (e.g. chocolates) as a show of thanks and appreciation for their time.

Staff quantitative surveys (Groups 1–6)

Staff will be invited to complete surveys on their experiences of working in the different models of care. The initial invitation to participate will be sent to staff via email with the option for them to complete electronic surveys via an email link or paper surveys distributed via team leaders from the research team. Staff will

receive face-to-face, text and email reminders to complete the survey.

Data collection

Routinely collected clinical and costing data

Data for each mother/infant dyad at the MMH will be collected from several sources. MMH obstetric (MatriX), neonatal database and expenditure data (Australian activity based funding Diagnosis Related Groups [DRG] codes) will provide detailed patient-level information on inpatient contacts for the mother and baby. Routinely collected data including expenditure data will be collected from the RBWH where it will be coded before being merged with the study database. Perinatal data will also be extracted from the Queensland Health database.

The IUIH (MMeX) and ATSICHS (Medical Director and Pracsoft; MMeX) routinely collect data on service delivery (access, clinical data, e.g. immunisations, and expenditure data) which will also be collected. The clinical and costing outcomes data will be derived from routinely collected information and survey data.

Women's surveys and infant assessments

Survey data collected at different time points will be used to measure program acceptability, sustainability and effectiveness; and infant growth and development. Women will be invited to complete face-to-face, postal or online surveys (their choice) at booking-in, 36 weeks of pregnancy, at two months and six months after birth. Maternal surveys will include questions related to women's maternity care experience and out-of-pocket costs incurred in accessing maternity or child health services (see Table 5 for list of survey items). At two and six months after the birth, women will be asked to provide information about their infant's development (Ages and Stages Questionnaire [36]). At six months postnatal, women and infants will be invited to participate in a face-to-face developmental assessment, and offered a developmental report on their infant's performance on the Bayley-III Scales of Infant and Toddler Development [37]. Referral to a specialist will be available for infants identified with developmental delays or who otherwise raise concerns. Additionally, if any woman is identified to be at risk of depression or psychological distress or self-harm, she will also be offered referral to appropriate services.

Participants will be provided with an AU$10 gift card after completing the booking-in and 36 weeks antenatal surveys and a large tote bag at 36 weeks. An AU$30 gift card and a small toy or bib/blanket will be given for the two and six-month postnatal surveys to thank women for their time. Women who participate with their infant

Table 5 Items included in Women's antenatal and postnatal surveys

Items	1	2	3	4
Socio-demographic characteristics				
Indigenous status, maternal and paternal	✓			
Maternal relationship status	✓			
Educational attainment, maternal and paternal	✓			
Employment status, maternal and paternal	✓			
Government pension main source of income	✓		✓	✓
Has healthcare concession card	✓			
Has private health insurance	✓			
Has access to vehicle/transport	✓			
Number of places of residence during pregnancy		✓		
Current housing	✓	✓		
Experienced homelessness during pregnancy		✓		
Financial insecurity	✓	✓	✓	✓
Self-reported health problems				
Experienced health problems, mother and infant			✓	✓
Baby admitted to hospital, date, reason, duration			✓	✓
Mother admitted to hospital, date, reason, duration			✓	✓
Number of visits with baby to child health nurse, reason			✓	✓
Number of visit with baby to paediatrician & reason			✓	✓
Pregnancy, birth/labour & care				
Gestation/age of baby	✓	✓	✓	✓
General feelings about pregnancy	✓	✓	✓	✓
Number of weeks first contact with care for pregnancy	✓			
Where was care received	✓			
Plans for birth location	✓			
Experience of staff behaviour		✓	✓	
Culturally safe aspects of care (importance, satisfaction)	✓		✓	
Felt respected & understood by hospital staff (by area)			✓	
Felt treated poorly or judged by staff			✓	
Satisfaction with care, recommend to others		✓		
Known midwife present during labour/birth			✓	
Attendance of group antenatal classes		✓		
Smoking				
Current smoking status, including number of cigarettes per day	D	✓	✓	✓
Attempts to quit	D	✓		
Advised to quit by health staff		✓		
Smoking support received, perceptions		✓		
Smoking household members	✓	✓		✓
Feeding baby				
Previous breastfeeding experiences, inc. difficulties	D	✓		
Intentions to breastfeed, inc. duration	D	✓		

Table 5 Items included in Women's antenatal and postnatal surveys *(Continued)*

Items	1	2	3	4
Confidence to breastfeed		✓		
Experience of breastfeeding, inc. initiation			✓	
Use of formula, inc. reasons, age of baby			✓	
What baby has been fed in past 24h			✓	✓
Where received feeding information			✓	
Use of commercial baby food				✓
Reasons for starting solids				✓
Partner involvement				
Partner's feelings about pregnancy	✓			
Baby's father & father figures (involvement, attended visits, support services)				✓
Social and emotional wellbeing				
Negative life events - full extended version	✓	✓		✓
Additional worries experienced	✓	✓		✓
Family separations			✓	
Positive wellbeing scale	✓	✓	✓	✓
Modified Kessler Psychological Distress Scale (K5)	✓	✓	✓	✓
Edinburgh Postnatal Depression Scale	D		✓	
Practical Social Support Scale	✓			
Social support available, inc. partner		✓		
Out-of-pocket costs				
Time spent, support person, carer, transport, food & drink		✓		
All services accessed for pregnancy/birth/baby, number of visits, out of pocket cost per visit (i.e. not refunded by Medicare)			✓	
Out of pocket cost of medicines during pregnancy/birth/baby			✓	
Infant development				
Ages and Stages Questionnaire			✓	✓
Bayley III Cognitive, Language and Motor Skills (face-to-face assessment)				✓

Note: D = clinical data available

in the Bayley assessment will receive an additional AU$10 gift card upon completion.

Tell My Story

Researchers will interview women and discuss family practices including lifestyle, stressors, social support, cultural practices and childrearing. There will be the option for women to do a one-off in-depth interview or to take part in repeated interviews antenatally and until the infant is six months old. Interviews will explore Indigenous perspectives of culturally safe care (acceptability) and what constitutes social, cultural and clinical risk and wellbeing for Aboriginal and Torres Strait Islander women. Women will be asked about their relationships with healthcare providers, their experiences with maternity services and how these impact engagement, health choices and outcomes.

Interviews will be recorded using a digital recorder and observations recorded using hand written notes. Antenatal and postnatal interviews will be conducted in a convenient location for women – in the home, clinic or hospital. Participants will be provided with a AU$30 gift voucher as a thank-you for their time.

Staff surveys, interviews and focus groups

Staff interviews and focus groups All staff who have provided specialised maternity care for women having Aboriginal and/or Torres Strait Islander babies at either the MMH (including Birthing in Our Community) or at the RBWH (including the Ngarrama Indigenous Service) will be invited to participate in staff interviews and focus groups. This includes but is not limited to exit interviews with staff leaving or who have left the service. These interviews will explore the experiences of staff working within the programs and identify any recommendations for future and existing services. This will assist with identifying the 'key ingredients' of a best practice model of maternity care as well as evaluating the acceptability, feasibility, and cost-effectiveness of the different models of care. Semi-structured interviews will be conducted over the phone, in person or in small groups. With the staff members' permission, these interviews will be audio-recorded.

Staff surveys In order to evaluate the sustainability of the models from a workforce perspective, annual quantitative surveys will be conducted with staff involved in the program. A comparison group of MMH and RBWH caseload midwives will also be invited to participate in selected surveys to assess whether there is a significant difference in workload, daily activities and work-related stress between the caseload midwifery teams. Online and anonymous surveys will be conducted with staff. These will be voluntary and confidential, and likely include the Maslach Burnout Inventory or Copenhagen Burnout Inventory [38], the Attitudes to Professional Role, Caseload Midwifery Industrial Agreement Questionnaire, Time in Motion Study, Kessler Psychological Distress and Wellbeing Scale as well as questions about team cohesion, meeting goals, cultural capability of staff, and suggestions for improvements.

Outcome measures
Primary outcome measures (all groups)

- Proportion of women giving birth preterm (< 37 weeks gestation)
- Proportion of women who attend five or more antenatal visits during pregnancy
- Proportion of women smoking after 20 weeks gestation
- Proportion of women exclusively breast-feeding at discharge from hospital.

Secondary outcome measures (all groups where reliable data is available)

- Gestation at first antenatal visit to a health provider, at booking into hospital (weeks, Mean, Median, Range, First trimester (Yes/No)), Number of total antenatal visits (Mean, SD, Median, Range, < 5 visits, 5 and more visits)
- The proportion of women with modifiable risk factors for preterm birth (i.e. inadequate antenatal care, smoking, stress and missing data in these fields)
- Smoking status at booking (Yes/No), during the first 20 weeks (Yes/No), and after the first 20 weeks (Yes/No), at discharge and six months postnatal, Number of cigarettes intake each day if smoking (Mean, SD)
- The proportion of women who attended antenatal education sessions (Yes/No)
- Pharmacological analgesia in labour (Epidural/spinal analgesia, Narcotic analgesia, Nitrous oxide gas)
- Onset of labour (Induced, No labour, Spontaneous)
- Mode of birth (Non-instrumental vaginal birth, Instrumental vaginal birth, Elective Caesarean section, Emergency Caesarean section)
- Management of third stage labour (Active, Physiological)
- Postpartum haemorrhage (< 500; 500–999; 1000-1499; 1500 ml and more or with blood transfusion)
- Perineal trauma status (Intact/1st degree tear, 2nd degree tear, 3rd/4th degree tear).
- Episiotomy (Yes/No)
- Women who had a known caregiver for labour and birth (Yes/No)
- Birth weight (grams, Mean, SD, < 2500 g, 2500 g or more)
- Apgar score 5 min (< 7, 7 or above)
- Admission to a separate neonatal nursery (Yes/No)
- Perinatal outcomes (Liveborn survived, Liveborn neonatal death prior to discharge from hospital, Stillbirth)
- Cause of perinatal deaths

- Antenatal intention to breastfeed (Yes/No) Women exclusively breastfeeding at discharge from hospital following birth (Yes/No), at two months postnatal (Yes/No), and six months postnatal (Yes/No)
- Mother readmission to hospital up to six months postpartum (Yes/No)
- Infant readmission to hospital up to six months of age (Yes/No)
- Length of stay in hospital for mothers and infants following birth (Mean, Median, Range)
- Cost of care per mother/infant pair during pregnancy, birth, postnatal until mother six weeks postpartum and baby 28 days after birth
- Negative life events scale – full extended version – at booking-in and six months postnatal (Yes/No, Number of events)
- Modified Kessler Psychological Distress Scale (K5) score at booking-in, 36 weeks gestation, two and six months postnatal
- Edinburgh Postnatal Depression Scale score at booking-in and six months postnatal
- Ages and Stages Questionnaire score at two and six months postnatal
- Bayley III Cognitive, Language and Motor Skills score at six months postnatal

Note, all tools will be scored according to their recommended guidelines and outcomes reported accordingly.

Data analysis and management
Quantitative
Clinical data will initially be collected in a reidentifiable form (via the unique patient identifier) so that it can be linked with data obtained from other sources (e.g. surveys), to enable the economic analyses to be undertaken. Once merged, identifiers will be removed and only the coded number will remain.

Quantitative analyses will compare the difference in clinical outcomes between Birthing in Our Community (intervention), the Ngarrama Service (concurrent control), standard care (historical and concurrent control), and also non-Indigenous women and babies (historical and concurrent control) at MMH and RBWH.

Data on all women attending either hospital during the study period will be extracted. Women transferring in from other hospital or rural and remote areas for higher-level services (variable available), and those with no antenatal care will be excluded from analysis. Analyses will be by birth model of care and women with multiple births and their infants with identified fetal anomaly will be excluded from analysis unless noted otherwise.

Initial bivariate analysis will investigate possible differences between the cohorts for baseline socio-demographic (socio-economic status), and clinical characteristics (e.g. age, parity, body mass index, smoking, obstetric history) that could affect outcome measures. Dependent on data type, analysis will be undertaken using an independent samples t-test, Mann-Whitney U test or chi-squared test. Outcome measures will be presented using relative risks with 95% confidence intervals. Multivariate logistic, linear regression models and propensity score matching will be used to adjust for confounders. Longitudinal outcomes (e.g. breastfeeding) will be analysed with generalized estimating equations to account for the correlation between observations repeated in the same person. To understand the mechanism or process that underlies the effect of model of care on outcomes, mediation analysis will be conducted to identify if and to what extent the other variables explains the relationship. All withdrawals, losses to follow-up, and deaths will be reported. Analysis will be performed with SPSS Version 22.0/Stata 14.0 and statistical significance will be at the 0.05 level.

Survey data will be uploaded from iPads/tablet computers, Qualtrics or other software tools such as Remark (for the printed versions) to a dedicated spreadsheet and subjected to simple descriptive analysis using SPSS/Stata. Bayley-III data at the six-month infant assessment will be scored by the research assistant in real time (i.e. as the assessment proceeds) using the age-standardized Bayley Record and Score Forms, and associated Tables to give norm-referenced scores. These scores will then be uploaded onto the project specific database. Staff surveys will be analysed using SPSS/Stata to test for significant trends and potential differences between groups.

Cost-effectiveness analysis
The cost-effectiveness analysis will be conducted to examine the direct costs, from a societal perspective, to women and their families, maternity and child health care services and other community services in relation to pregnancy and birth. We will compare the mean costs per mother/infant pair between Birthing in Our Community (Group 1) and the Ngarrama Service (Group 4) to standard care group (Group 2 and 5) up to 6 weeks postpartum. Costs will be calculated for both mother and baby to include: women and family's out-of-pocket expenses related to clinic appointments, outpatients (ultrasound, pathology, etc.) and prescribed medicines, and hospitalisation costs. Data will be collected through routinely collected information as well as questions embedded in the 36-week antenatal and 2 month postnatal surveys. Average costs for each mother and infant for the duration of the maternity episode (i.e. from when she first confirmed her pregnancy to 6 weeks postnatal) will be calculated and compared to determine the cost effectiveness of a model of care.

Qualitative

Qualitative interview data from the Tell My Story study will be audiotaped, as will staff focus groups and interviews. Data will be analysed using Interpretative Phenomenological Analysis (IPA), a qualitative method of analysis which draws knowledge from everyday experiences and is descriptive. Transcripts will be read by a minimum of two team members who will identify key themes and independently create a coding system. Codes will be compared, inconsistencies discussed and reconciled, and a final coding scheme agreed before entry into NVivo Version 8. The analysis will comprise of: Firstly, coding of initial interview transcripts to identify themes and develop a coding framework. Secondly, identification and categorisation of women and staff experiences using the coding framework. The coding framework will be revised and refined as new themes emerge. Finally, key findings will be used to inform the development future Birthing on Country services. Data will be saved on the computer hard drive and transcribed verbatim.

Discussion

This study will test the impact of two maternity models of care for one of Australia's highest priority health populations: Aboriginal and Torres Strait Islander mothers and babies. The model and economic impact assessment have been derived from international best-practice and service evaluations in Australia and our study has the statistical power to detect a difference in preterm birth. The multi-agency approach to implementing a Birthing on Country Service Model at one site has been recommended in Aboriginal and Torres Strait Islander policy documents and will be evaluated. The economic impact assessment aims to quantify the impact of the model by articulating the process by which research leads to impacts on the end-user and/or the broader community. If the model is successful and demonstrates a good return on investment, we will have developed and evaluated a culturally safe service model transferable to other settings for trialling in a broader context.

Abbreviations

ATSICHS: Aboriginal and Torres Strait Islander Community Health Service Brisbane Ltd; BiOC: Birthing in Our Community; IBUS : Indigenous Birthing in an Urban Setting; IUIH: Institute for Urban Indigenous Health; MMH: Mater Mothers' Hospital; NHMRC: National Health and Medical Research Council (Australia); RBWH: Royal Brisbane & Women's Hospital

Funding

Funding from partner organisations was used to establish the Birthing in Our Community program. The Queensland Government funded an increase in service capacity and a community-based Hub with the funds administered through IUIH. The Queensland Government also fund the Ngarrama Indigenous Maternity Service. National Health and Medical Research Council Partnership Grant (APP1077036) funds are used to conduct the IBUS Study, with further support from partner organisations and universities for members of the investigator team, research support and infrastructure. The National Health and Medical Research Council did not have any role in the study design, data collection, data analysis, data interpretation, or writing of this manuscript.

Authors' contributions

SKi was the primary author of the grant application with primary assistance from YR, SKr, CN, ST and MP, ACl, RW, JW, DW. SH has been primary author of the protocol and amendments, with minor edits from SKi, YG, RW, MP and ACl. SKi, CN, ACr, JC, MR, KW, SKr, RB, SW and MK have significantly contributed to service implementation and design. All authors read and approved the final manuscript.

Competing interests

The authors declare that they have no competing interests.

Author details

[1]Midwifery Research Unit, Mater Research Institute-University of Queensland, Brisbane, QLD, Australia. [2]School of Nursing, Midwifery and Social Work, University of Queensland, Brisbane, Australia. [3]Institute for Urban Indigenous Health, Brisbane, QLD, Australia. [4]Aboriginal and Torres Strait Islander Community Health Service Brisbane Limited, Brisbane, QLD, Australia. [5]Mater Misericordia Limited, Brisbane, QLD, Australia. [6]The University of Sydney, Sydney, NSW, Australia. [7]Griffith University, First Peoples Health Unit Queensland, Brisbane, Australia. [8]Department of Health, Aboriginal and Torres Strait Islander Health Branch, Brisbane, QLD, Australia. [9]Australian Catholic University, Sydney, QLD, Australia. [10]National Centre of Research Excellence in Nursing Interventions, Griffith University, Menzies Health Institute, Brisbane, QLD, Australia.

References

1. Australian Institute of Health and Welfare: Maternal deaths in Australia 2012–2014. *Cat. No. PER 92.* Canberra: AIHW; 2017.
2. Australian Institute of Health and Welfare: Australia Mothers and Babies 2015 - In Brief. *Perinatal* statistics *series no 33*, Cat. no. PER 91. Canberra: AIHW; 2017.
3. Li Z, et al: Australia's mothers and babies 2010. Canberra: AIHW National Perinatal Epidemiology and Statistics Unit; 2012.
4. Gotsch F, et al. The preterm parturition syndrome and its implications for understanding the biology, risk assessment, diagnosis, treatment and prevention of preterm birth. J Matern Fetal Neonatal Med. 2009;22:5–23.
5. Lumley J, Chamberlain C, Dowswell T, Oliver S, Oakley L, WatsonL. Interventions for promoting smoking cessation during pregnancy. Cochrane Database Syst Rev. 2009;(3):CD001055. https://www.ncbi.nlm.nih.gov/pmc/articles/PMC4090746/.
6. Gluckman PD, Hanson M, Pinal C. The developmental origins of adult disease. Maternal & Child Nutrition. 2005;1:130–41.
7. Johnston T, Coory M. Reducing perinatal mortality among Indigenous babies in Queensland: should the first priority be better primary health care or better access to hospital care during confinement? Australian and New Zealand Health Policy. 2005;2:11.

8.   Freemantle C, et al. Patterns, trends, and increasing disparities in mortality for Aboriginal & non-Aboriginal infants born in WA, 1980-200. Lancet. 2006; 367:1758–66.

9.   Moutquin J. Socio-economic and psychosocial factors in the management and prevention of preterm labour. BJOG. 2003;110:56–60.

10. Sangkomkamhang U, et al. Antenatal lower genital tract infection screening and treatment programs for preventing preterm delivery. Cochrane Database Syst Rev. 2008:CD006178.

11. British Medical Association. Smoking and reproductive life: the impact of smoking on sexual, reproductive and child health. London: British Medical Association; 2004.

12. Muglia L, Katz M. The enigma of spontaneous preterm birth. N Engl J Med. 2010;2010(11):529–35.

13. Steering Committee for the Review of Government Service Provision: Overcoming Indigenous disadvantage: key indicators. Canberra: steering Committee for the Review of government service provision, Productivity commission; 2009.

14. Kildea S, Van Wagner V: 'Birthing on country,' Maternity service delivery models: a review of the literature. Canberra: maternity services inter-jurisdictional Committee for the Australian Health Minister's advisory council, brokered by the sax institute; 2013.

15. Herceg A: Improving health in Aboriginal & Torres Strait Islander mothers, babies and young children: a literature review. Canberra: Australian Government Department of Health & ageing; 2005.

16. Rumbold A, Cunningham J. A review of the impact of antenatal care services for Australian Indigenous women and attempts to strengthen these services. Matern Child Health J. 2008;12:83–100.

17. AHMAC: National maternity services plan, 2011. Canberra: Australian health ministers advisory council, Commonwealth of Australia; 2011.

18. Kildea S, Stapleton H, Magick Dennis F: Birthing on Country Workshop Report, Alice Springs, 4th July. Brisbane: ACU and Mater Medical Research Institute; 2013.

19. Kildea S, Lockey R, Roberts J, Magick Dennis F: Guiding Principles for Developing a Birthing on Country Service Model and Evaluation Framework, Phase 1. Brisbane: Mater Medical Research Unit and the University of Queensland on behalf of the Maternity Services Inter-Jurisdictional Committee for the Australian Health Ministers' Advisory Council; 2016.

20. Kruske S: Culturally competent maternity Care for Aboriginal and Torres Strait Women Report. Brisbane: September 2012 – prepared on behalf of the maternity services inter-jurisdictional Committee for the Australian Health Ministers' advisory council; 2013.

21. Hartz D, Foureur M, Tracy SK. Australian caseload midwifery: the exception or the rule. Women and Birth. 2012;25:39–46.

22. McLachlan HL, et al. Effects of continuity of care by a primary midwife (caseload midwifery) on caesarean section rates in women of low obstetric risk: the COSMOS randomised controlled trial. BJOG. 2012;119:1483–92.

23. Tracy SK, et al. Caseload midwifery care versus standard maternity care for women of any risk: M@NGO, a randomised controlled trial. Lancet. 2013; 382(9906):1723-32.

24. Homer C, et al. It's more than just having a baby' women's experiences of a maternity service for Australian Aboriginal and Torres Strait islander families. Midwifery. 2012;28:e509–15.

25. Stamp G, et al. Aboriginal maternal and infant care workers: partners in caring for Aboriginal mothers and babies. Rural Remote Health. 2008;8:883.

26. Kildea S, Tracy S, Sherwood J, Magick-Dennis F, Barclay LM. Improving maternity services for Indigenous women in Australia: moving from policy to practice. Med J Aust. 2016;205:374–9.

27. Biddle N: CAEPR Indigenous population project: 2011 census papers. Canberra: Centre for Aboriginal Economic Policy Research, Australian National University; 2013.

28. Kildea S, Hickey S, Nelson C, Currie J, Carson A, Reynolds M, Wilson K, Kruske S, Passey M, Roe Y, et al. Birthing on country (in our community): a case study of engaging stakeholders and developing a best-practice Indigenous maternity service in an urban setting. Aust Health Rev. 2017. https://doi.org/10.1071/AH16218.

29. Campbell N, et al. Designing and evaluating complex interventions to improve health care. BMJ. 2007;334:455–9.

30. Craig P, et al.: Developing and evaluating complex interventions: new guidance. Medical Research Council; 2008.

31. Stringer E. Action Research 2nd Edition. California: SAGE; 1999.

32. NHMRC. Values and Ethics: Guidelines for Ethical Conduct in Aboriginal and Torres Strait Islander Health Research. Canberra: National Health and Medical Research Council; 2003.

33. Kildea S, Stapleton H, Murphy R, Kosiak M, Gibbons K. The maternal and neonatal outcomes for an urban Indigenous population compared with their non-Indigenous counterparts and a trend analysis over four triennia. BMC Pregnancy and Childbirth. 2013;13:167.

34. Panaretto K, et al. Sustainable antenatal care services in an urban Indigenous community: the Townsville experience. Med J Aust. 2007; 187:18–22.

35. National Statement on Ethical Conduct in Human Research. The National Health and Medical Research Council, the Australian Research Council and universities Australia. Commonwealth of Australia, Canberra; 2007 (updated 2018).

36. Squires J, Twombly E, Bricker D, Potter L. ASQ-3 User's guide. Baltimore, Maryland: Brookes Pub; 2009.

37. Bayley N: Bayley scales of infant and toddler development, third edition (BAYLEY-III). Pearsons Clinical; 2005.

38. Kristensen T, Borritz M, Villadsen E, Christensen K. The Copenhagen burnout inventory: a new tool for the assessment of burnout. Work & Stress. 2005;19: 192–207.

39. NHMRC. Keeping research on track: A guide for Aboriginal and Torres Strait Islander people about about health research ethics. Canberra: National Health and Medical Research Council; 2005.

Permissions

The contributors of this book come from diverse backgrounds, making this book a truly international effort. This book will bring forth new frontiers with its revolutionizing research information and detailed analysis of the nascent developments around the world.

We would like to thank all the contributing authors for lending their expertise to make the book truly unique. They have played a crucial role in the development of this book. Without their invaluable contributions this book wouldn't have been possible. They have made vital efforts to compile up to date information on the varied aspects of this subject to make this book a valuable addition to the collection of many professionals and students.

This book was conceptualized with the vision of imparting up-to-date information and advanced data in this field. To ensure the same, a matchless editorial board was set up. Every individual on the board went through rigorous rounds of assessment to prove their worth. After which they invested a large part of their time researching and compiling the most relevant data for our readers.

The editorial board has been involved in producing this book since its inception. They have spent rigorous hours researching and exploring the diverse topics which have resulted in the successful publishing of this book. They have passed on their knowledge of decades through this book. To expedite this challenging task, the publisher supported the team at every step. A small team of assistant editors was also appointed to further simplify the editing procedure and attain best results for the readers.

Apart from the editorial board, the designing team has also invested a significant amount of their time in understanding the subject and creating the most relevant covers. They scrutinized every image to scout for the most suitable representation of the subject and create an appropriate cover for the book.

The publishing team has been an ardent support to the editorial, designing and production team. Their endless efforts to recruit the best for this project, has resulted in the accomplishment of this book. They are a veteran in the field of academics and their pool of knowledge is as vast as their experience in printing. Their expertise and guidance has proved useful at every step. Their uncompromising quality standards have made this book an exceptional effort. Their encouragement from time to time has been an inspiration for everyone.

The publisher and the editorial board hope that this book will prove to be a valuable piece of knowledge for researchers, students, practitioners and scholars across the globe.

Contributors

Mary McCauley, Valentina Actis Danna and Nynke van den Broek
Centre for Maternal and Newborn Health, Liverpool School of Tropical Medicine, Pembroke Place, Liverpool L3 5QA, UK

Dorah Mrema
Kilimanjaro Christian Medical Centre, Moshi, Kilimanjaro, Tanzania

Roselyter Monchari Riang'a
School of Arts and Social Sciences, Moi University, Eldoret, Kenya
Athena Institute, Faculty of Science, Vrije Universiteit Amsterdam, De Boelelaan 1085, 1081 HV Amsterdam, The Netherlands

Anne Kisaka Nangulu
School of Arts and Social Sciences, Moi University, Eldoret, Kenya
Commission for University Education, Red Hill Road, off Limuru Road, Gigiri, Nairobi, Kenya

Jacqueline E. W. Broerse
Athena Institute, Faculty of Science, Vrije Universiteit Amsterdam, De Boelelaan 1085, 1081 HV Amsterdam, The Netherlands

Lisa Peberdy, Jeanine Young and Debbie Louise Massey
School of Nursing, Midwifery and Paramedicine, University of the Sunshine Coast, Locked Bag 4, Maroochydore DC, QLD 4558, Australia

Lauren Kearney
School of Nursing, Midwifery and Paramedicine, University of the Sunshine Coast, Locked Bag 4, Maroochydore DC, QLD 4558, Australia
Sunshine Coast Hospital and Health Service, Maroochydore DC, Queensland, Australia

Nirmala Chandrasekaran, Leanne R De Souza and Howard Berger
Department of Maternal and Fetal Medicine, St Michaels Hospital, 30 Bond street, Toronto, ON M5B 1W8, Canada

Marcelo L Urquia
Li Ka Shing Knowledge Institute, St Michael's Hospital, Toronto, Canada

Beverley Young
Perinatal Mental Health Program, Mount Sinai Hospital, Toronto, Canada

Anne Mcleod
Sunnybrook Health Sciences, Toronto, Canada

Rory Windrim
Mt Sinai Hospital, Toronto, Canada

Roy M Nilsen, Eline S Vik and Vigdis Aasheim
Faculty of Health and Social Sciences, Western Norway University of Applied Sciences, Inndalsveien 28, 5063 Bergen, Norway

Svein A Rasmussen
Department of Clinical Science, University of Bergen, Bergen, Norway

Rhonda Small
Judith Lumley Centre, School of Nursing and Midwifery, La Trobe University, Melbourne, Australia
Reproductive Health, Department of Women's and Children's Health, Karolinska Institute, Stockholm, Sweden

Erica Schytt
Reproductive Health, Department of Women's and Children's Health, Karolinska Institute, Stockholm, Sweden
Centre for Clinical Research Dalarna, Uppsala University, Falun, Sweden

Dag Moster
Department of Paediatrics, Haukeland University Hospital, Bergen, Norway
Department of Global Public Health and Primary Care, University of Bergen, Bergen, Norway

Shankar Prinja, Aditi Gupta, Pankaj Bahuguna and Ruby Nimesh
School of Public Health, Post Graduate Institute of Medical Education and Research, Sector-12, Chandigarh 160012, India

Tesfaye Assebe Yadeta
School of Nursing and Midwifery, College of Health and Medical Sciences, Haramaya University, Harar, Ethiopia
School of Public Health, College of Health and Medical Sciences, Haramaya University, Harar, Ethiopia
Department of Medical Laboratory Sciences, College of Health and Medical Sciences, Haramaya University, Harar, Ethiopia

Alemayehu Worku
Department of Epidemiology and Biostatistics, School of Public Health, Addis Ababa University, Addis Ababa, Ethiopia

Gudina Egata
School of Public Health, College of Health and Medical Sciences, Haramaya University, Harar, Ethiopia

Berhanu Seyoum and Dadi Marami
Department of Medical Laboratory Sciences, College of Health and Medical Sciences, Haramaya University, Harar, Ethiopia

Yemane Berhane
Department of Epidemiology, Addis Continental Institute of Public Health, Addis Ababa, Ethiopia

Stuart James Fischbein
Birthing Instincts, Inc., Los Angeles, CA, USA

Rixa Freeze
Wabash College, 211 Center Hall, Crawfordsville, IN 47933, USA

Milene Saori Kassai and Roseli Oselka Saccardo Sarni
Department of Pediatrics, Faculdade de Medicina do ABC, Avenida Lauro Gomes, 2000. Vila Sacadura Cabral, Santo André, São Paulo 09060-870, Brazil

Fabíola Isabel Suano-Souza
Department of Pediatrics, Faculdade de Medicina do ABC, Avenida Lauro Gomes, 2000. Vila Sacadura Cabral, Santo André, São Paulo 09060-870, Brazil
Department of Pediatrics, Universidade Federal de São Paulo – Escola Paulista de Medicina, Rua Botucatu, 898, Vila Clementino, São Paulo 04023-062, Brazil

Fernanda Ramirez Cafeo and Fernando Alves Affonso-Kaufman
Department of Pediatrics, Universidade Federal de São Paulo – Escola Paulista de Medicina, Rua Botucatu, 898, Vila Clementino, São Paulo 04023-062, Brazil

M.A. Ag Ahmed
Université Laval, 1050 Avenue de la Médecine, room 3696, Québec G1V 0A6, Canada

L. Hamelin-Brabant
Faculty of Nursing Sciences, Université Laval, 1050 Avenue de la Médecine, room 3447, Québec G1V 0A6, Canada

M.P. Gagnon
Faculty of Nursing Sciences, Université Laval, 1050 Avenue de la Médecine, room 1426, Québec G1V 0A6, Canada

Xingchen Zhou, Huihui Chen, Xuhong Fang and Xipeng Wang
Department of Gynecology, Xinhua Hospital affiliated with Shanghai Jiaotong University, 1665 Kong Jiang Rd, Yang Pu District, Shanghai 200092, China

Xiaoqian Yang
Department of Gynecology, Shanghai First Maternity and Infant Hospital, Affiliated to Tongji University, Shanghai, China

Fouzia Khanam, Belal Hossain, Sabuj Kanti Mistry and Mahfuzar Rahman
Research and Evaluation Division, BRAC Center, Dhaka 1212, Bangladesh

Dipak K. Mitra
Department of Public Health, North South University, Dhaka, Bangladesh

Wameq Azfar Raza
Poverty and Equity, The World Bank, Dhaka, Bangladesh

Mahfuza Rifat and Kaosar Afsana
Health, Nutrition and Population Program, BRAC Center, Dhaka, Bangladesh

Maryam Nesari and Joanne K Olson
Faculty of Nursing, University of Alberta, Edmonton, AB, Canada

Ben Vandermeer
Alberta Research Centre for Health Evidence, Department of Pediatrics, University of Alberta, Edmonton, AB, Canada

Linda Slater
John W. Scott Health Sciences Library, University of Alberta, Edmonton, AB, Canada

David M Olson
Departments of Obstetrics and Gynecology, Pediatrics and Physiology, University of Alberta, Edmonton, AB T6G 2S2, Canada

Blair C. McNamara
Yale School of Medicine, 333 Cedar Street, New Haven, CT 06510, USA

Abigail Cutler
Department of Obstetrics, Gynecology and Reproductive Sciences, Yale School of Medicine, New Haven, CT, USA

Lisbet Lundsberg
Department of Obstetrics Gynecology and Reproductive Sciences, Yale School of Medicine, New Haven, CT, USA

Holly Powell Kennedy
Yale School of Nursing, West Haven, CT, USA

Aileen Gariepy
Department of Obstetrics, Gynecology and Reproductive Sciences, Yale School of Medicine, New Haven, CT, USA

Maria Ekelin
Department of Health Sciences, Lund University, S-22100 Lund, Sweden

Hanne Kristine Hegaard
Department of Health Sciences, Lund University, S-22100 Lund, Sweden
Department of Obstetrics, Copenhagen University Hospital, Rigshospitalet, Copenhagen, Denmark
The Research Unit Women's and Children's Health, The Juliane Marie Centre, Copenhagen University Hospital, Rigshospitalet, Blegdamsvej 9, 2100 Copenhagen, Denmark
The Institute of Clinical Medicine, Faculty of Health and Medical Sciences, University of Copenhagen, Blegdamsvej 3, Copenhagen, Denmark

Mette Grønbæk Backhausen
Department of Obstetrics, Copenhagen University Hospital, Rigshospitalet, Copenhagen, Denmark
The Research Unit Women's and Children's Health, The Juliane Marie Centre, Copenhagen University Hospital, Rigshospitalet, Blegdamsvej 9, 2100 Copenhagen, Denmark

Department of Gynecology and Obstetrics, Zealand University Hospital, Sygehusvej 10, 4000 Roskilde, Denmark

Madalitso Khwepeya
School of Nursing, College of Nursing, Taipei Medical University, Taipei, Taiwan
Maternity Department, Machinga District Hospital, Liwonde, Malawi

Gabrielle T Lee
Applied Psychology, Faculty of Education, Western University, London, ON, Canada

Su-Ru Chen and Shu-Yu Kuo
School of Nursing, College of Nursing, Taipei Medical University, 250 Wuxing Street, Taipei 11031, Taiwan

Mali Abdollahian and Kaye Marion
1School of Science (Mathematical and Geospatial Sciences), College of Science, Engineering and Health, RMIT University, GPO, Melbourne, VIC 3001, Australia

Dewi Anggraini
School of Science (Mathematical and Geospatial Sciences), College of Science, Engineering and Health, RMIT University, GPO Melbourne, VIC 3001, Australia
2Study Program of Statistics, Faculty of Mathematics and Natural Sciences, University of Lambung Mangkurat (ULM), Ahmad Yani Street, Km. 36, Banjarbaru, South Kalimantan 70714, Indonesia

Markus Fleisch
Clinic for Gynecology and Obstetrics, Helios University Hospital Wuppertal, University Witten/Herdecke, Heusnerstr 40, 42283 Wuppertal, Germany

Philip Hepp
Clinic for Gynecology and Obstetrics, Helios University Hospital Wuppertal, University Witten/Herdecke, Heusnerstr 40, 42283 Wuppertal, Germany

Clinic for Gynecology and Obstetrics, Heinrich-Heine-University, Düsseldorf, Germany

Carsten Hagenbeck, Julius Gilles, Percy Balan and Tanja Fehm
Clinic for Gynecology and Obstetrics, Heinrich-Heine-University, Düsseldorf, Germany

Oliver T. Wolf
Department of Cognitive Psychology, Institute of Cognitive Neuroscience, Faculty of Psychology, Ruhr-University Bochum, Bochum, Germany

Wolfram Goertz
Musikerambulanz, Heinrich-Heine-University, Düsseldorf, Germany

Wolfgang Janni
Clinic for Gynecology and Obstetrics, University Hospital Ulm, Ulm, Germany

Nora K. Schaal
Department of Experimental Psychology, Heinrich-Heine-University, Düsseldorf, Germany

A. Kater-Kuipers, E. M. Bunnik and I. D. de Beaufort
Department of Medical Ethics and Philosophy of Medicine, Erasmus MC, University Medical Centre Rotterdam, Room 24.17, Wytemaweg 80, 3015 CN Rotterdam, The Netherlands

R. J. H. Galjaard
Department of Clinical Genetics, Erasmus MC, University Medical Centre Rotterdam, Wytemaweg 80, 3015 CN Rotterdam, The Netherlands

Rebecca Delafield
Department of Native Hawaiian Health, John A. Burns School of Medicine, University of Hawai'i at Mānoa, 677 Ala Moana Blvd., Suite 1015, Honolulu, HI 96813-5401, USA

Catherine M. Pirkle
Office of Public Health Studies, University of Hawai'i at Mānoa, 1960 East-West Road, BioMed T102, Honolulu, HI 96822-2319, USA

Alexandre Dumont
Research Institute for Development, Université Paris Descartes, Sorbonne Paris Cité, Research Unit 196 (CEPED), Paris, France

Sophie Hickey and Yvette Roe
Midwifery Research Unit, Mater Research Institute-University of Queensland, Brisbane, QLD, Australia

Carmel Nelson, Adrian Carson and Sue Kruske
Institute for Urban Indigenous Health, Brisbane, QLD, Australia

Jody Currie and Renee Blackman
Aboriginal and Torres Strait Islander Community Health Service Brisbane Limited, Brisbane, QLD, Australia

Maree Reynolds, Kay Wilson and Shannon Watego
Mater Misericordia Limited, Brisbane, QLD, Australia

Megan Passey and Sally Tracy
The University of Sydney, Sydney, NSW, Australia

Roianne West
Griffith University, First Peoples Health Unit Queensland, Brisbane, Australia

Daniel Williamson
Department of Health, Aboriginal and Torres Strait Islander Health Branch, Brisbane, QLD, Australia

Machellee Kosiak
Australian Catholic University, Sydney, QLD, Australia

Yu Gao and Sue Kildea
Midwifery Research Unit, Mater Research Institute-University of Queensland, Brisbane, QLD, Australia
School of Nursing, Midwifery and Social Work, University of Queensland, Brisbane, Australia

Joan Webster
National Centre of Research Excellence in Nursing Interventions, Griffith University, Menzies Health Institute, Brisbane, QLD, Australia

Index

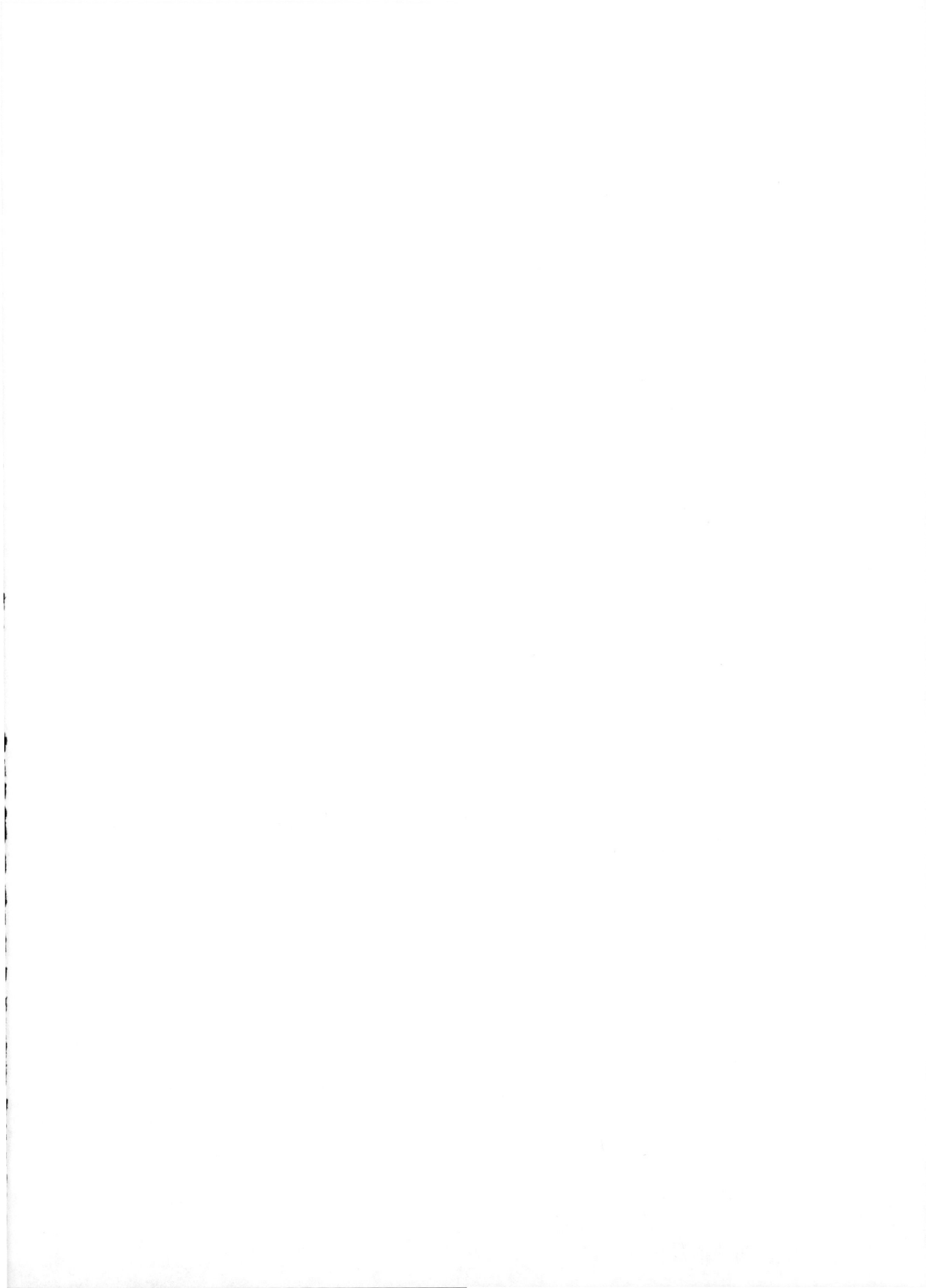